Self-Assessment Color Review

Avian Medicine and Surgery

Second Edition

Self-Assessment Color Review

Avian Medicine and Surgery

Second Edition

Edited by

Neil A. Forbes
Great Western Exotics
Swindon, U.K.

David Sanchez-Migallon Guzman
School of Veterinary Medicine, UC Davis
California, U.S.A.

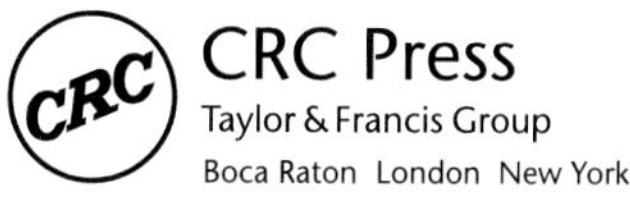

CRC Press
Taylor & Francis Group
Boca Raton London New York

CRC Press is an imprint of the
Taylor & Francis Group, an **informa** business

CRC Press
Taylor & Francis Group
6000 Broken Sound Parkway NW, Suite 300
Boca Raton, FL 33487-2742

Printed on acid-free paper

International Standard Book Number-13: 978-1-4987-0351-2 (Paperback)

Visit the Taylor & Francis Web site at
http://www.taylorandfrancis.com

and the CRC Press Web site at
http://www.crcpress.com

Contents

Preface

The first edition of *Avian Medicine SACR* was published in 1998 and has proven to not only have been popular, but many current key workers in the field have reported that this was the text that inspired their careers in avian medicine.

Since the first edition, the whole movement of 'evidence-based medicine', advancing recognition of 'specialization in avian medicine' and improved training in exotic medicine at an undergraduate level in many veterinary schools has thankfully advanced the discipline further. Concurrently, owners now have a greater understanding of diagnostics and potential treatments, which in turn fuels a greater expectation in respect of outcomes. So the time has come to update and renew this fun and simulating text.

There are many quality reference texts on avian medicine and surgery that offer detailed in-depth information; however, accessing this information can be laborious and time consuming. This book, along with others in the self-assessment color review series, is designed to assess one's level of knowledge and offers comprehensive, clinically-oriented information that can be quickly accessed, easily understood, and applied. The book covers a wide range of disciplines, organ systems, and species, but is not as all-inclusive as a text would be. The questions are presented in the same way clinical cases would be presented on a daily basis, challenging the reader to real clinical situations and, in most cases, offering a comprehensive solution to the question.

In this edition we have attempted to cover all the currently important and salient clinical conditions. In comparison with the first edition, greater emphasis is paid to recent diseases, techniques and treatments (e.g. endoscopy, cardiology, therapeutics, virology, PCR testing, and new surgical techniques). Whilst many readers found the previous format with questions on one page and answers on the next easy to follow and use, this newer format has questions at the beginning and answers at the end. This new format has removed any 'answer length restraints', enabling us to provide more complete and thorough answers, which we believe will be appreciated by readers. In addition, many of the answers are now referenced, giving readers the opportunity to follow up with further investigation and reading on specific topics.

The book is designed to be fun to read while at the same time being instructive. This type of learning has proven to be most effective for neophyte avian practitioners as well as experienced clinicians by guiding the reader through the main decision-making processes.

In compiling this book we have enlisted contributions from leading international authorities with diverse fields of expertise. We are sure that there will be varying opinions on some of the material presented and that products discussed will not be available in all countries. References are included at the end of most of the answers.

We hope that the reader will find this book a useful learning tool and at the same time enjoy the learning process.

Neil A. Forbes
David Sanchez-Migallon Guzman

Contributors

Roberto F. Aguilar
Institute of Veterinary, Animal and Biomedical Sciences
Massey University
Palmerston North, New Zealand

Alberto Rodriguez Barbon
Durrell Wildlife Conservation Trust
Trinity, Jersey, U.K.

Hugues Beaufrère
Ontario Veterinary College
University of Guelph
Guelph, Ontario, Canada

R. Avery Bennett
Veterinary Clinical Sciences
Louisiana State University
Baton Rouge, Louisana, U.S.A.

Alan Beynon
St David's Poultry Team
Dorrington, U.K.

João Brandão
Center of Veterinary Health Sciences
Oklahoma State University
Stillwater, Oklahoma, U.S.A.

Terry W. Campbell
Colorado State University
Fort Collins, Colorado, U.S.A.

Laurel Degernes
NCSU College of Veterinary Medicine
Raleigh, North Carolina, U.S.A.

Mathias Dislich
Parque das Aves
Foz do Iguaçu, Brazil

Stephen Divers
University of Georgia
Athen, Georgia, U.S.A.

Bob Doneley
School of Veterinary Science
University of Queensland
Brisbane, Australia

Neil Forbes
Great Western Exotics
Swindon, U.K.

Ady Y. Gancz
Koret School of Veterinary Medicine
Hebrew University of Jerusalem
Bet-Dagan, Israel

Jennifer Graham
Tufts Cummings School of Veterinary Medicine
North Grafton, Massachusetts, U.S.A.

Cheryl Greenacre
The University of Tennessee
Knoxville, Tennessee, U.S.A.

Claire Grosset
Veterinary Medicine
University of Montréal
Montréal, Canada

Vanessa L. Grunkemeyer
University of New Hampshire College of Life Sciences and Agriculture
Durham, New Hampshire, U.S.A.

David Sanchez-Migallon Guzman
School of Veterinary Medicine
UC Davis, California, U.S.A.

Minh Huynh
Centre Hospitalier Vétérinaire Fregis
Paris, France

Michael Jones
The University of Tennessee
Knoxville, Tennessee, U.S.A.

Krista Keller
University Hills Animal Hospital
Denver, Colorado, U.S.A.

Isabelle Langois
Veterinary Medicine
University of Montréal
Montréal, Canada

Crosta Lorenzo
Veterinari Montevecchia
Montevecchia, Italy

Christoph Mans
University of Wisconsin-Madison
Madison, Wisconsin, U.S.A.

Ricardo de Matos
College of Veterinary Medicine
Cornell University
Ithaca, New York, U.S.A.

Deborah Monks
Brisbane Bird and Exotics Veterinary Service
Macgregor, Australia

Glen Olsen
USGS Patuxent Wildlife Research Center
Patuxent Veterinary Hospital
Laurel, Maryland, U.S.A.

Joanne Paul-Murphy
School of Veterinary Medicine
UC Davis, California, U.S.A.

Christal Pollock
Lafeber Company, Cornell
Illinois, U.S.A.

Julia Ponder
The Raptor Center
University of Minnesota
St. Paul, Minnesota, U.S.A.

Shane Raidal
Charles Sturt University
Wagga Wagga, Australia

Drury Reavill
Zoo/Exotic Pathology Service
Carmichael, California, U.S.A.

April Romagnano
Avian & Exotic Clinic of Palm City
Palm City, Florida, U.S.A.

Mikel Sabater
Avian Reptile and Exotic Pet Hospital
University of Sydney
Sydney, Australia

Jaime Samour
Wildlife Division
Wrsan, Abu Dhabi, U.A.E.

Peter Sandmeier
Kleintier- und Vogelpraxis
Baden, Switzerland

Nico Schoemaker
Utrecht University
Utrecht, The Netherlands

Izidora Sladakovic
University of Georgia
Athens, Georgia, U.S.A.

Dale Smith
Ontario Veterinary College
University of Guelph
Guelph, Ontario, Canada

Stephen Smith
Tiggywinkles Wildlife Hospital
Haddenham, Bucks, U.K.

Brian Speer
Medical Center for Birds
Oakley, California, U.S.A.

Jonathan Stockman
Waltham Centre for Pet Nutrition
Melton Mowbray, U.K.

Jens Straub
Animal Clinic Dr. Krauss Duesseldorf GmbH
Department of Avian and Reptile Medicine
Duesseldorf, Germany

Morena Bernadette Wernick
ExoticVet GmbH
Jona, Switzerland

Nicole Wyre
Zodiac Pet & Exotic Hospital
Hong Kong, China

Yvonne van Zeeland
Utrecht University
Utrecht, The Netherlands

Dedications

To my wife Karen for her support and tolerance and my daughters Katrina and Sarah-Jane, acknowledging the many hours when their father was too busy to be with them.

NF

To Oma, with all my love. To my parents, Pilar and Alfonso, and my siblings Francisco, Ester, and Alberto, for their love and support even in the distance. To those who inspired me, intentionally or unintentionally, to be the person and the veterinarian that I am today. To the future generation of avian veterinarians who will care for our feathered friends.

DG

Acknowledgments

My eternal thanks to my mentor, Professor John E Cooper, for his initial encouragement and introduction into avian medicine at the start of my career, and his support and enthusiasm throughout my career. To all those who have assisted in the development and recognition of Veterinary Specialization.

NAF

I would like to thank all the authors for their effort and contribution to this issue, as well as the residents, students, and technicians that participated in some of the cases illustrated. Also, I would like to thank my colleagues Joanne, Michelle, and Jessica, who I share with all the daily challenges at work; without their continuous support, I would not have been able to accomplish this task. Lastly, I would like to thank the CRC Press team and Neil for the opportunity given to serve as co-editor of this book, and for their support and guidance.

DG

Photo Credits

24a, b	Dr. J. Brandão
48	Dr. Stephen Divers
58	Dr. Stephen Divers
60a–c	Dr. Noemie Summa
73	Dr. Jens Straub
77	Dr. Thereza Rizzi
79	Dr. Stephen Divers
111	Dr. Stephen Divers
125	Dr. Stephen Divers
146	Dr. Stephen Divers
153	Dr. Matthew Grabovsky
162	Dr. Neil Forbes
165	Dr. Stephen Divers
184	Dr. Marisa Pérez

186	Dr. Stephen Divers
189	Dr. N. Chai
192	Dr. J. Samour
193	Dr. Eduardo Huguet
195	Dr. Peter Coutteel
197	Dr. T. Dutton
199	Dr. Stephen Divers
220	LafeberVet
256	Dr. Stephen Divers
266	LafeberVet

Abbreviations

ALP	alkaline phosphatase
AST	aspartate aminotransferase
BUN	blood urea nitrogen
BW	bodyweight
CBC	complete blood count
CK	creatine kinase
COX	cyclooxygenase
CPR	cardiopulmonary resuscitation
CRI	constant rate infusion
CT	computed tomography
DNA	deoxyribonucleic acid
ECG	electrocardiography/ electrocardiogram
EDTA	ethylenediaminetetraacetic acid
ELISA	enzyme-linked immunosorbent assay
ESF	external skeletal fixator
GGT	gamma-glutamyltransferase
GLDH	glutamate dehydrogenase
GnRH	gonadotropin-releasing hormone
Hb	hemoglobin
IM	intramuscular/intramuscularly
IN	intranasal/intranasally
IO	intraosseous
IV	intravenous/intravenously
LDH	lactate dehydrogenase
LDL	low-density lipoprotein
MCH	mean corpuscular hemoglobin
MCHC	mean corpuscular hemoglobin concentration
MCV	mean corpuscular volume
MRI	magnetic resonance imaging
NaCl	sodium chloride
NSAID	nonsteroidal anti-inflammatory drug
OD	oculus dexter (right eye)
OS	oculus sinister (left eye)
PCR	polymerase chain reaction
PCV	packed cell volume
PO	per os/orally
RBC	red blood cell
RT-PCR	real-time polymerase chain reaction
SC	subcutaneous/subcutaneously
UV	ultraviolet
WBC	white blood cell

Broad Classification of Cases

(Cases may be classified under more than one category)

Anesthesia/analgesia
8, 33, 58, 65, 88, 95, 97, 131, 147, 173, 191, 203, 208, 211, 228, 230, 231, 234, 241

Anatomy
11, 19, 24, 47, 48, 52, 56, 64, 83, 89, 102, 111, 117, 119, 131, 132, 137, 141, 148, 165, 176, 179, 183, 189, 211, 214, 228, 233, 246, 256, 257, 259, 264, 270

Bacterial infection
10, 34, 40, 48, 52, 62, 83, 102, 110, 111, 119, 129, 144, 145, 149, 161, 164, 171, 178, 202, 215, 219, 225, 237, 242, 244, 255, 262

Basic procedures
10, 14, 15, 21, 50, 89, 167, 189, 209, 216, 220, 266

Beak and head kinetics
21, 96, 102, 130, 141, 160, 228, 252

Behavior
9, 38, 51, 75, 103, 118, 133, 265, 267, 271

Biochemistry
3, 4, 10, 15, 18, 26, 35, 36, 41, 46, 50, 63, 67, 76, 109, 198, 206, 209, 243

Bumblefoot
59, 74, 251

Cardiovascular
22, 26, 39, 56, 73, 87, 88, 93, 201, 239, 254, 269

Chlamydia
82, 133, 145, 226, 262

Clinical pathology
3, 4, 10, 14, 15, 18, 26, 29, 35, 36, 40, 41, 44, 46, 58, 59, 61, 63, 67, 69, 76, 77, 78, 99, 101, 107, 109, 134, 140, 155, 161, 164, 176, 177, 178, 198, 206, 209, 219, 243, 263

Cytology
14, 16, 20, 37, 40, 53, 58, 77, 78, 82, 101, 123, 140, 155, 163, 164, 188, 215, 244, 248, 255, 259

Dermatology
3, 17, 21, 25, 49, 72, 96, 104, 121, 122, 133, 158, 160, 178, 180, 190, 198, 204, 213, 216, 224, 240, 245, 247, 251, 266, 270

Diagnostics
1, 3, 4, 7, 10, 12, 14, 15, 16, 18, 20, 22, 26, 30, 31, 34, 35, 40, 44, 45, 50, 53, 57, 58, 59, 61, 63, 67, 68, 72, 76, 80, 82, 87, 90, 93, 95, 96, 101, 104, 109, 113, 114, 123, 125, 129, 134, 135, 138, 140, 143, 158, 161, 178, 181, 187, 195, 198, 206, 209, 215, 237, 248, 249, 268

Emergency and critical care
15, 36, 50, 55, 73, 106, 147, 151, 231, 241, 242, 250

Endocrinology
24, 148, 198, 243

CASE 1 An adult male red-breasted toucan (*Ramphastos dicolorus*) underwent a routine health examination, which included a coelioscopy (**1a–c**). The liver appeared enlarged but, most noticeable, the surface of the organ was replaced with generalized yellow–brown discoloration.

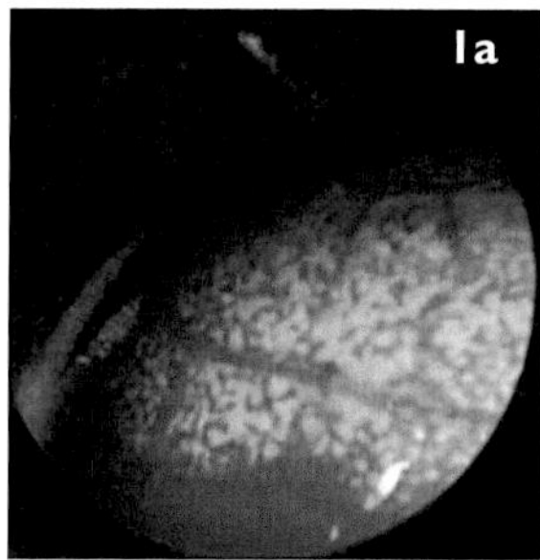
1a

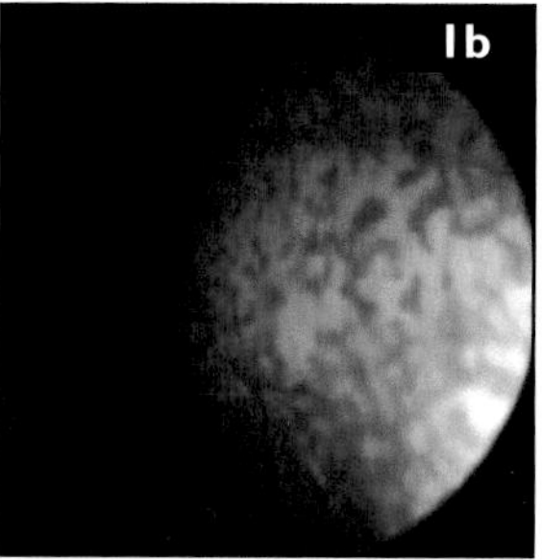
1b

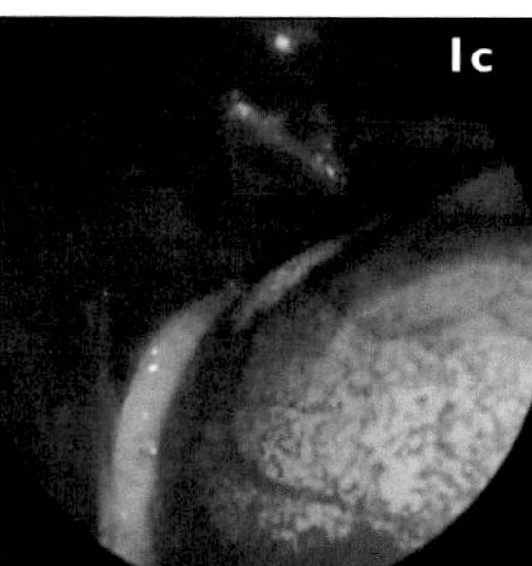
1c

1. What are the main differential diagnoses?
2. What complementary test would you request or perform?
3. How would you treat this condition?

CASE 2 A local zoo is housing a flock of 15 Chilean flamingos (*Phoenicopterus chilensis*). They have held the birds for 4 years. The birds have access to a pond and a large beach with soil substrate (**2**). The zoo would like to breed them; however, to date, they have not been successful.

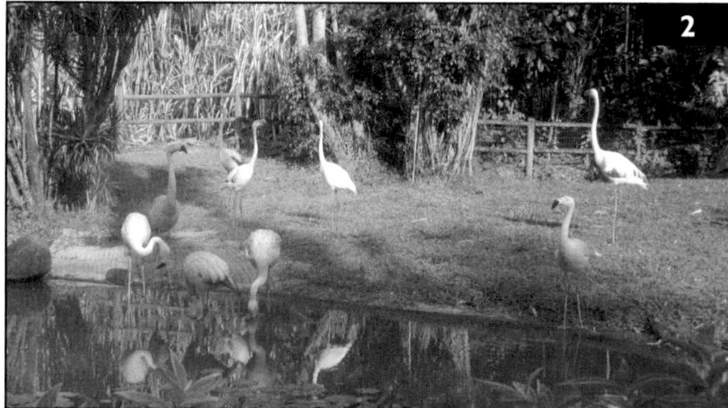
2

1. What advice could you give to improve reproductive success in this collection?
2. List some possible causes of low egg fertility in flamingo flocks? What management techniques can be used to overcome this difficulty?
3. What management actions can be taken to reduce hand-reared chick mortality during the first days of life?

CASE 3 A 10-year-old male sulphur-crested cockatoo (*Cacatua galerita galerita*) is presented with a history of intermittent vomiting (2–3 times weekly), reduced appetite, and feather damaging behavior. The client reports that the bird is fed nothing but sunflower seed and a vitamin–mineral supplement occasionally in its drinking water. On physical examination the bird is obese, weighing 1,140 g (normal weight 800–1,000 g) and with substantial fat deposits over the flanks and ventral body. The crop contains a mixture of fluid and soft ingesta. There is feather loss over the back and ventral body. There is no coelomic distension, but palpation elicits a painful response from the bird. You collect blood from the bird and submit it for hematology and biochemical analysis. The results are shown below. Erythrocyte morphology normal; heterophils show 3+ toxic changes.

Analyte	Result	Reference intervals
Hematology		
Packed cell volume (%)	52	40–55
Estimated white cell count (× 10^9/L)	33	8–15
Heterophils (%)	54	50–70
Lymphocytes (%)	28	30–50
Eosinophils (%)	0	0–1
Monocytes (%)	12	0–4
Basophils (%)	6	0–1
Biochemistry		
AST (U/L)	220	140–360
CK (U/L)	450	147–418
Bile acids (μmol/L; μg/mL)	39 (15.0)	70–80 (28.6–32.7)
GLDH (U/L)	2	1–4
Amylase (U/L)	5,617	200–876
Uric acid (μmol/L; mg/dL)	590 (10.03)	160–500 (2.72–8.5)
Urea (mmol/L; mg/dL)	0.9 (2.53)	0.45–1.13 (1.26–3.18)
Glucose (mmol/L; mg/dL)	16.5 (297)	7.40–22.70 (133–408)
Calcium (mmol/L; mg/dL)	1.56 (6.2)	1.83–2.31 (7.3–9.3)
Phosphorus (mmol/L; mg/dL)	0.5 (1.55)	Unknown
Cholesterol (mmol/L; mg/dL)	9.3 (359.6)	3.50–7.30 (135–282)
Triglyceride (mmol/L; mg/dL)	3.7 (327)	1.39–9.40 (123–832)
Total protein (g/L; g/dL)	46 (4.6)	21–39 (2.1–3.9)

1 What is your problem list, differential diagnosis, and most likely diagnosis?
2 What further diagnostics could be used to confirm your tentative diagnosis?
3 How would you treat this patient?

CASE 4 An adult female blue-crowned conure (*Thecocercus acuticaudata*) presented for lethargy, anorexia, and reluctance to open the eyes. Whole body radiographs indicated hepatomegaly. The plasma chemistry profile revealed a mild increase in creatine kinase of 1,413 IU/L, an aspartate aminotransferase of 407 IU/L, and a normal total protein of 22 g/L (2.2 g/dL). The complete blood cell count is as follows:

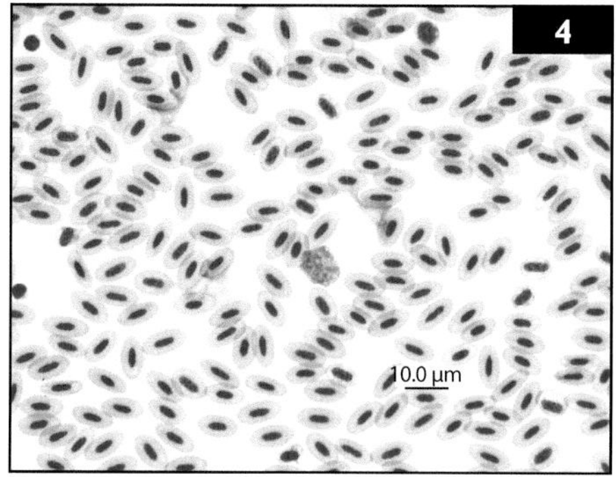

WBC × 10⁹/L	Heterophils × 10⁹/L	Lymphocytes × 10⁹/L	Monocytes × 10⁹/L	Eosinophils × 10⁹/L	Basophils × 10⁹/L	PCV %	Total protein g/L (g/dL) (by refractometer)
	18%	60%	16%	2%	4%	15	
1.1	0.198	0.66	0.176	0.022	0.044		64
(1,100/μL)	(198/μL)	(660/μL)	(176/μL)	(22/μL)	(44/μL)		(6.4)

1 How should one interpret the complete blood cell count?
2 How should one interpret the image of the blood film (4)?
3 What is the significance of the cells in the image of the blood film?

CASE 5

1 Describe suitable endoscopy instrumentation required for the following procedures:
   - Coelioscopy with kidney and liver biopsies in a 1 kg raptor.
   - Tracheoscopy in a 400 gram parrot.
   - Air sac tube placement in a 400 gram parrot.
   - Cloacoscopy in a 3 kg goose.
2 Contrary to reptile and mammal coelioscopy/laparoscopy, why is CO_2 insufflation contraindicated and not required for avian coelioscopy?
3 When performing endoscopy and endosurgery within the avian air sac system, why is it important to ensure that there is a snug skin–endoscope interface and that all sheath ports are closed?

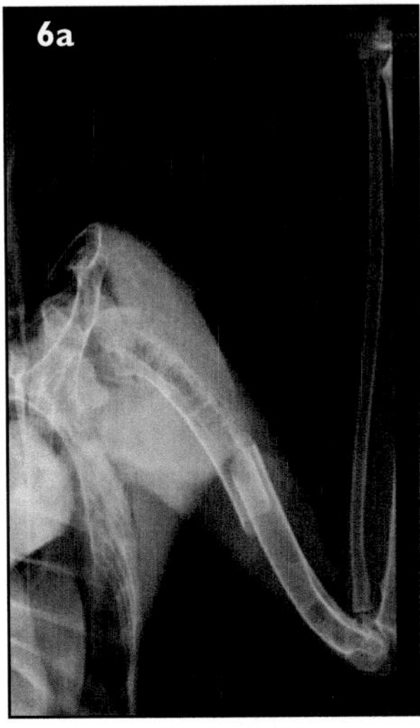

CASE 6 A 4.3 kg adult female bald eagle (*Haliaeetus leucocephalus*) presents to your clinic after being hit by a bus. The bird is depressed and currently not a good anesthetic candidate. Radiographs are obtained (**6a, b**).

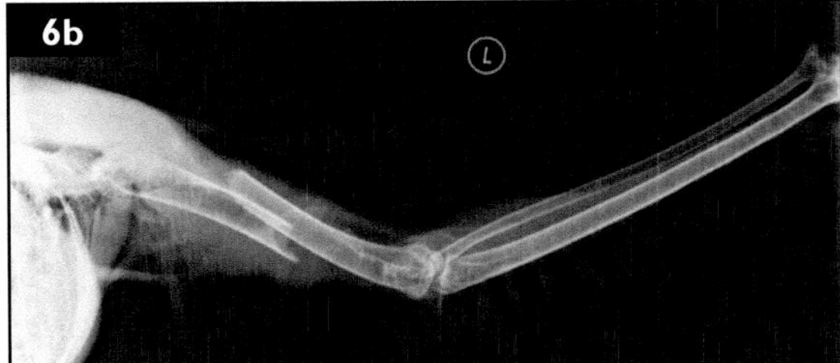

1 What are your main concerns on initial evaluation?
2 Describe how you would initially stabilize this fracture.
3 What fixation method would you use for surgical repair?

CASE 7 You are presented with a backyard chicken for evaluation of decreased appetite and activity level, lack of egg production, and coelomic distension. On physical examination, the most relevant finding is severe coelomic distension. The coelom is relatively soft and no masses can be palpated.

An ultrasound image of the coelomic cavity is shown (**7a**). On further evaluation of the coelom, a mixed echogenicity structure was identified dorsal to the ventriculus and caudodorsal to the liver and heart (**7b**). The results of a postmortem examination are shown (**7c**).

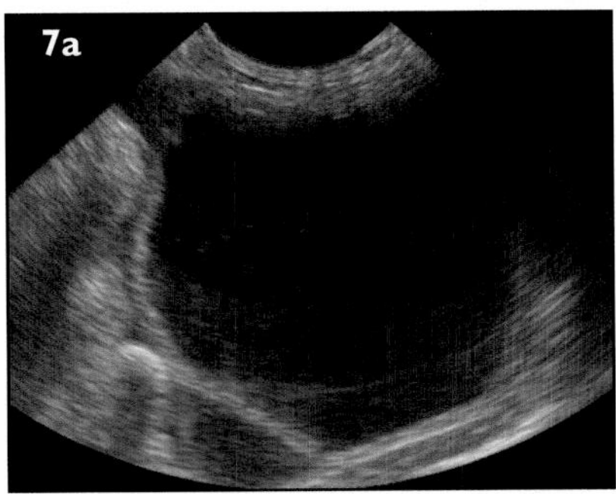

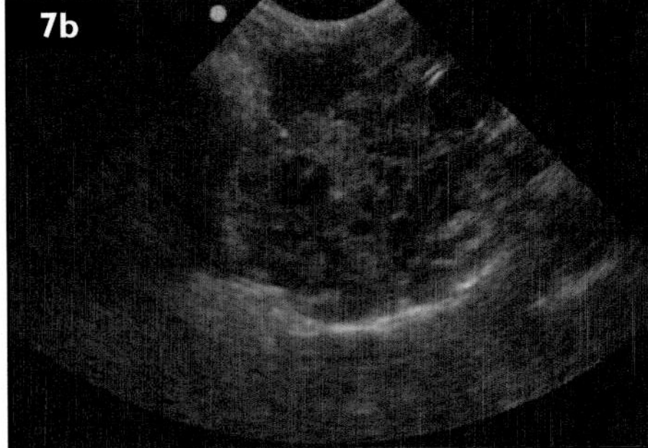

1 Based on the physical examination findings and the features of **7a**, what is the cause of the coelomic distension in this hen?
2 Based on the clinical history, physical examination findings, ultrasound findings, and postmortem findings, what is the most likely diagnosis for this case?
3 What are the treatment options (medical and/or surgical) for this case?

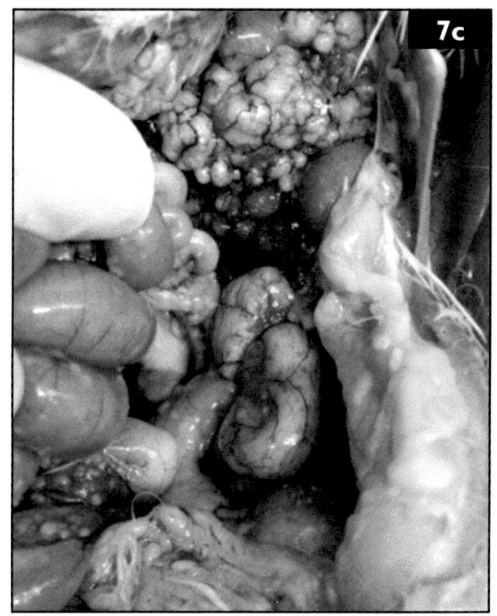
7c

CASE 8 A double yellow-headed Amazon parrot (*Amazona orathrix*) is presented with a left tibiotarsal fracture. The owner reports that this happened this morning during playing. The bird appears quiet but responsive, and is lame and not weight bearing on the left leg. The owner expresses interest in surgical repair of the fracture and hospitalization during the initial postoperative period (**8**).

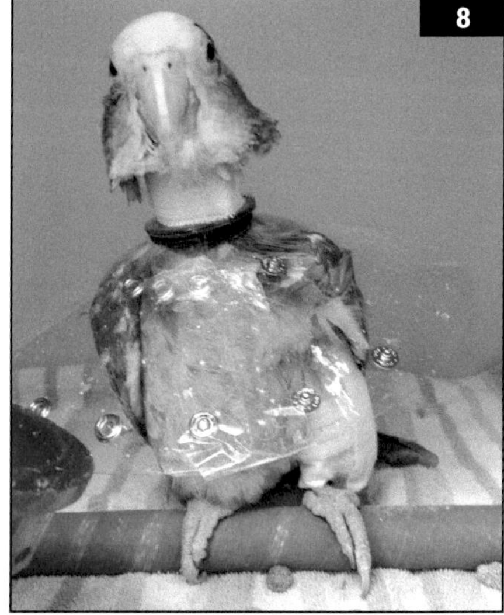
8

1 How would you manage pain in this patient (1) during the preoperative period, (2) during the intraoperative period, and (3) during the postoperative period?

CASE 9 An owner consults you because she has been having difficulties with getting her African grey parrot (*Psittacus erithacus*) to step up onto her hand so that she can place it back into its cage. The problem has progressed to such an extent that she now cannot even approach the bird with her hand when it is sitting on top of the cage, without the bird lunging towards her and biting her (**9**). She is desperate and would appreciate your advice on how to improve this situation, as the biting has become progressively worse and more forceful, resulting in serious bite injuries to her fingers.

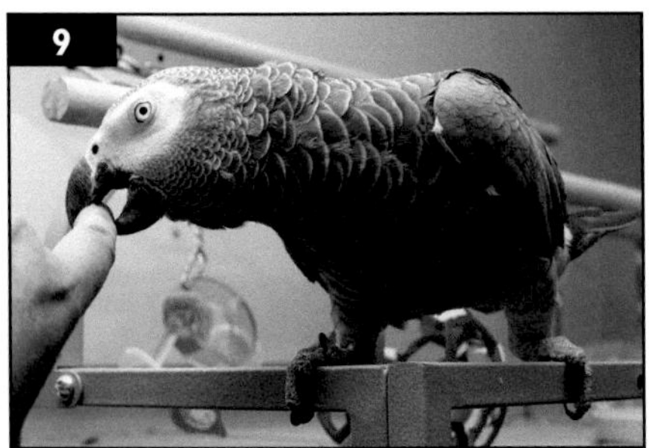

To better understand problem behavior and be able to design a suitable treatment plan, a so-called functional assessment, which describes the functional relationship between the parrot's behavior (B), its antecedents (A), and consequences (C), and predicts the parrot's future behavior on the basis of this relationship, is deemed essential.

1 Conduct a functional assessment of this African grey parrot's behavior. Include a description of the ABCs as well as a prediction of the parrot's behavior in your analysis.

In the situation as described above, so-called operant learning has taken place by which the bird has learned that by its behavior it is able to operate (control) its environment to obtain a certain effect. Four types of operant learning can be distinguished (i.e. positive and negative reinforcement, and positive and negative punishment).

2 Which of the following types has taken place in this situation?
3 Describe the different interventions that could be considered in this behavior modification plan to reduce the biting and/or prevent injury to the owner's hand.

CASE 10 Many avian focused practices have in-house laboratories providing hematologic and biochemical results for their patients. This represents a significant investment in both capital and labor for the practice, and the purchase and use of such equipment has to be carefully considered.

1 List the advantages and disadvantages of in-house laboratory testing.
2 List the advantages and disadvantages of external laboratory testing.

CASE 11 A flesh footed shearwater (*Puffinus carneipes*) is presented for rehabilitation following a storm with heavy winds. The bird is bright, alert, and responsive, feather examination shows good water proofing, and it appears ready for release. The bird was windblown on to land, and otherwise appears healthy. Survey radiographs show a bilateral elongated mineral opacity cranial to the elbow in the propatagium (**11a, b**).

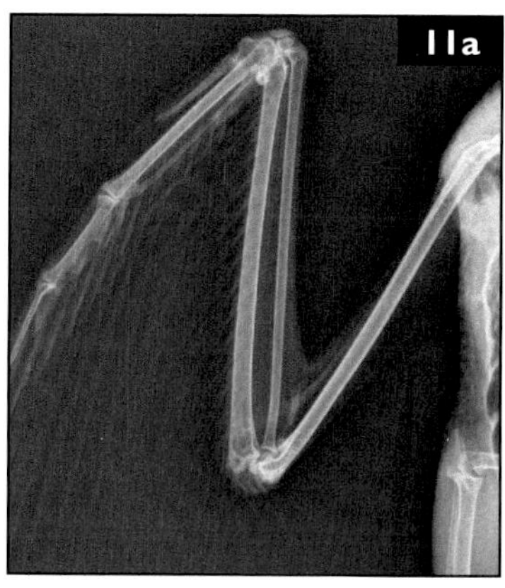
11a

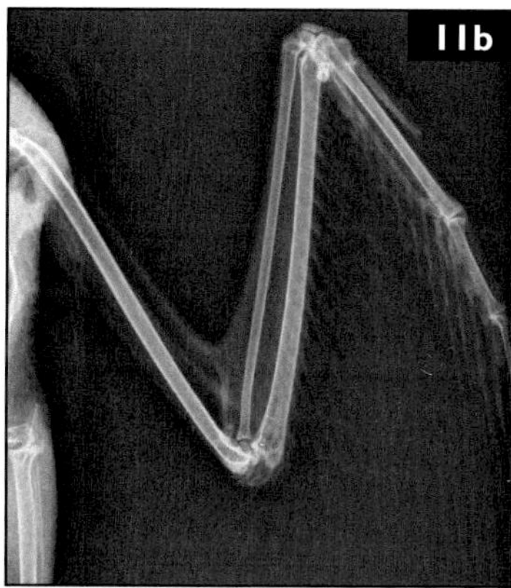
11b

1 What is the clinical significance of these radiographic findings?
2 What is the name for this structure?
3 What is its function?

CASE 12 A reproductively active 1-year-old Rhode Island Red hen (*Gallus gallus domesticus*) presented on account of a decrease in egg laying, lethargy, and anorexia for a period of 5 days. The owner had noticed a white to yellow thick discharge from the cloaca (**12**).

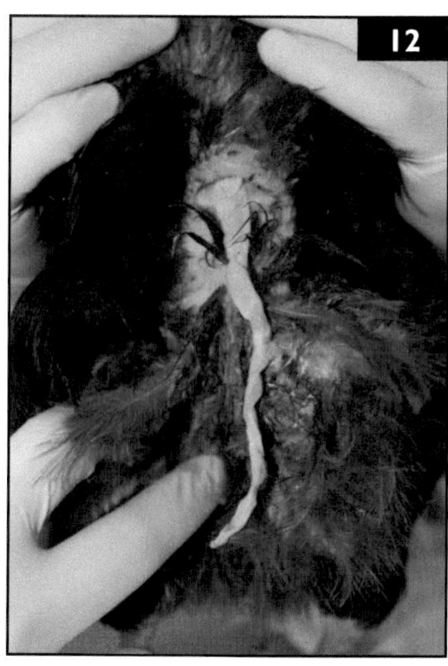
12

1 What is the most likely organ system involved and the cause of the presentation?
2 What are the recommended diagnostic tests?
3 What is the suggested treatment and underlying agent?

CASE 13 The police are investigating a suspected wildlife poisoning incident and seek your advice. After three red kites (*Milvus milvus*) have been found poisoned locally over the last 4 months, they visit a local farmer and locate six illegal poisons. The aged farmer (84 years old) reiterates that he hates raptors, stating that the kites pick up and fly off with his piglets, but denies having poisoned them. Two of the three dead birds were located on his property, but one was found dead some 2 km away. Each bird was submitted to a full postmortem examination. Mevinphos was found in the mouth or crop of each bird, at 6×, 7×, and 6.5× LD50 levels. The third bird died in April (springtime, **13**). It was a female, was missing some feathers on the back of its neck, and showed marked follicular development on the ovary. The question posed to you, in relation to the bird that was found dead 2 km away from the farm, is whether it could have ingested poison from the farm, the point being that if the third bird was poisoned by someone else, then there is a possibility that the first two could also have been poisoned by someone else and as such a prosecution would be unrealistic.

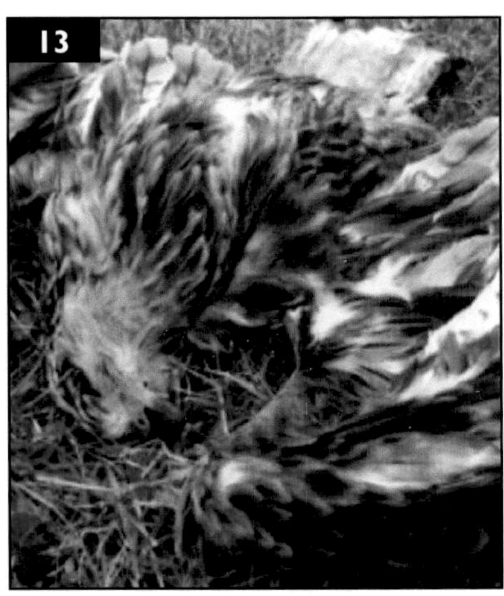

1 Would a red kite be able to carry away piglets?
2 Would the red kite that had consumed a 6–7× LD50 of Mevinphos be able to fly 2 km following ingestion? If not, what other explanations are possible, and what further action would you take to investigate the case?
3 What relevance have the findings on the third bird?

CASE 14 A 2-year-old African penguin (*Sphenicus demersus*) housed in an outdoor enclosure is presented for lethargy, biliverdinuria, and anorexia. The physical examination is unremarkable. Radiographs are obtained under general anesthesia and are normal. You want to collect a blood sample for a CBC and biochemistry panel.

1 Where are the blood sampling sites located in Spheniciformes?
2 Which hemoparasites might be causing these clinical signs?
3 What diagnostic tests can be performed to screen for these hemoparasites?

CASE 15 A 10-year-old female African grey parrot (*Psittacus erithacus*) is presented to your practice with a history of nonspecific signs of illness, duration 2–3 days, including a reduction in food and water intake, severe depression, a fluffed and ruffled appearance, as well as vomiting or regurgitation. The bird weighs 390 g. Although the owner reports a history of diarrhea, on physical examination the fecal component of the droppings is normal while the urine component is larger than normal. During the physical examination, the parrot is estimated to be approximately 8% dehydrated.

Hematology	Units	Patient value	Reference interval
PCV	%	60	40–55
RBC	$10^6/\mu L$	4.5	2.4–4.5
Hb	g/dL	13	11–16
MCV	fl	160	90–180
MCH	pg	47	28–52
MCHC	g/dL	30	23–33
WBC	$10^9/L$	8.2	5–15
Heterophils	$10^9/L$	6.2	4.6–7.5
Lymphocytes	$10^9/L$	1.8	1.9–5.1
Monocytes	$10^9/L$	0.12	0–0.2
Eosinophils	$10^9/L$	0.08	0–0.1
Basophils	$10^9/L$	0	0–0.1

Biochemistry	SI units	Patient value	Reference interval	Old units	Patient value	Reference interval
ALP	U/L	120	12–160			
Amylase	U/L	470	415–626			
AST	U/L	257	100–350			
Calcium	mmol/L	2.4	2–3.25	mg/dL	9.6	8–13
Chloride				mEq/L	140	
Cholesterol	mmol/L	10.36	4.14–11	mg/dL	400	160–425
CK	U/L	57.5	123–875			
Glucose	mmol/L	22	10.45–19.25	mg/dL	400	190–350
LDH	U/L	398	150–450			
Phosphorus	mmol/L	1.91	1–1.74	mg/dL	5.9	3.2–5.4
Uric acid	μmol/L	536	238–595	mg/dL	9	4–10
Sodium	mmol/L	160	134–152	mEq/L	160	134–152
Potassium	mmol/L	3.1	2.6–4.2	mEq/L	3.1	2.6–4.2
Protein (total)	g/L	33	30–50	mg/dL	3.3	3–5
Albumin	g/L	15	15.7–32.3	g/dL	1.5	1.57–3.23
Globulin	g/L	18		g/dL	1.8	
A:G ratio		0.8	1.6–4.3			
Osmolality	mOsm/kg	334	228–324			

1 What route would you use to administer fluids in this patient?

2 What type of fluid, how much volume, and at what rate would be most appropriate?

CASE 16 A female gyrfalcon (*Falco rusticolus*) was taken to a veterinary hospital for clinical examination. The falcon had been maintained in a captive breeding facility, having been recently imported into the UK from the Middle East. The owner reported the passing of pistachio green urates for the past 10 days, reduced appetite, and progressive weight loss. On examination, the falcon showed a body condition of 3/5 and was bright and alert. The falcon was admitted for treatment and boarding. Unfortunately, the falcon died overnight prior to any diagnostic analyses or any treatment being provided. On postmortem examination the liver was grossly enlarged, mottled in color, and looked firm and waxy in appearance (**16**). Histopathology revealed extensive amorphous eosinophilic extracellular deposits (95%), consistent with amyloid, across the parenchyma of the liver and other organs, notably the spleen and kidneys. This was confirmed after staining the slide using Congo red stain technique. The results suggest the amyloid was amyloid AA.

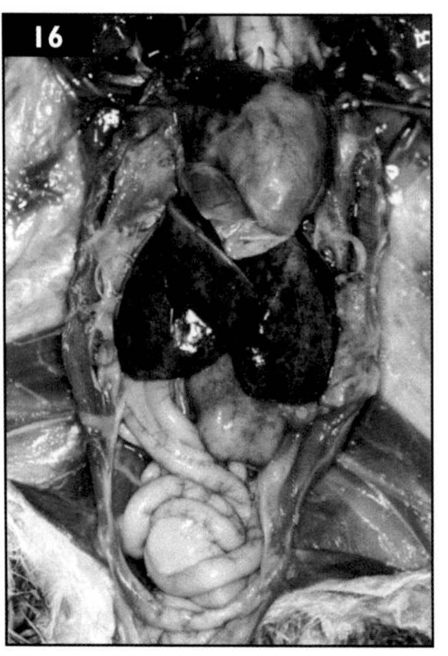
16

1 Based on the clinical history and gross postmortem findings, what are your differential diagnoses?
2 What diagnostic test would you perform to confirm the diagnosis?
3 Is amyloidosis likely to be the cause of death? How can you treat amyloidosis? Can amyloidosis be prevented?

CASE 17 The feather of an ostrich (*Struthio camelus*) is shown (**17**).

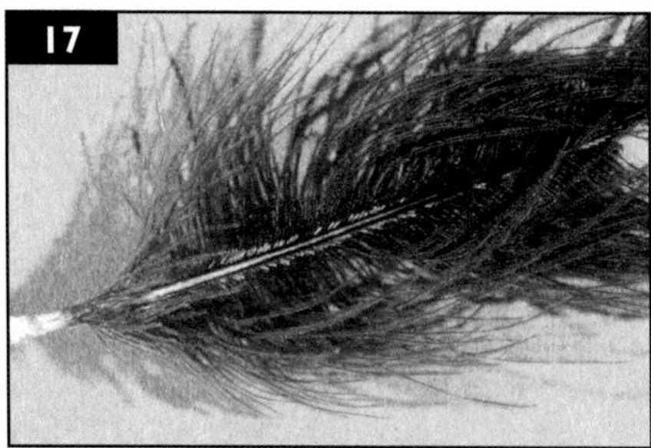
17

1 What abnormality is visible on this feather, and what is its cause?
2 What is the significance to the individual ostrich and to the flock?
3 What management actions are required to deal with the problem illustrated?

CASE 18 A 7-year-old female intact Congo African grey parrot (*Psittacus erithacus*) presents because she has had a seizure at home. She is on a commercial seed diet with some table food as well. When presented at the hospital, she is no longer seizuring but is weak and unable to perch. A blood sample is collected for a biochemistry panel.

Parameter	Value	Reference interval
AST (U/L)	523	100–350
Bile acid (μmol/L)	22	18–71
Calcium, total (mmol/L) (mg/dL)	1.7 (6.8)	2–3.24 (8–13)
Cholesterol (mmol/L) (mg/dL)	6.47 (251)	3.88–10.99 (160–425)
CK (U/L)	1,348	123–875
Glucose (mmol/L) (mg/dL)	19.04 (343)	10.55–19.43 (190–350)
Phosphorus (mmol/L) (mg/dL)	1.07 (3.3)	1.03–1.74 (3.2–5.4)
Potassium (mEq/L)	3.9	2.6–4.2
Protein, total (g/L) (g/dL)	46 (4.6)	30–50 (3–5)
Albumin (g/L) (g/dL)	31 (3.1)	15.7–32.3 (1.57–3.23)
Globulin (g/L) (g/dL)	15 (1.5)	14.3–17.7 (1.43–1.77)
Sodium (mEq/L)	142	134–152
Uric acid (μmol/L) (mg/dL)	333 (5.6)	238–595 (4–10)

1 What is the most likely cause of this bird's seizure?
2 If hypocalcemia is suspected based on clinical signs and history, but total calcium levels are within normal limits, what additional test should be considered?
3 What other analyte should be evaluated in this patient if initial treatment to increase the calcium level is not effective?
4 What treatment should be given immediately to prevent another seizure?

CASE 19 In some avian species (e.g. owls, falcons, bitterns, gannets) one claw is modified into a comb-like structure (**19**).

1 What is the name of this claw? In which digit is it found?
2 How many phalanges integrate this digit?
3 What are the two main anatomic structures in the claws of birds of prey?

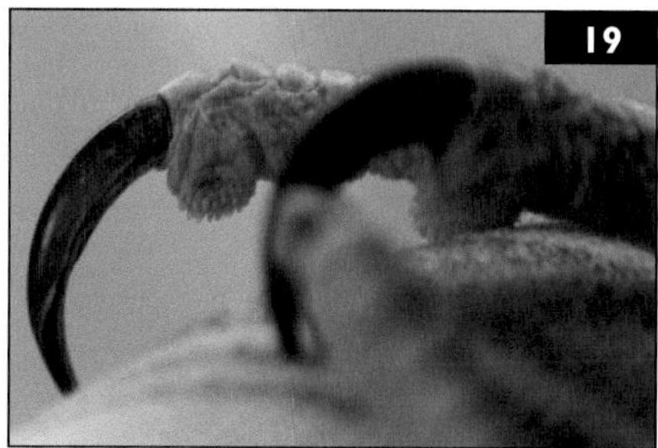
19

CASE 20 A young blue crown conure (*Thectocercus acuticaudatus*) presented with unilateral blepharospasm, reddened conjunctiva, corneal edema, and multiple 0.25–0.5 mm vascularized anterior stromal nodules (**20a**). After an ophthalmic evaluation, a corneal cytology sample was collected with the back end of a No. 15 Bard-Parker scalpel (**20b**).

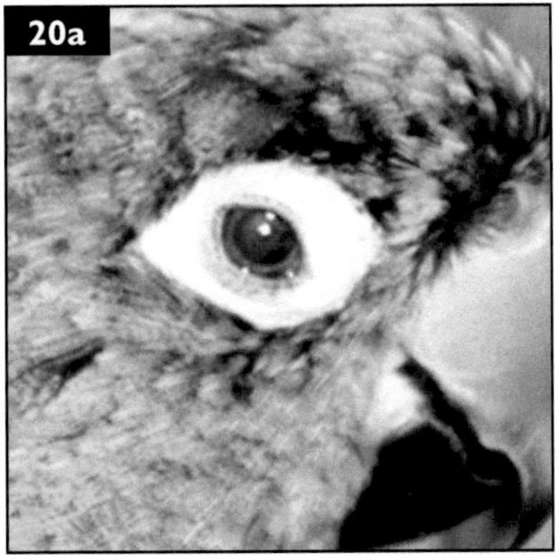
20a

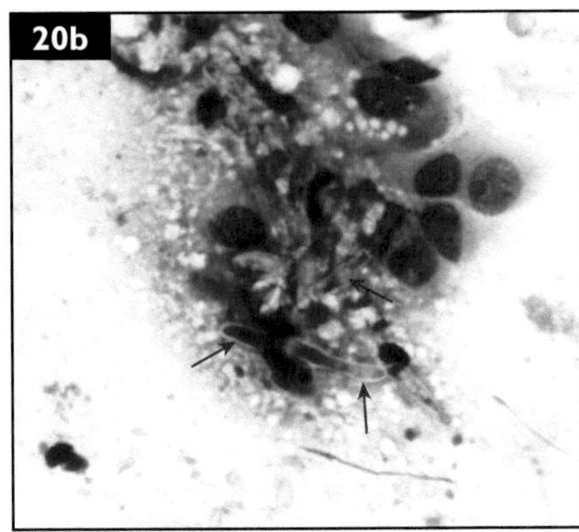
20b

1 What would be the differential diagnoses based on the clinical presentation?
2 What is your diagnosis based on the corneal cytology?
3 What additional diagnostics and treatment would you pursue in this case?

CASE 21 An 8-year-old blue and gold macaw (*Ara ararauna*) is presented for an overgrown beak (**21**). The condition has been evolving for years. Physical examination of the bird shows a severe overgrown rhinotheca in length and thickness.

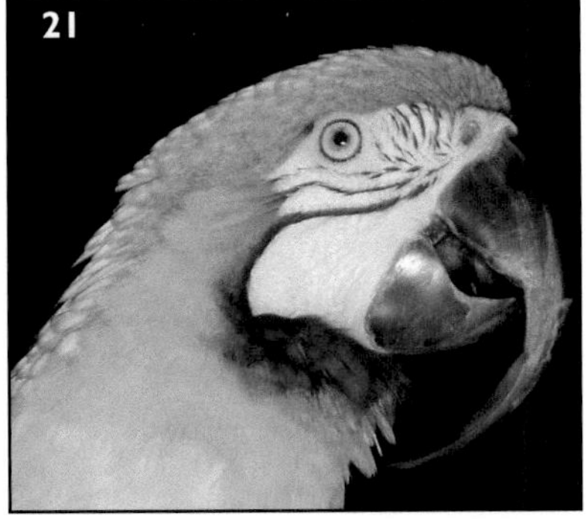
21

1 What additional examination could you perform to assess the thickness of the overgrown keratin layer?
2 How would you treat this condition?
3 What pathologies may result in excessive beak growth in psittacine birds?

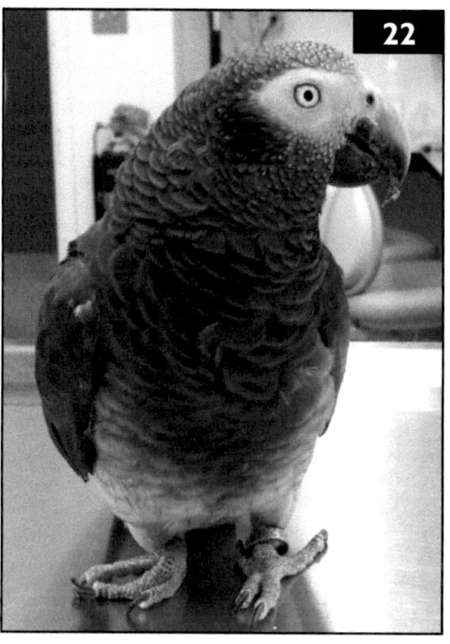

CASE 22 A 17-year-old male Timneh African grey parrot (*Psittacus erithacus timneh*) was presented on emergency for seizure episodes. When the owner returned from work on the night of presentation, the bird was at the bottom of the cage standing strangely (22). He was able to step up, but when the owner put him back in the cage, he began seizing in the cage and this occurred again outside on the floor. During these episodes, his eyes were open, his wings and right pelvic limb shook, and he leaned over. When the bird recovered, he appeared to have right-sided weakness and knuckling of the right foot with decreased gripping. The bird was fed a balanced pelleted diet and had lived indoors without being exposed to other birds for all his life. The neurologic examination revealed a quiet but responsive bird, ataxic, and weak on the right foot. Menace was absent in the right eye, with decreased vision. Proprioceptive deficits were absent in the right leg. The ophthalmic examination was unremarkable other than partial vision loss in the right eye. CBC and biochemistry panel were normal apart from a stress leukogram and moderate elevation of cholesterol and LDL. Radiographs showed increased opacity of great vessels of the heart. A heavy metal panel was negative for lead, zinc, and copper.

1 What is the most likely diagnosis?
2 What additional test would you perform to confirm your diagnosis?
3 How would you treat this bird?

CASE 23 A new client requests a wellness examination for his female (DNA-sexed) Hispaniolan Amazon parrot (*Amazona ventralis*). The bird's current diet is composed of a combination of sunflower seeds, bananas, corn, broccoli, strawberries, commercial pellets formulated for psittacines, and peanut butter as a treat. The owner estimates that the commercial pellets comprise about 20–25% of the bird's daily intake.

1 What is your assessment of this diet?
2 What are the potential nutritional deficiencies that psittacines fed such a diet may be presented with? How would they manifest clinically?
3 What would be your recommendation in terms of this bird's diet?

CASE 24 Two radiographic images (**24a, b**) were obtained from a wild adult male barred owl (*Strix varia*) found on the ground unable to fly. A poorly defined soft tissue opacity can be seen in the area of the right thoracic inlet.

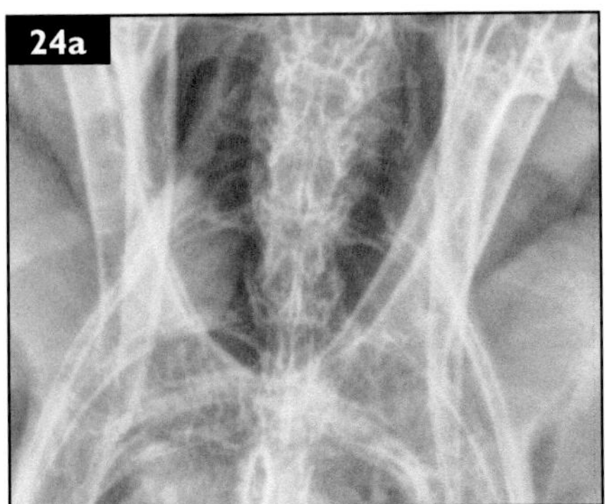
24a

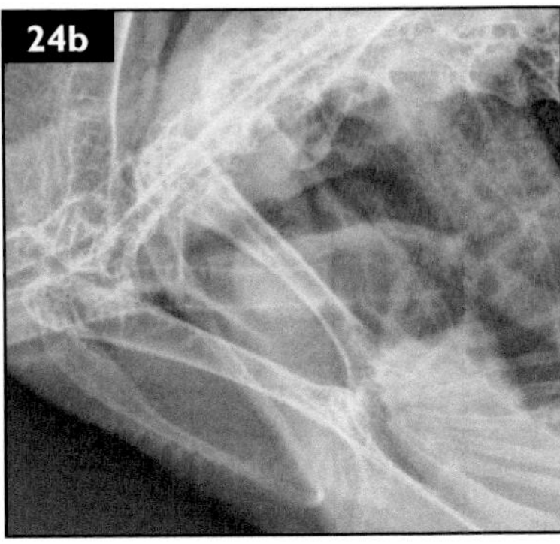
24b

1 Describe the normal anatomic structures that can be found in the area of the soft tissue structure, taking into consideration both radiographic views. List five differential diagnoses for the soft tissue structure seen in the radiographs.
2 What other diagnostic tests should be considered to further evaluate the nature and identity of the soft tissue structure seen on the image?
3 If the mass affects the thyroid gland, what is the most likely diagnosis?

CASE 25 A saker falcon (**25a**) (*Falco cherrug*) and a raven (**25b**) (*Corvus corax*) are each presented for evaluation with digital lesions of unknown duration.

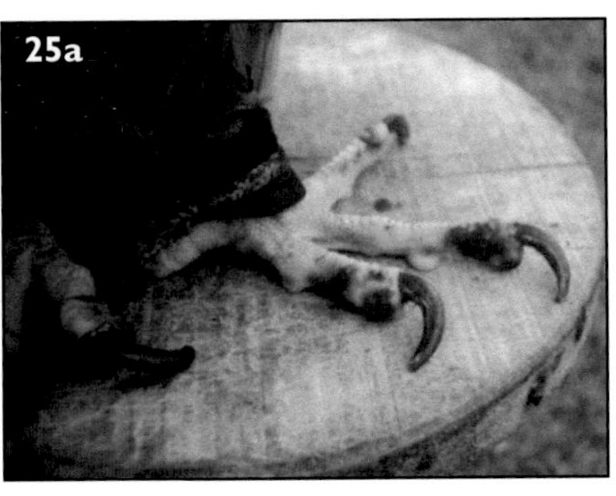
25a

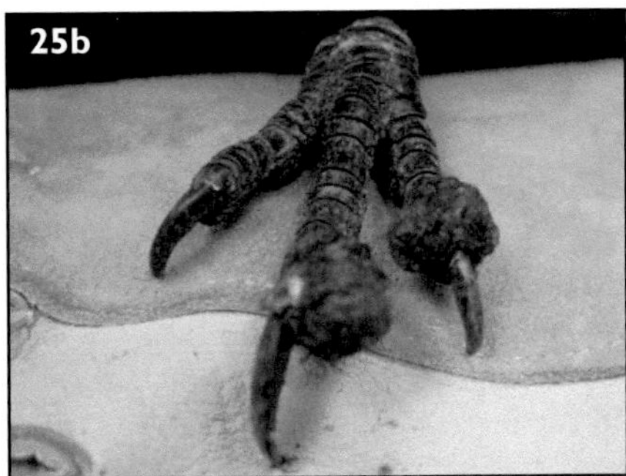
25b

1 What disease is demonstrated in each image?
2 What is the etiology?
3 What treatment and preventive actions should be taken?

CASE 26 A 4-year-old galah cockatoo (*Eolophus roseicapilla*) is referred to you. The referring veterinarian initially saw the bird when it was fluffed up and anorexic, with increased green coloration in the urates. Supportive therapy was provided and antibiotic, antifungal, and NSAID treatment was commenced. The patient initially improved, but never returned to its former self. Blood testing was carried out a month later; hematologic parameters were within reference values except for an elevated hematocrit of 58%. Biochemistry indicated elevated AST and GLDH and normal CK and bile acid. All other parameters were within reference values. In subsequent weeks, the owners noted marked exercise intolerance and the bird was referred for further diagnostic tests. The CBC and plasma biochemistry panel were repeated. The hematocrit had increased to 61%, all other parameters had normalized. Radiographs were taken (**26a, b**). In the lateral view, the heart length is 2.83 cm and the sternal length is 4.79 cm, while on the ventrodorsal view the heart width is 2.11 cm and the thorax width is 3.49 cm. Using those measurements, the heart is 60% of the chest width and the heart length is 44% of the sternal length.

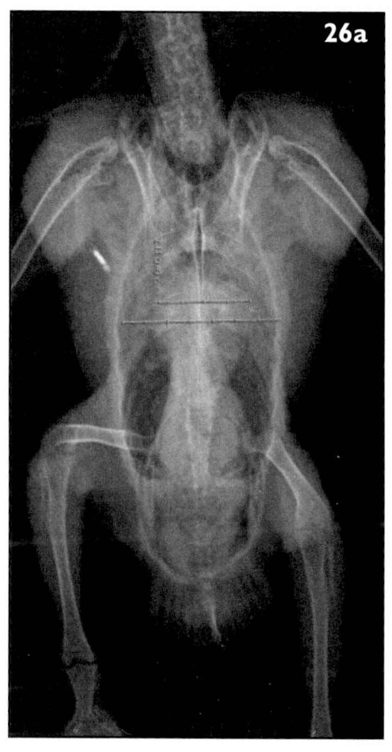
26a

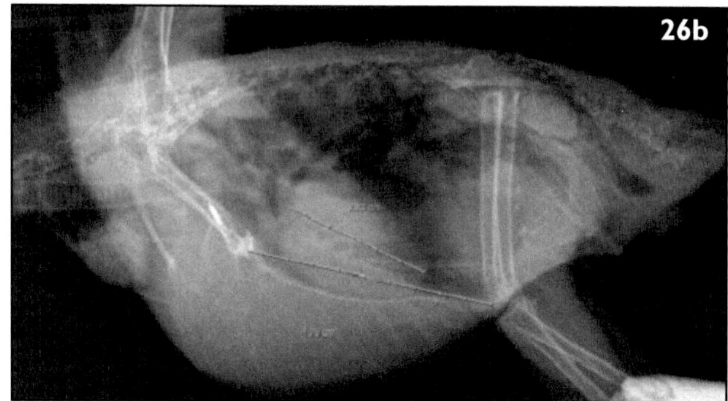
26b

1 What are the abnormal radiographic findings?
2 How do these findings explain the clinical pathology finding?
3 What further diagnostic tests might be beneficial?

CASE 27 Two 2-year-old barred Plymouth rock hens (*Gallus gallus domesticus*) presenting with a 2-day history of progressively worsening respiratory disease consisting of varying degrees of mild serous nasal discharge, rales, mild coughing, periorbital swelling, and edema of the head are shown (27). These hens and about 20 others of the same age had been purchased as a group 6 days previously from a private breeder. At presentation approximately half the birds had died showing similar signs, and some hens also had laid eggs with irregular shells. The owner brought these two for euthanasia and testing.

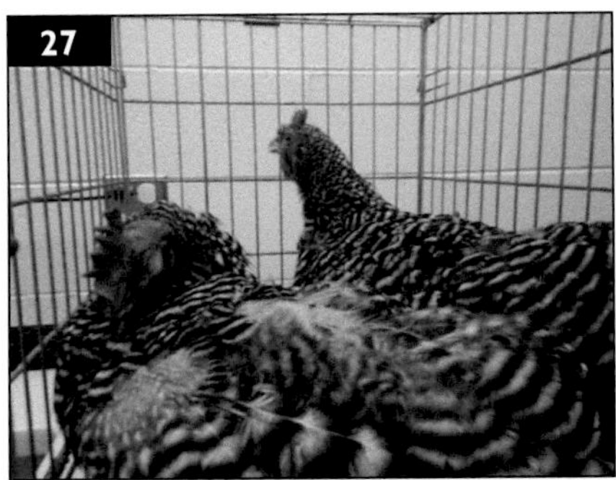

1 What diseases could cause these clinical signs? Which one is most likely?
2 How would you euthanize these birds?
3 What diagnostic test would you perform?

CASE 28 Radiowave radiosurgical instruments (28) use electron waves at a specific radiofrequency to cause ionic agitation in the cells at the tip of the electrode when the electrode is in contact with tissue, resulting in heating of the tissue with vaporization of tissue fluid, thus causing incision and coagulation. This heat causes collagen denaturation and tissue shrinkage with thrombosis of associated blood vessels, which manifests as improved incisional hemostasis.

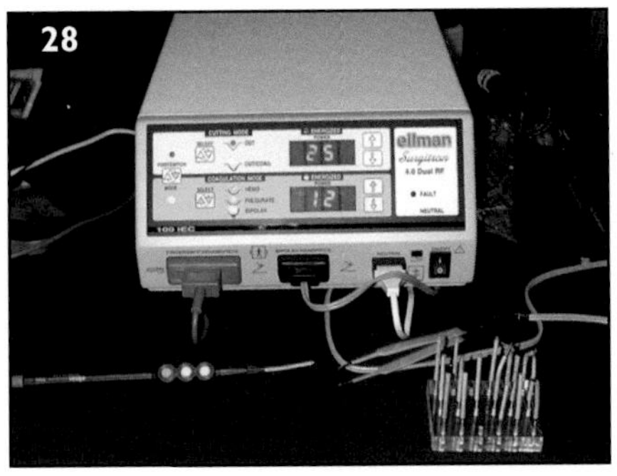

1 List the five principal factors that control the amount of lateral heat damage occurring in a radiosurgical incision.
2 What are the advantages of bipolar over monopolar radiosurgery?
3 What special considerations occur during the preparation of a potential surgical field if radiosurgery is to be used?

CASE 29 A 5-month-old African grey parrot (*Psittacus erithacus*) presents because of lethargy, decrease vocalization and inappetence. The bird was mildly dehydrated but otherwise the physical examination was fairly unremarkable. During the physical examination, the bird passed bright yellow urates. Hematologic findings indicated that the bird had a moderate anemia that appeared nonregenerative and severe leukopenia with absence of heterophils.

Erythrocyte parameters	Result
Red blood cells	2.11 M/μL (2.11 × 10^{12}/L)
Hematocrit	29% (0.29 L/L)
Mean corpuscular volume	137.4 fl
Red blood cell morphology	
Anisocytosis	Slight
Leukocyte parameters	
White blood cells	1,400/μL (1.4 × 10^9/L)
Neutrophils	0/μL (0 × 10^9/L)
Lymphocytes	1,176/μL (1.176 × 10^9/L)
Monocytes	224/μL (0.224 × 10^9/L)
Eosinophils	0/μL (0 × 10^9/L)
Basophils	0/μL (0 × 10^9/L)
Other parameters	
Plasma protein	3.2 g/dL (32 g/L)
Plasma fibrinogen	200 mg/dL (5.88 μmol/L)
Protein:fibrinogen ratio	15

1 What is the most likely diagnosis?
2 What additional test would you perform to confirm your diagnosis?
3 How would you treat this disease? What is the prognosis?

CASE 30
1 What is *Hexamita meleagridis* (*Spironucleus meleagridis*)?
2 What are the clinical signs observed in partridges and pheasants, and why do these signs occur?
3 How is this disease diagnosed and controlled?

CASE 31 A domestic egg laying hen (*Gallus gallus domesticus*) is presented for evaluation of lack of egg production despite broody behavior. The owner reported that the bird is also eating less, appears thin, and has a distended but firm coelom, both of which you confirm during your physical examination. Two ultrasound images are shown (**31a**, dorsocaudal coelom; **31b**, dorsal mid-coelom just cranial to **31a**).

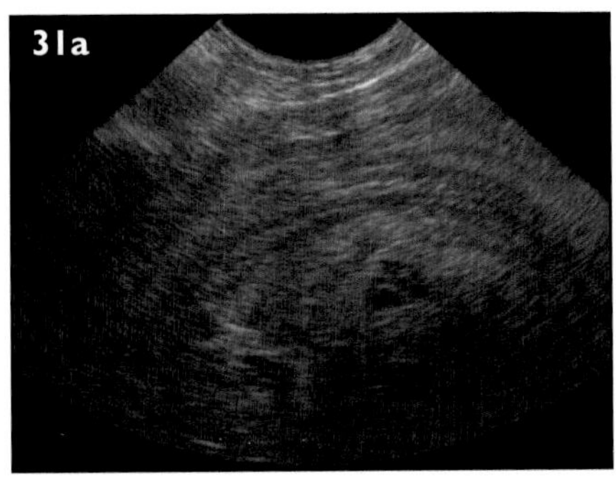

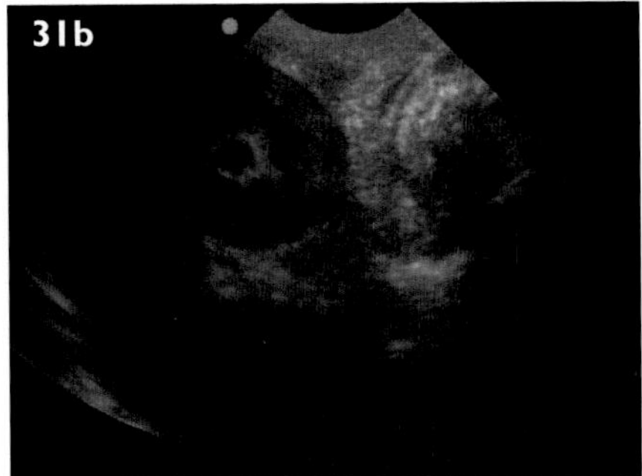

1 Based on the physical examination findings and the features of the ultrasound images, what is the cause of the coelomic distension in this hen?
2 What is the proposed pathophysiology of this condition in laying hens?
3 Describe the treatment options (medical and/or surgical) for this case.

CASE 32 A red-breasted toucan (*Ramphastos dicolorus*) was found severely depressed on the floor of its aviary, with fluffed feathers. Supportive care and enrofloxacin were administered but the bird was found dead soon afterwards. At gross necropsy the bird showed severely hemorrhagic lungs (**32a**) and several other organs were congested with petechiae.

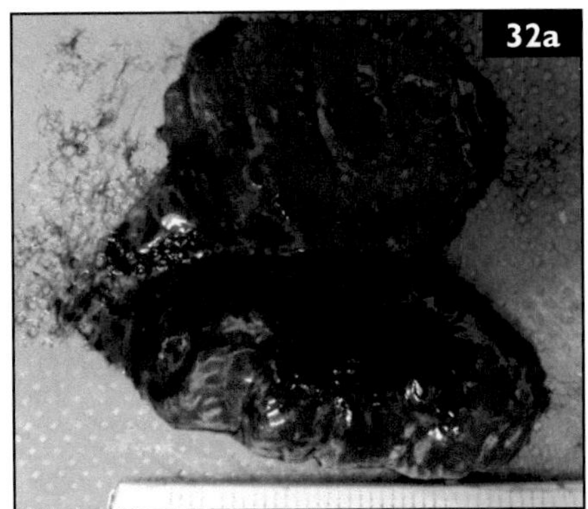

1 What are your main differential diagnoses?
2 How would you confirm them?
3 How would you treat this condition?

CASE 33 An adult Hispaniolan Amazon parrot (*Amazona ventralis*) is being manually restrained in a towel for induction of anesthesia, prior to diagnostic work up. Isoflurane is delivered in oxygen via a facemask tightly fitting around the bird's face to decrease exposure of personnel to anesthetic gas (**33**).

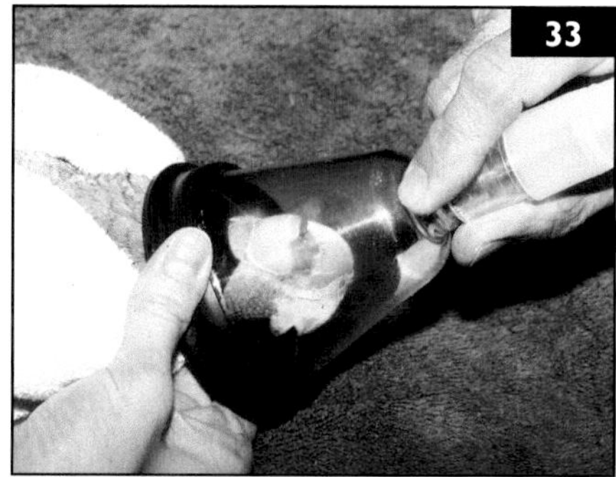

1 How long should avian patients be fasted prior to anesthesia?
2 What preanesthetic evaluation should be considered?
3 What premedication may be considered?

CASE 34 A saker falcon (*Falco cherrug*) was presented with a history of progressive weight loss and reduced appetite. The owner reported that for the past week the falcon had been trying to eat but appeared to have difficulty tearing and swallowing its food. On examination the tongue was found to be significantly enlarged, containing numerous white caseous foci on its dorsal and lateral aspects. Similar caseous foci were also seen on the hard palate (**34**). Abundant clear mucus could be observed on the choana and under the tongue. Food remains were plastered on both sides of the upper and lower beaks.

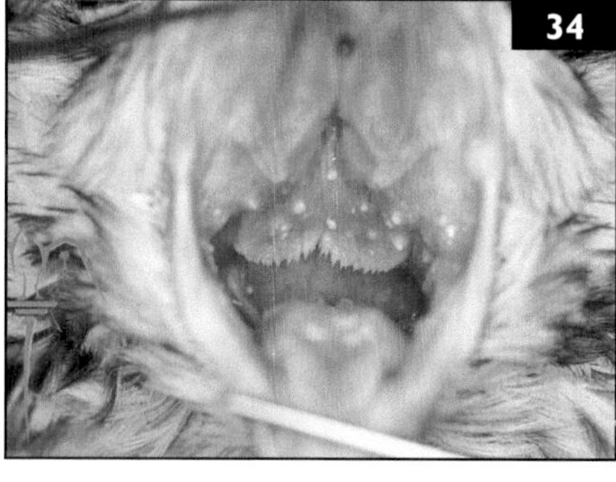

1 Based on the history and clinical findings described, list three significant differential diagnoses.
2 What diagnostic tests would you perform to confirm the diagnosis?
3 Microbiological cultures yielded pure growths of *Pseudomonas aeruginosa*, which were suspected to have occurred subsequent to a prior *Trichomonas* infection. What therapeutic management would you establish for the *Pseudomonas* spp. infection?

CASE 35 An adult female peregrine falcon (*Falco peregrinus*) was presented to a veterinary clinic for general examination with a history of anorexia for the past 2 days and the passing of green stained urates. The falcon was imported into the country as a juvenile (<9 months old) bird the previous year. The presenting falconer was its second owner and the bird had not been taken outside the country during the past year. The bird was mildly dehydrated and weak, but otherwise relatively bright and responsive.

1 What common diseases could produce anorexia and the passing of green urates in falcons?
2 What laboratory diagnostic tests you would require to establish a definitive diagnosis?

The falcon was placed in an isolation room but was found dead the following morning. Postmortem examination showed a distended ventriculus with petechial hemorrhages at the isthmus. The liver was slightly enlarged and congested. There was also hydropericardium with mild pericarditis. Both lungs were slightly congested. No significant growth was observed on bacterial culture. Histopathology findings included myocardial necrotic foci with some cells showing intranuclear inclusions, marked hemosiderosis of hepatocytes with some necrotic foci, marked perivascular edema of the lungs, and meningeal congestion. Inoculation of macerated tissues into the allantoic cavity of 10–12-day-old embryonated chicken eggs and onto monolayers of chicken embryo fibroblast (CEF) cell cultures was carried out. The embryonated chickens died 3 days after inoculation and acute cytopathogenic effect developed 3 days after inoculation of CEF. Fluid from the allantoic cavity and the cell cultures were subjected to hemagglutination inhibition testing. In addition, an influenza A antigen ELISA test was used. The samples showed a strong positive reaction to the avian influenza virus. Consequently, samples were sent to a specialized laboratory for further virology identification studies. The results showed that the virus isolated was the highly pathogenic avian influenza virus phenotype H5N1. The closest relatives of this particular strain were recent H5N1 isolates from Novosibirsk in Russia and Mongolia.

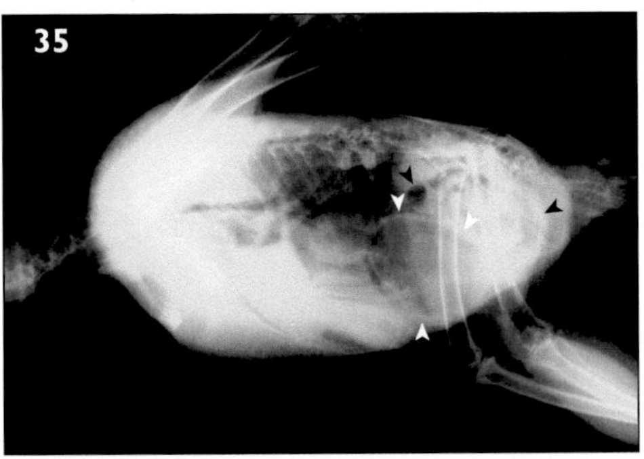

Radiology examination showed a distended ventriculus with apparent thickening of the ventricular wall (**35**, white arrowheads) in addition to mild enlargement of the liver and the spleen. The intestinal tract was filled with gas (black arrowheads). Hematology assays revealed a total white blood cell count within normal range (7.1×10^9/L [normal value $5.7 \pm 0.31 \times 10^9$/L]) and a mild heterophilia (6.6×10^9/L [normal value $4.14 \pm 0.24 \times 10^9$/L]). Approximately 50% of the heterophils showed loss of granulation. The only significant finding in the blood chemistry analyses was a severely elevated AST (242 U/L [reference interval 45–95 U/L]). More specific testing using antigen capture tests, virus isolation, and/or PCR would be required to establish a definite diagnosis.

3 How would you proceed in the light of these findings?

CASE 36 A 22-year-old female intact Congo African grey parrot (*Psittacus erithacus*) presents as an emergency having been attacked by a dog in the household. She has several bite wounds, bruises, and damage to her wing (**36**). Blood is collected for hematology and plasma biochemistry panel.

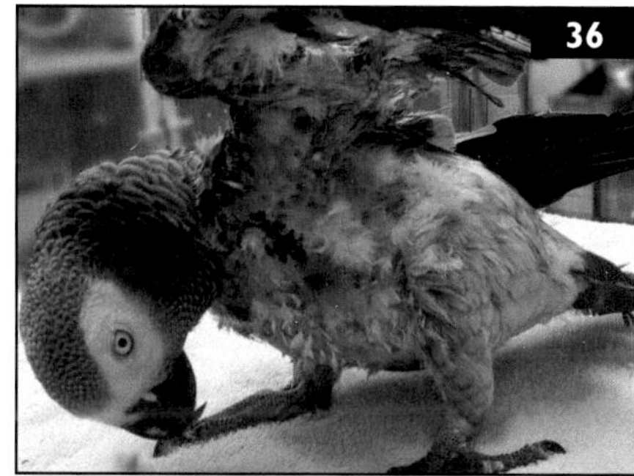

Parameter	Value	Reference interval
AST (U/L)	854	100–350
Calcium, total (mmol/L) (mg/dL)	2.27 (9.1)	2–3.24 (8–13)
CK (U/L)	3,439	123–875
Glucose (mmol/l) (mg/dL)	19.32 (348)	10.55–19.43 (190–350)
Phosphorus (mmol/L) (mg/dL)	1.26 (3.9)	1.03–1.74 (3.2–5.4/2.4–5.3)
Potassium (mEq/L)	3.1	2.6–4.2
Protein, total (g/L) (g/dL)	38 (3.8)	30–50 (3–5)
Albumin (g/L) (g/dL)	23 (2.3)	15.7–32.3 (1.57–3.23)
Globulin (g/L) (g/dL)	15 (1.5)	14.3–17.7 (1.43–1.77)
Sodium (mEq/L)	147	134–152
Uric acid (μmol/L) (mg/dL)	268 (4.5)	238–595 (4–10)

1 What is the most likely cause for the elevated AST in this patient?
2 Can liver disease be ruled out as a cause for the elevated AST? What other values could be tested to rule in or out liver disease?
3 Apart from muscle trauma such as a dog bite, in what other situations is it common to see elevated CK levels in avian patients?

CASE 37 An African grey parrot (*Psittacus erithacus*) was presented with severe respiratory signs, voice changes, decreased weight, and change in behavior. Ventrodorsal and lateral radiographs revealed increased linear opacities consistent with thickened air sacs and distinct soft tissue opacities within the caudal thoracic air sacs and lungs (**37a, b**). Endoscopy and cytology confirmed the presence of an aspergilloma within the caudal thoracic air sacs.

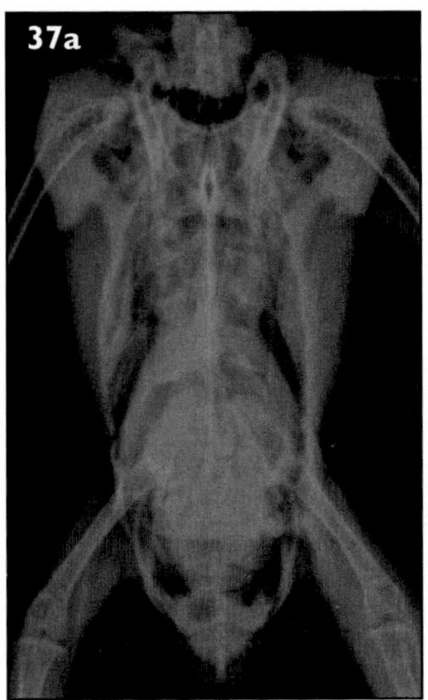
37a

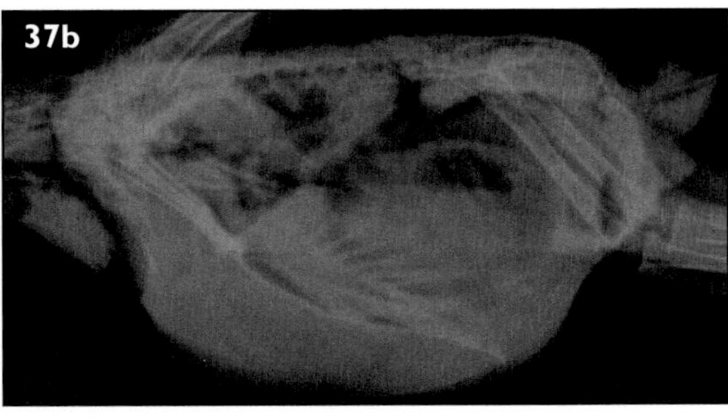
37b

1 Which species of *Aspergillus* are causative agents of respiratory aspergillosis in psittacine birds? What is the commonest source of infection?

2 How you would treat a psittacine bird with respiratory aspergillosis? What should be considered regarding the different drugs?

3 Which antifungal drug has been shown to cause adverse reactions in African grey parrots suffering from aspergillosis? Which alternate systemic antifungal drugs may be used for aspergillosis in these birds?

CASE 38 A 2-year-old budgerigar (*Melopsittacus undulatus*) is presented for regurgitating food immediately after eating, accompanied by progressive increased inspiratory effort and a noticeable enlargement in the crop area that has progressed over the past 7 days. While collecting the history and visually examining the bird and cage, you note that it is being fed millet seed.

1 What would be included in your differential diagnoses for this case?

2 What diagnostic tests could be of aid in diagnosis?

3 What would be included in your treatment plan?

CASE 39 A 10-year-old umbrella cockatoo (*Cacatua alba*) was presented for acute dyspnea responsive to oxygen therapy. Physical examination revealed a grade 3/5 systolic heart murmur. The CBC was within reference values. Ventrodorsal and lateral radiographs are shown (**39a, b**), as well as horizontal four-chamber view echocardiography through a median transcoelomic approach (**39c**).

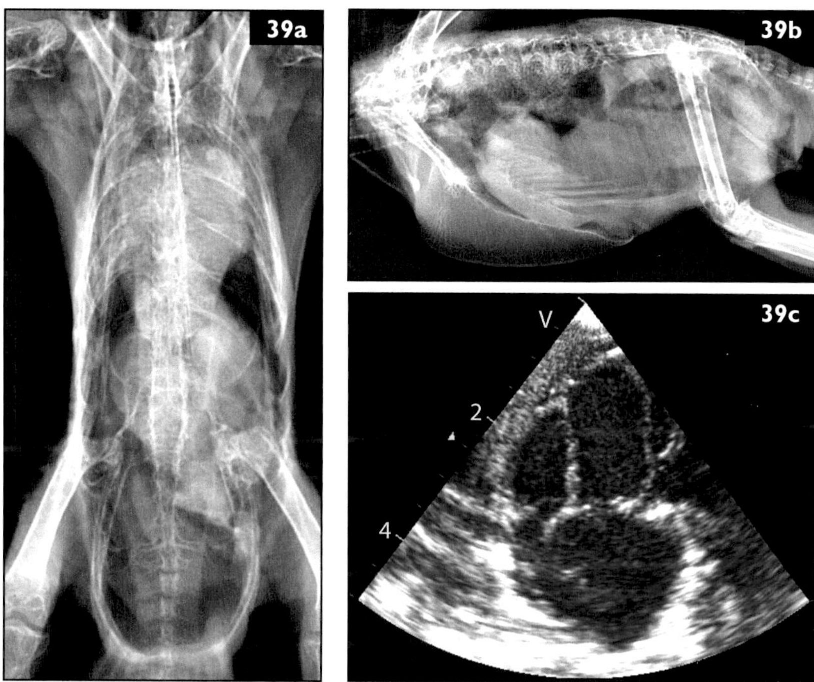

1 Describe the radiographic findings. What should the radiographic size for the heart be in medium to large-size parrots? What is the radiographic appearance of the heart in cockatoos?
2 Describe the echocardiographic findings. What do you know about the reliability of echocardiographic measurements in birds? What is the differential diagnosis for these findings? What is the likely cause for the respiratory signs?
3 What other clinical signs are common in companion psittacine birds with this condition?

CASE 40 An adult toco toucan (*Ramphastos toco*) was presented at the clinic with acute-onset severe diarrhea. The stools had a foul smell and a significant amount of fresh blood was mixed with the feces (**40a**). Cytology of the feces using a Romanowsky stain (Diff-Quik™) was performed (**40b**).

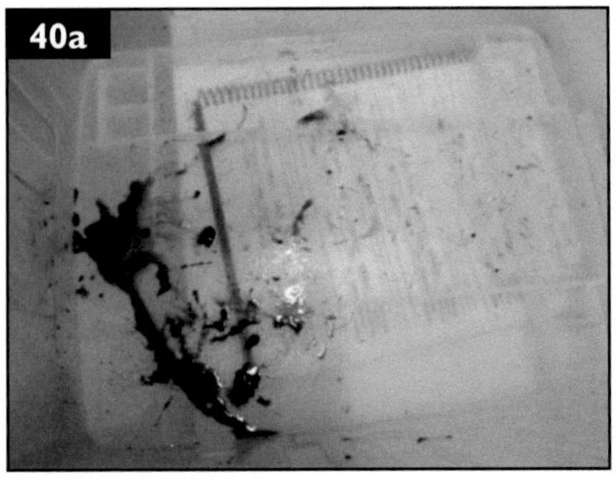
40a

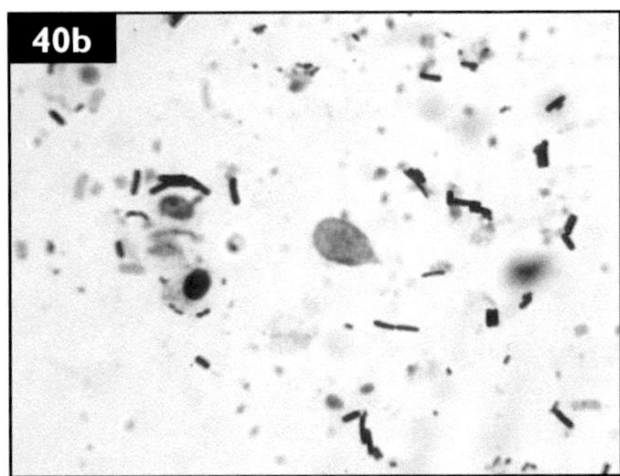
40b

1 What is your presumptive diagnosis?
2 What additional examination would you request?
3 How would you treat this condition?

CASE 41 A gyrfalcon (*Falco rusticolus*) breeder client, despite having a flight exclusion over his property, is twice overflown by two chinook helicopters (**41**) at a height of 50 m within 1.5 hours during the breeding season, resulting in significant losses to incubating eggs. The military accept they were present and you are required to prove a loss occurred and calculate an accurate quantum of losses. The client breeds gyr and gyr hybrids. He has white, black, and gray gyrs, with a number of imprint semen donors. While he has breeding plans, when a falcon requires insemination, he will use what semen is available on the day. This could be peregrine, saker, or gyr (black, white, gray). The client incubates eggs artificially and under parents. It is reported that only the eggs under the parents are affected.

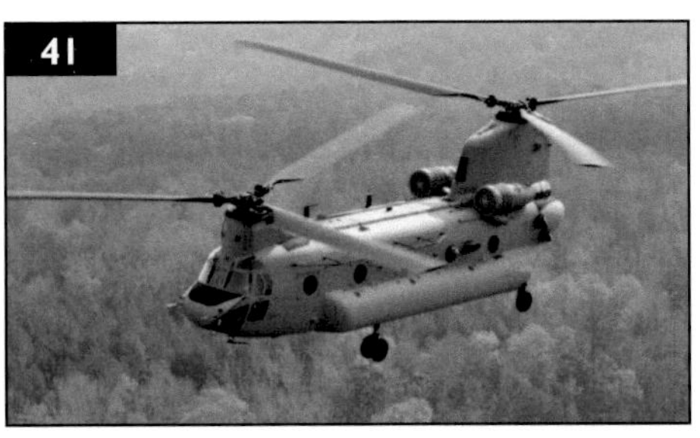
41

1 What initial data, information, and material do you request?
2 At what stage of incubation are eggs most likely to suffer?
3 You realize that you cannot accurately calculate the losses. Why?

CASE 42 A 12-year-old African grey parrot (*Psittacus erithacus*) is presented for hyporexia, red coloration of the urine, strabismus, and seizures. Whole body radiographs are obtained (**42a, b**).

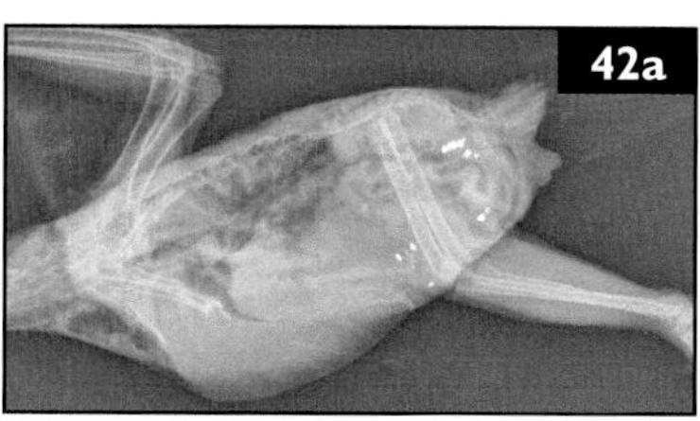

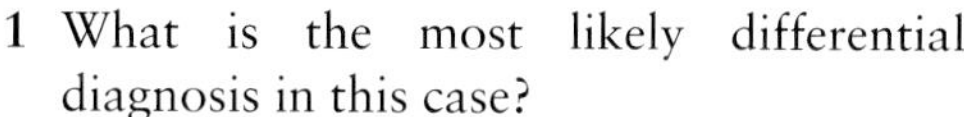

1 What is the most likely differential diagnosis in this case?
2 What complementary test do you perform to confirm this suspicion?
3 What treatment would you recommend?

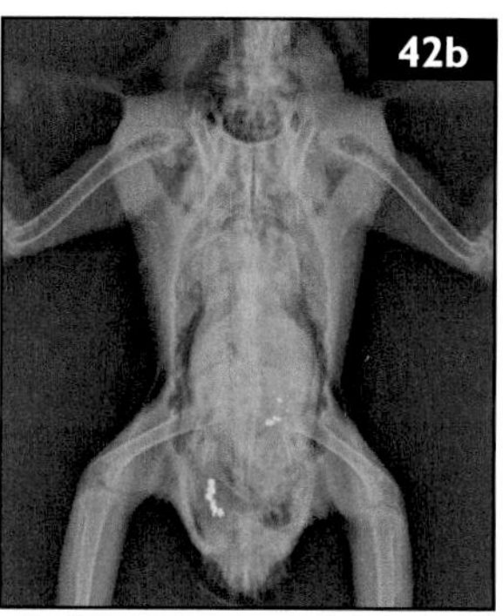

CASE 43 An ESF-intramedullary (ESF-IM) pin tie-in fixator was applied to a complex segmental tibiotarsus fracture in a 4.75 kg juvenile female bald eagle (*Haliaeetus leucocephalus*) approximately 4 weeks ago. The IM pin was removed as part of dynamic destabilization of the fracture, and a complication was noted on follow-up radiographs (**43a, b**).

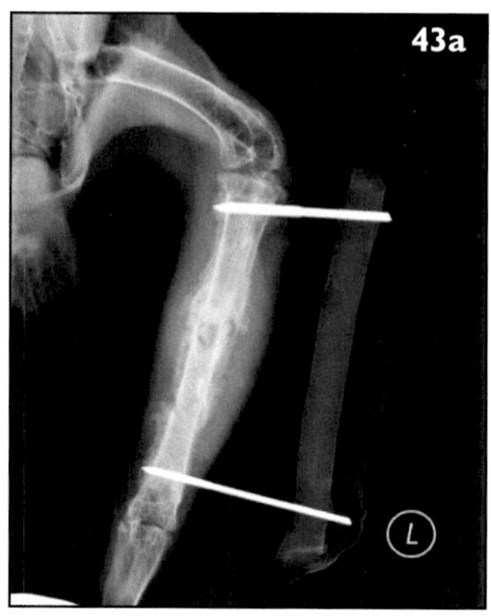

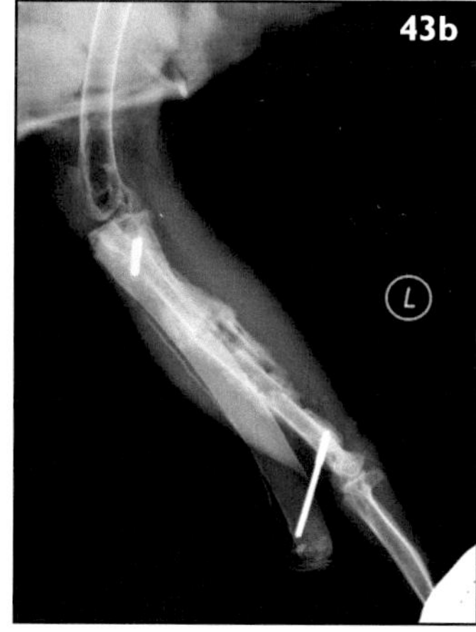

1 Name the primary bony abnormality present.
2 How would you treat this problem?
3 How would you minimize the risk of developing this problem?

CASE 44 A blue-crowned laughing thrush (*Dryonastes courtoisii*) is presented for postmortem examination. During the gross examination you observe small white granular-shaped lesions in the pectoral muscles and heart, hepatomegaly, splenomegaly, and intestinal distension (**44a**). You perform a blood smear (**44b**).

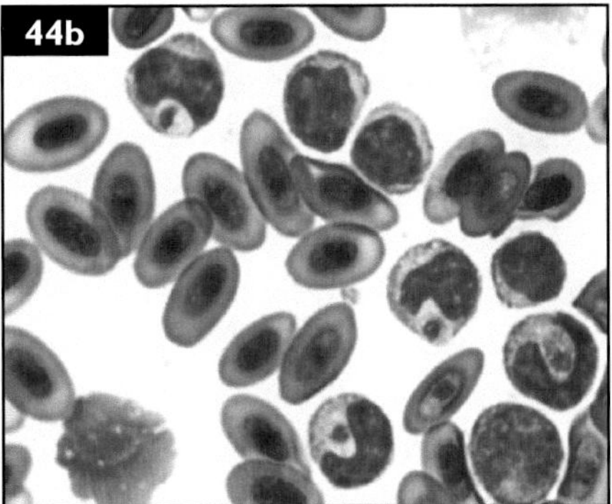

1 Which protozoal organism would you consider as a differential diagnosis?
2 How would you evaluate whether the rest of the flock is affected by the same parasite?
3 What treatment would you consider, and what is the main limitation of this treatment?

CASE 45 A 6-week-old scarlet macaw (*Ara macao*) is presented because of failure to thrive. The chick has been hand-reared from hatching on a home-prepared liquid formula. The diet is comprised of peanut butter, banana, yogurt, applesauce, baby creamed corn, and baby food. On examination the bird is bright and alert but seems stunted in comparison to what you would expect in a chick of this age.

1 What would be your nutritional assessment of this diet?
2 What would be your dietary recommendation in light of the presentation?
3 List the important considerations in the diet preparation and feeding regimen of a young macaw chick?

CASE 46 A 32-year-old male double yellow-headed Amazon parrot (*Amazona oratrix*) presents for lethargy, regurgitation, anorexia, and abnormal droppings. At home, he is on an all seed diet. On physical examination he is obese, has several suspected lipomas, and produces droppings with yellow tinged urates (**46a**). Blood is collected for a biochemistry panel and it is severely lipemic (**46b**).

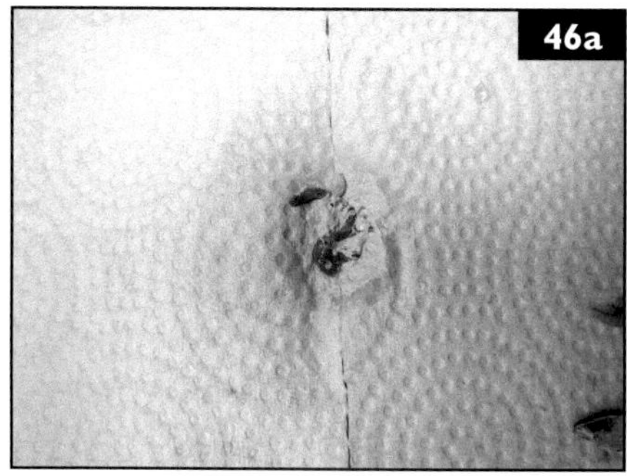
46a

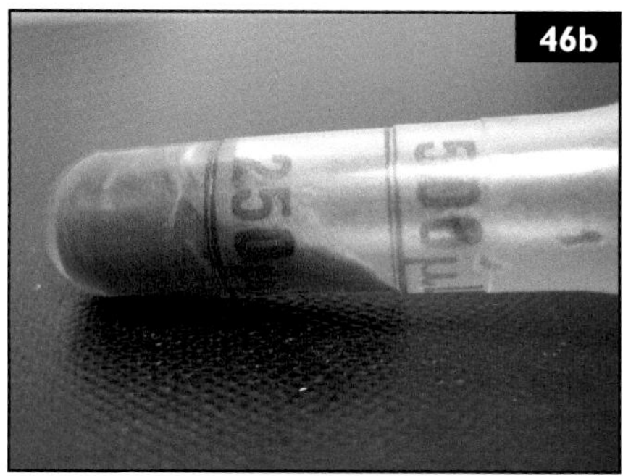

46b

Parameter	Value	Reference interval
AST (U/L)	1,488	130–350
Calcium (mmol/L) (mg/dL)	2.22 (8.9)	2–3.24 (8–13)
Cholesterol (mmol/L) (mg/dL)	24.47 (946)	5.17–8.35 (200–323)
CK (U/L)	245	45–265
Glucose (mmol/L) (mg/dL)	17.98 (324)	12.21–19.43 (220–350)
LDH (U/L)	1,616	160–420
Phosphorus (mmol/L) (mg/dL)	1.36 (4.2)	1–1.78 (3.1–5.5)
Potassium (mEq/L)	3.8	3–4.5
Protein, total (g/L) (g/dL)	48 (4.8)	30–50 (3–5)
Albumin (g/L) (g/dL)	34 (3.4)	19–35 (1.9–3.5)
Globulin (g/L) (g/dL)	14 (1.4)	11–15 (1.1–1.5)
Sodium (mEq/L)	149	136–152
Uric acid (µmol/L) (mg/dL)	364 (6.1)	119–595 (2–10)

1 What disease process is suspected in this patient? Is there an additional biochemical analyte that should be checked?
2 How do the yellow urates correlate with the blood work findings?
3 What additional diagnostic tests could be performed to confirm the suspected disease in this patient?

CASE 47 An adult yellow-eyed penguin (*Megadyptes antipodes*) was presented with hind limb paralysis, depression, and sternal recumbency. Neurologic examination revealed absence of deep pain perception, withdrawal of the lower limbs, and patellar reflexes. Whole body ventrodorsal and laterolateral radiographic views are taken (**47a, b**).

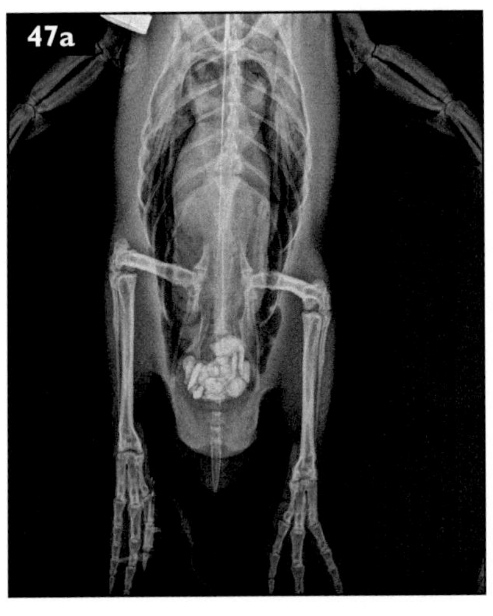
47a

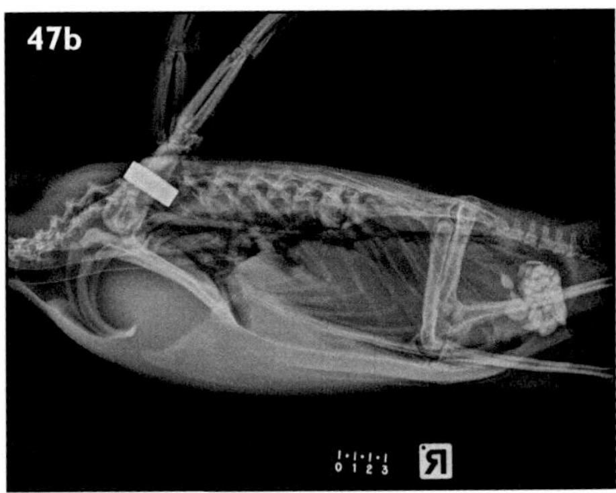
47b

1 What is the most likely diagnosis?
2 What is the prognosis for this condition?
3 What is the most likely etiology?

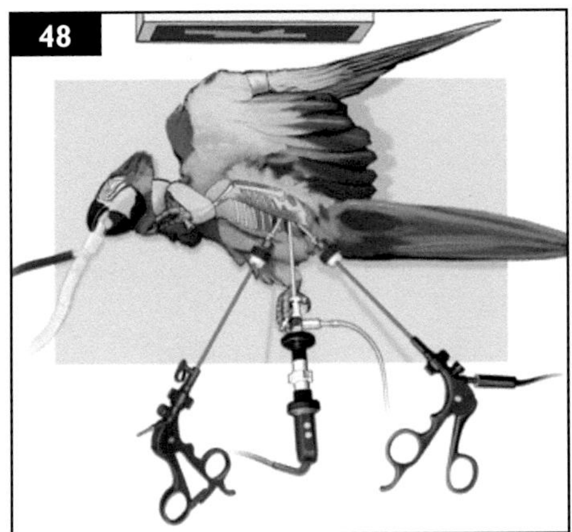
48

Courtesy of Educational Resources, UGA

CASE 48 The surgical positioning and instrument use for performing a three-port endosurgical salpingectomy in a macaw is shown (**48**).

1 List some disadvantages and advantages associated with endosurgery compared with the more traditional open coeliotomy.

CASE 49 A 2-year-old saker falcon (*Falco cherrug*) is presented with a grade 1/5 unilateral bumblefoot of the left foot (**49a**), a 4-year-old peregrine falcon (*Falco peregrinus*) is presented with a grade 3/5 lesion (**49b**), and a 7-year-old peregrine falcon is presented with a bilateral grade 4–5/5 lesion (**49c**).

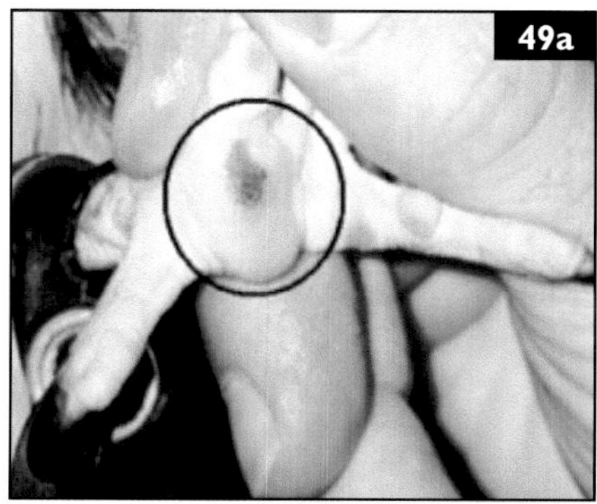
49a

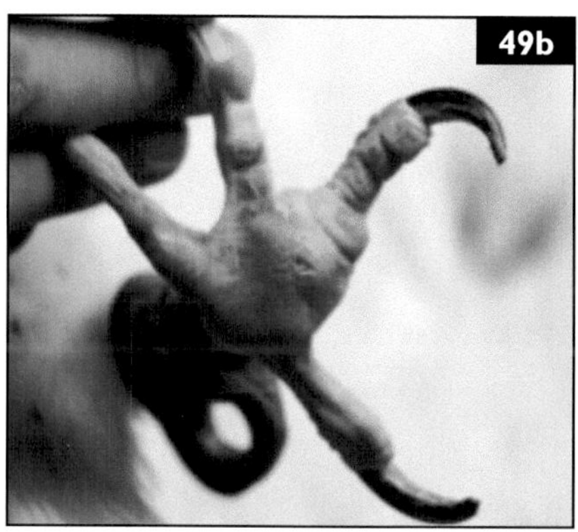
49b

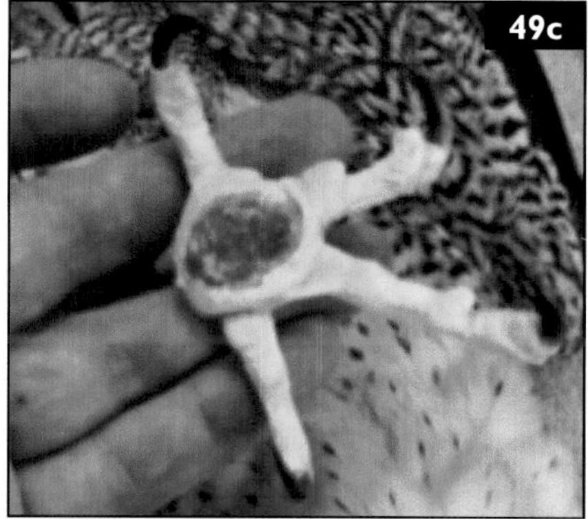
49c

1 How you would treat the grade 1/5 lesion?
2 How would you treat the grade 3/5 lesion?
3 How would you treat the grade 4–5/5 lesion?

CASE 50 An adult African grey parrot (*Psittacus erithacus*) is presented with a history of anorexia for 24 hours. During the physical examination, the parrot appears to be moderately to severely dehydrated, which you estimate to be approximately 8–10%. Determination of the hydration status of a bird can be challenging.

1 What physical examination findings can you use to estimate the hydration status?
2 What laboratory findings can help you confirm your findings from the physical examination?

CASE 51 Cloacal prolapse is a condition that is commonly encountered in adult umbrella (*Cacatua alba*) and Moluccan cockatoos (*Cacatua moluccensis*) (**51**). Although various medical causes (e.g. cloacitis, egg yolk peritonitis, salpingitis, bacterial, fungal or parasitic enteritis) may underlie the condition, cloacal prolapse is commonly thought to be behavioral in origin in these species, as a result of prolonged or recurrent straining.

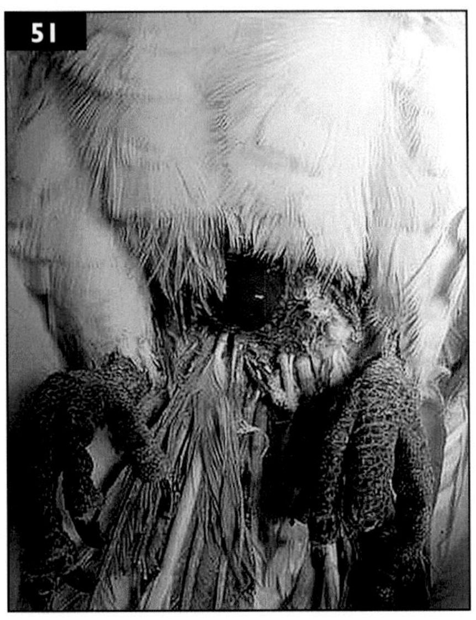

1 Provide at least three characteristic historical findings that are noted in many of the cockatoos presented with cloacal prolapse.
2 Describe the various treatment options that may be considered for these patients.
3 Which complication may commonly be seen in cockatoos with chronic cloacal prolapse, and how would this condition best be treated?

CASE 52 The head of a *Falco* spp. bird is shown (**52**). The routine task of trimming the beaks of falconry birds is usually carried out in the West by trained falconers. However, in the Middle East, falconers tend to take their falcons to local specialized falcon hospitals where technicians or veterinary surgeons carry out this procedure.

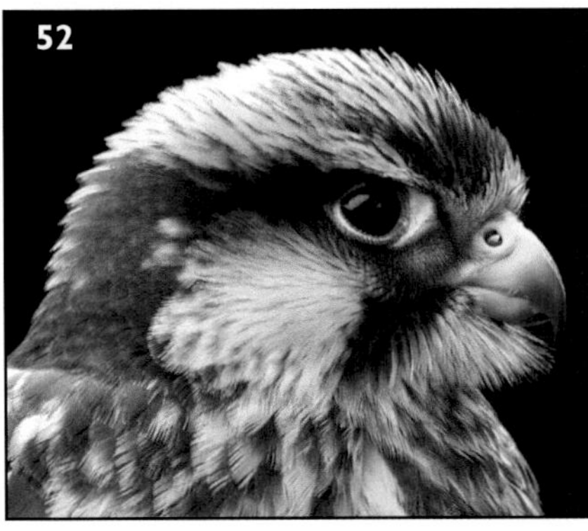

1 What anatomic structure of the beak is present in *Falco* spp., but is absent in *Accipiter* spp. and *Buteo* spp.?
2 This structure allows members of the Falconiformes to perform what task when hunting?
3 What is the ancient falconry term used for trimming the beak of falconry birds?

CASE 53 A flock of pigeons (*Columba livia domestica*) was treated for capillariasis using fenbendazole (Panacur 10%, 100 mg/ml; 50 mg/kg PO once daily for 5 days). On the last day of treatment the birds developed anorexia, vomiting, and lethargy. Blood work revealed leukopenia with marked heteropenia. In the bone marrow cytology, there was a severe depletion of the erythrocytic and leukocytic cell series (**53**, arrow indicates macrophage erythrocytosis and the * is an osteoclast, ×40).

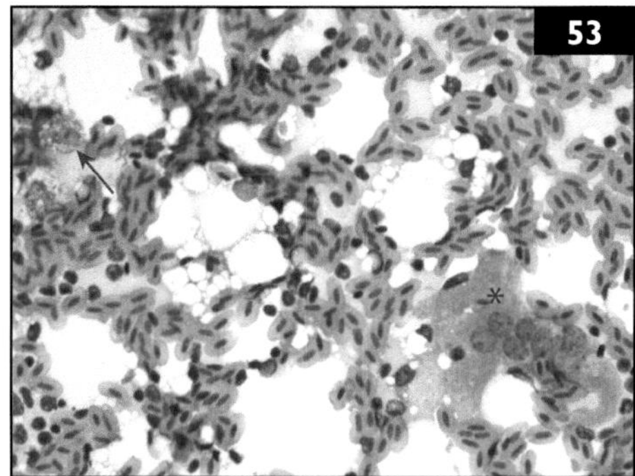

1 What is the possible cause for the bone marrow suppression?
2 What other system may be affected?
3 What other condition could enhance the toxicity of fenbendazole?

CASE 54 A 2-year-old male cockatiel (*Nymphicus hollandicus*) is presented with a 48-hour history of regurgitation and depression. The animal is single housed and allowed to fly free in the owner's house for 1–2 hours each day. The diet consists of a commercial seed mix. The animal has no previous medical history. Physical examination reveals moderate dehydration, good body condition, and dried saliva around the beak commissure. The owner is concerned that the bird may have chewed on a plant, thereby causing the illness. The leaves of the indoor plant are shown for evaluation (**54**).

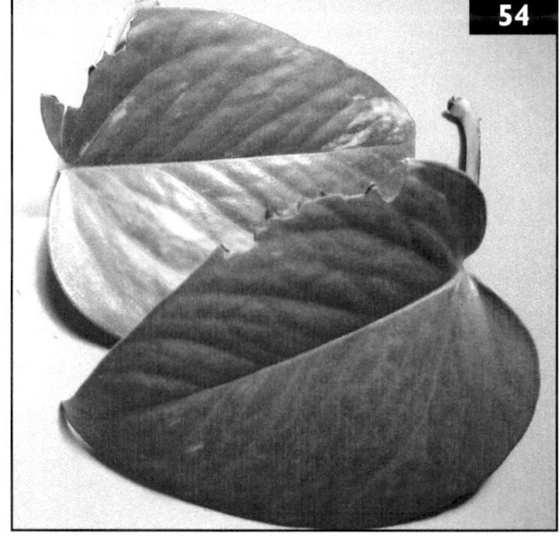

1 What type of plant is shown?
2 What is the mechanism of toxicity for this plant? What are the expected clinical signs?
3 What is the recommended treatment?

CASE 55 An adult great horned owl (*Bubo virginianus)* presents after being found on the side of the road unable to fly. On presentation the bird is dull but responsive. On physical examination mild bruising over the notarium is noted (55). A complete neurologic examination reveals no cranial nerve deficits, but the bird is unable to perch or stand and has severe proprioceptive deficits in the pelvic limbs. Spinal reflexes, including the vent sphincter reflex and pedal flexor reflex, are present, but the patellar reflex and wing withdrawal reflex are difficult to elicit and evaluate. The owl responds to deep pain stimulation in both extremities. You suspect spinal cord trauma. Radiographs are consistent with increased soft tissue opacity over the 4th thoracic vertebra, which appears slightly shorter with a mild ventral radiolucency. You suspect a compression fracture of the 4th thoracic vertebra and spinal cord trauma.

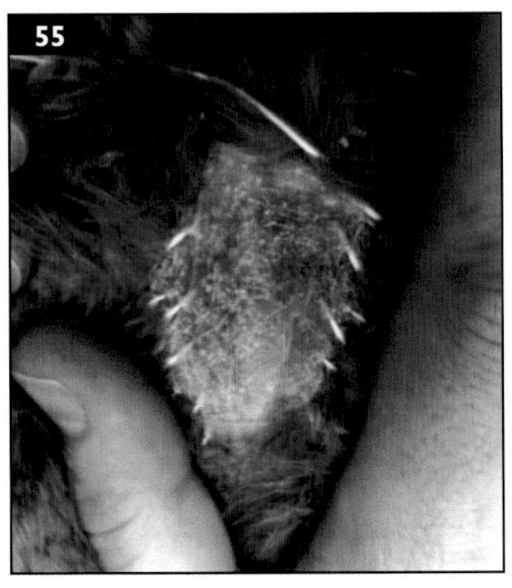

1 How would you confirm your diagnosis?
2 How would you treat this bird?
3 What is the prognosis?

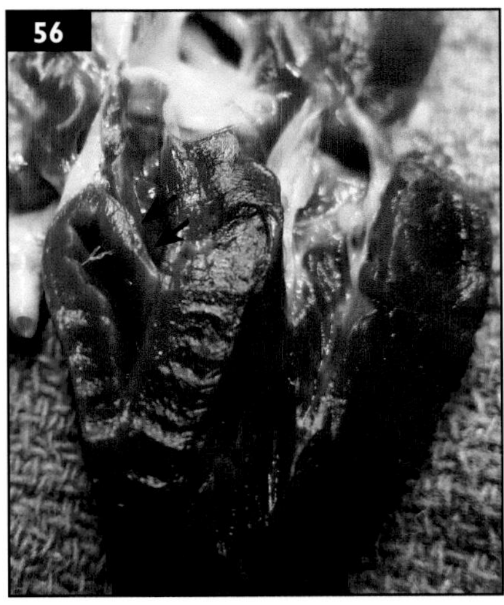

CASE 56

1 What anatomic structure is depicted by the arrows in this parrot's heart (56)?
2 What other anatomic differences are there between the avian and mammalian heart?
3 What are the clinical implications of these differences for diagnostic tests?

CASE 57 A research facility had a group of approximately 50 white Leghorn chicks at 3 weeks of age with a history of most chicks showing variable degrees of lethargy, stunting, and death over the previous week (57). No necropsies have been performed on the dead chicks. Some had mild diarrhea, but on physical examination they were found to have varying degrees of dyspnea due to coelomic effusion. Two were humanely euthanized after obtaining a blood sample, and then submitted for necropsy, which confirmed the coelomic effusion and an exudative diathesis. No signs of heart disease were present.

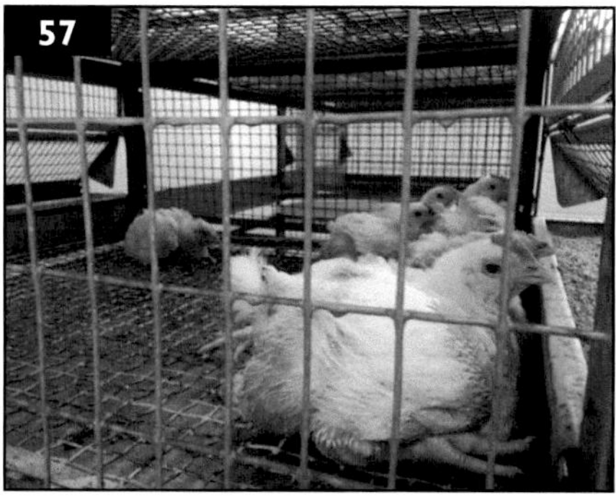

1 What could cause the clinical signs seen in these chicks?
2 How would you confirm the diagnosis?

CASE 58

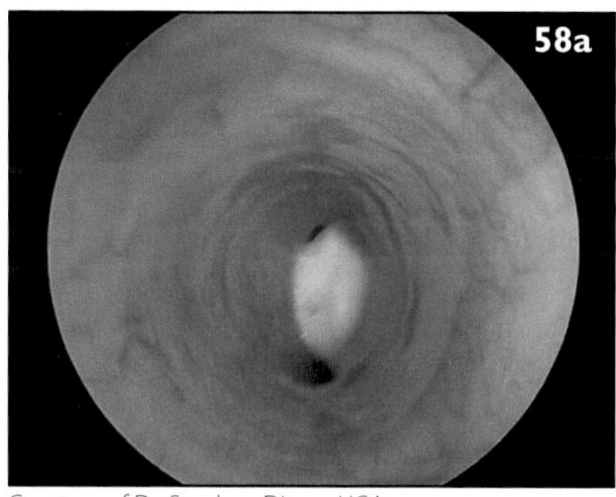

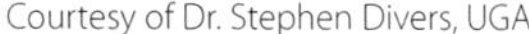
Courtesy of Dr. Stephen Divers, UGA

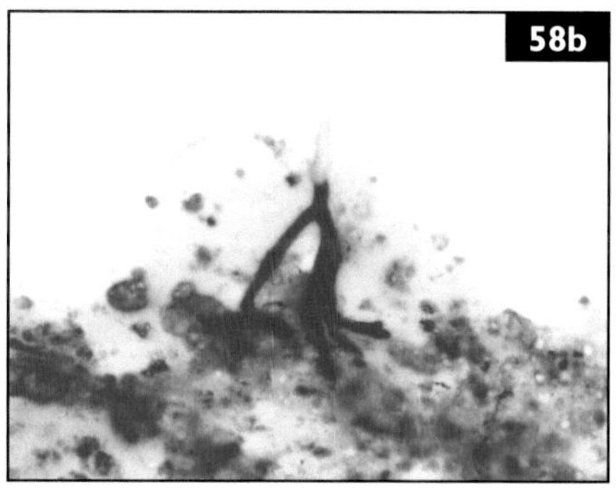

1 What are the preanesthetic considerations for a tracheoscopy?
2 A tracheoscopy is being performed in this cockatoo. An abnormal finding is encountered (**58a**). What are the differential diagnoses for this finding?
3 What are the immediate diagnostic and therapeutic steps that should be undertaken?
4 An intraoperative impression smear was evaluated in this case (**58b**). Describe the cytologic finding. What is the most likely diagnosis?

CASE 59 At the Doha Raptor Medicine Conference in 2014, Ali *et al.* presented data representing the incidence of various pathogens on culture from sick falcons (**59**) treated in the Souq Wakif Falcon Hospital in the previous 2 years. *Pseudomonas* spp. were isolated from 25.7% of cases, *E. coli* from 17.1% of cases, and *Staphylococcus* spp. from 5.8% of cases. These pathogens are all considered to be preventable and collectively comprise 48.6% of all pathogens isolated from sick falcons.

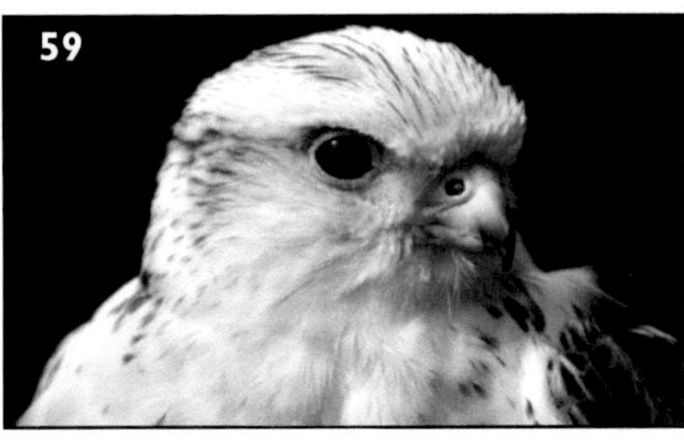
59

1 What is the likely origin of the *Pseudomonas* spp. infections, and how could this be best prevented?
2 What is the likely origin of the *E. coli* infections, and how could this be best prevented?
3 What is the likely origin of the *Staphylococcus* spp. infections, and how could this be best prevented?

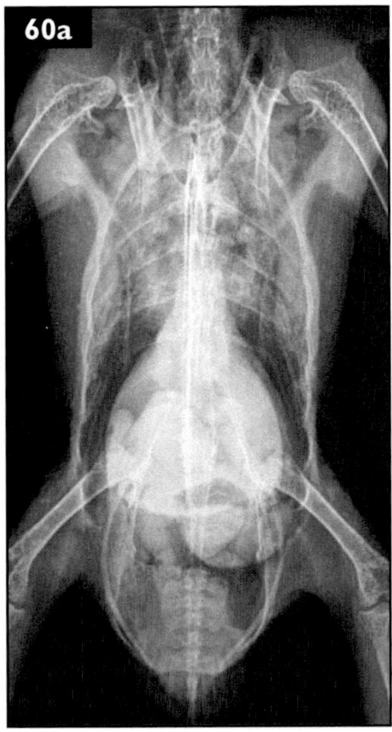
60a

CASE 60 A 2-year-old female African grey parrot (*Psittacus erithacus*) presented with a chronic history of lethargy, weight loss, and regurgitation. You obtain radiographs (**60a, b**) under sedation and manual restraint.

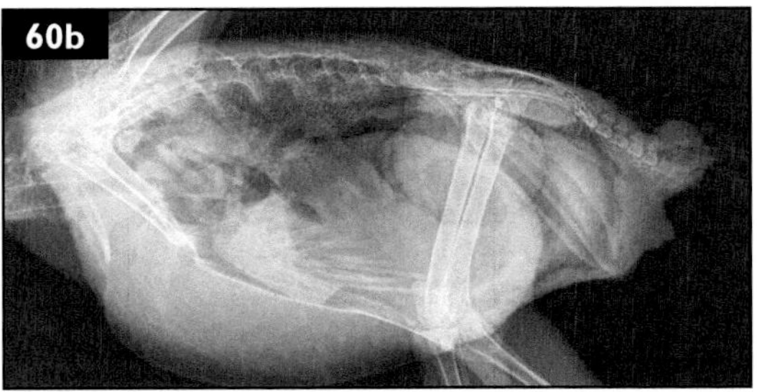
60b

1 What radiographic abnormalities are shown?
2 How can proventricular size be evaluated radiographically in psittacines?
3 What diseases could result in similar abnormal radiographic findings?

CASE 61 A 14-year-old male black swan (*Cygnus atratus*) belonging to a private collection was presented for routine health examination. Hematologic findings indicated that the bird had a severe lymphocytic leukocytosis, consistent with chronic lymphocytic leukemia. Radiographs showed the presence of multiple soft tissue masses within the caudal coelomic cavity.

Erythrocyte parameters	Result
Red blood cells	1.90 M/μL (1.9×10^{12}/L)
Hematocrit	34% (0.34 L/L)
Mean corpuscular volume	178.9 fl
Red blood cell morphology	
Anisocytosis	Slight
Leukocyte parameters	
White blood cells	1,375,000/μL ($1{,}375 \times 10^9$/L)
Neutrophils	13,750/μL (13.75×10^9/L)
Lymphocytes	1,361,250/μL ($1{,}361 \times 10^9$/L)
Monocytes	0/μL (0×10^9/L)
Eosinophils	0/μL (0×10^9/L)
Basophils	0/μL (0×10^9/L)
Other parameters	
Plasma protein	5.0 g/dL (50 g/L)
Plasma fibrinogen	500 mg/dL (14.7 μmol/L)
Protein:fibrinogen ratio	9

1 What is the most likely diagnosis?
2 What additional test would you perform to confirm your diagnosis?
3 How would you treat this disease?

CASE 62 Vaccination is one of the most important ways of preventing infectious diseases in pigeons.

1 Vaccines exist for protection against four different infectious agents in pigeons. What is known about the preventive efficacy of each of these vaccines?
2 Which routes are used for administration of the aforementioned vaccines in pigeons?
3 What are 'the recommended vaccination protocols' for each vaccine?

CASE 63 A 5-year-old female intact cockatiel (*Nymphicus hollandicus*) presents for a distended coelom. On physical examination, a hard structure is palpated in her coelom. Whole body radiographs are taken (**63a, b**) and a blood sample is collected for hematology and a plasma biochemistry panel.

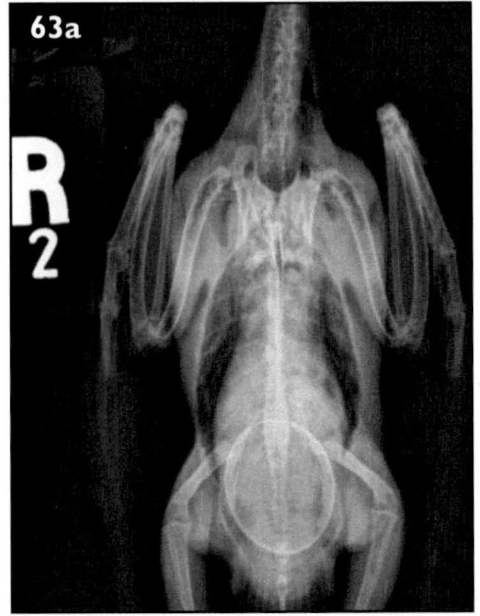

63a

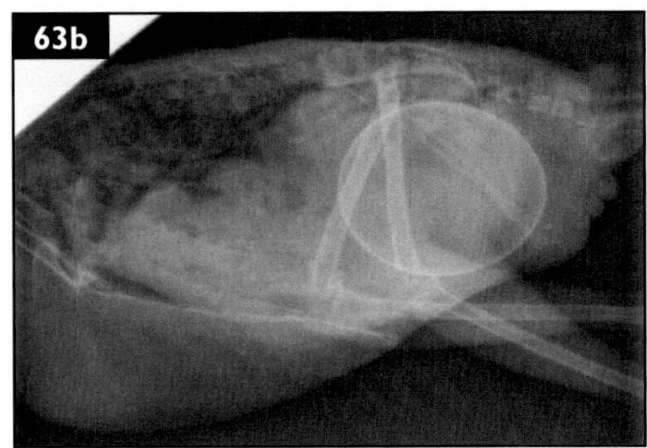
63b

Parameter	Value	Reference interval
AST (U/L)	302	100–396
Calcium (mmol/L) (mg/dL)	4.49 (18)	2.12–3.24 (8.5–13)
CK (U/L)	231	30–245
Glucose (mmol/L) (mg/dL)	19.65 (354)	11.1–24.98 (200–450)
Phosphorus (mmol/L) (mg/dL)	1.29 (4.0)	1.03–1.55 (3.2–4.8)
Potassium (mEq/L)	3.8	2.5–4.5
Protein, total (g/L) (g/dL)	52 (5.2)	24–41 (2.4–4.1)
Albumin (g/L) (g/dL)	25 (2.5)	7–18 (0.7–1.8)
Globulin (g/L) (g/dL)	27 (2.7)	17–23 (1.7–2.3)
Sodium (mEq/L)	144	132–150
Uric acid (µmol/L) (mg/dL)	232 (3.9)	208–654 (3.5–11)

1 What is the most likely cause of the hypercalcemia and hyperproteinemia seen in this cockatiel?
2 What other parameter could be measured to evaluate this bird's calcium status?
3 Does this cockatiel still require calcium supplementation even though her serum calcium levels are so high?

CASE 64 Excretion of water and nitrogenous wastes by birds (**64a**) combines processes of the kidneys and the intestines and, in some species, the action of salt secreting glands (**64b**).

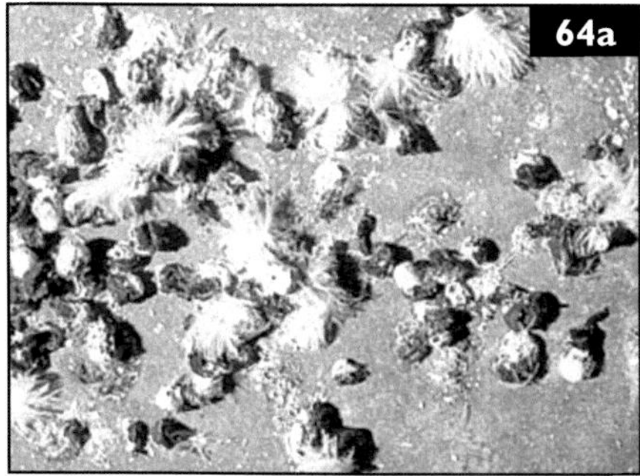

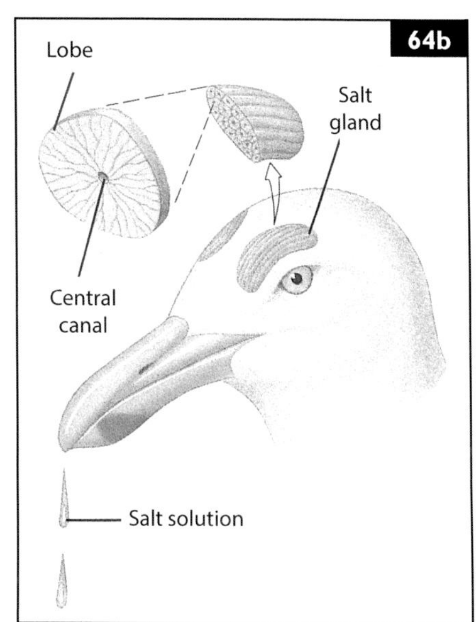

1 Is there any advantage of urine mixing with feces in the lower intestine?
2 What is the advantage of excretion of nitrogen wastes in the form of uric acid in birds, as opposed to the excretion of nitrogen as urea in mammals?

CASE 65 A 30-year-old African grey parrot (*Psittacus erithacus*) is presented for evaluation of a mature cataract (**65**). Following a complete ophthalmic evaluation including electroretinography (ERG) and ocular ultrasound, it was decided that the parrot was a good surgical candidate. CBC, chemistry panel, and radiographs did not show any significant abnormalities. The ophthalmologist requested that the patient was paralyzed intraoperatively to prevent any movements during the procedure.

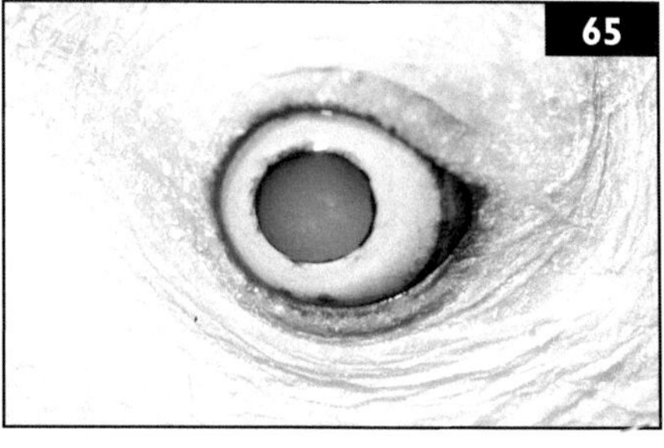

1 What is your anesthetic plan for premedication, induction, and maintenance of this patient?
2 How would you paralyze and monitor systemically the bird intraoperatively?
3 What are the potential anesthetic complications associated with ocular surgery?

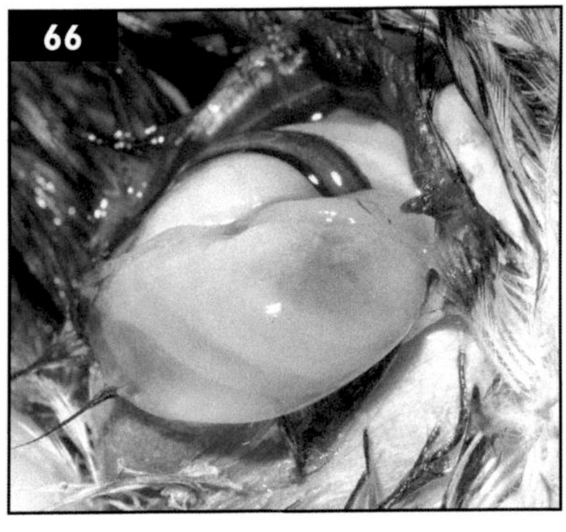

66

CASE 66 A juvenile Western screech owl (*Megascops kennicottii*) was presented with a perforated right globe (**66**). The animal was otherwise bright and responsive and well hydrated, and without any other significant abnormalities. The lesion appears to be relatively recent, but the damage to the globe is beyond surgical repair. The owl is crepuscular and is nonvisual on its right side.

1 What is the preferred surgical treatment for this condition?
2 Why is this technique recommended?
3 What are the release criteria once the procedure is completed?

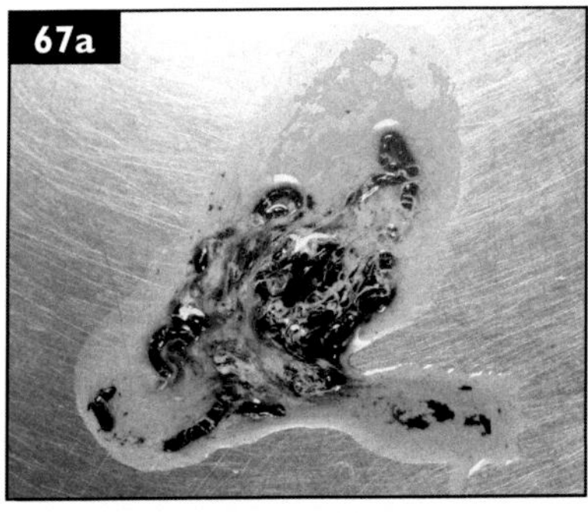

67a

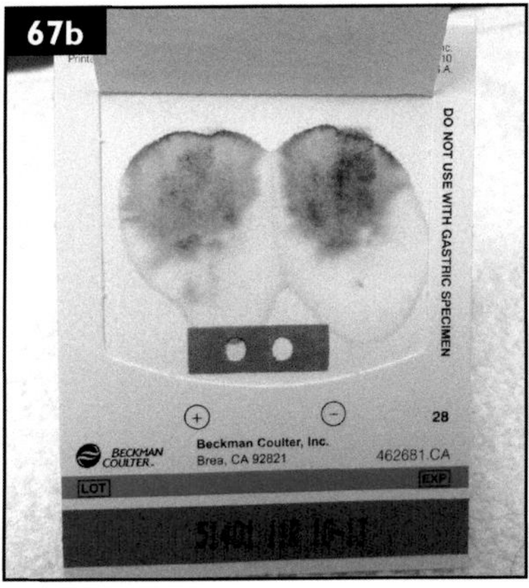

67b

CASE 67 An 8-year-old African grey parrot (*Psittacus erithacus*) is presented for evaluation for anorexia and lethargy of 5 days' duration. Physical examination reveals mild dehydration. A CBC reveals reduced hematocrit (32%, reference interval: 41–53%) and low total protein (21 g/L [2.1 g/dL], reference interval: 28–46 g/L [2.8–4.6 g/dL]) and plasma bile acids of 170 µmol/L (reference interval: 10–85 µmol/L). A fecal sample produced in the examination room is shown (**67a**).

1 What is the clinical diagnosis based on the available information?
2 You perform an occult fecal blood test. How do you interpret the result (**67b**), and what is the mechanism of action of this test? How sensitive and specific are commercially available occult fecal blood tests in birds?
3 What factors can interfere with fecal occult blood test results?

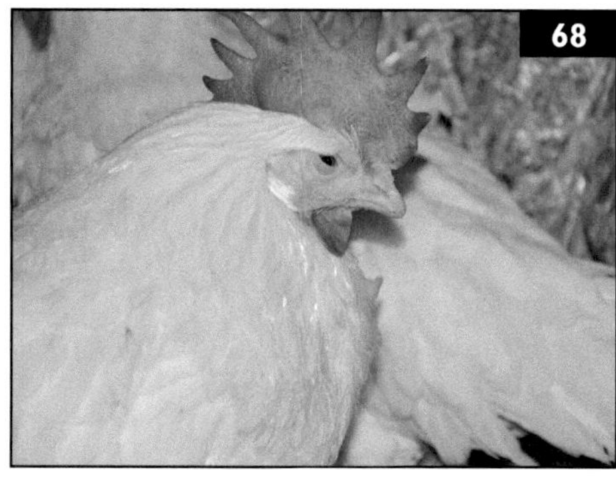

CASE 68 The owner of a small flock of free-range white leghorn chickens requests a consultation to investigate an ongoing problem with the flock (68). Egg production has decreased and the eggs are softer. Some of the birds appear weaker, more lethargic, with a few becoming acutely lame. The diet consists of 60% foraged greens and 40% of a maintenance chicken pelleted diet mixed with chopped greens.

1 Based on the history provided, what is the most likely diagnosis? What are the predisposing factors for this condition in this flock?
2 What other clinical signs may be seen with this condition? What gross lesions would you expect to see on postmortem examination in an affected bird?
3 What recommendations would you provide to the owner of this flock?

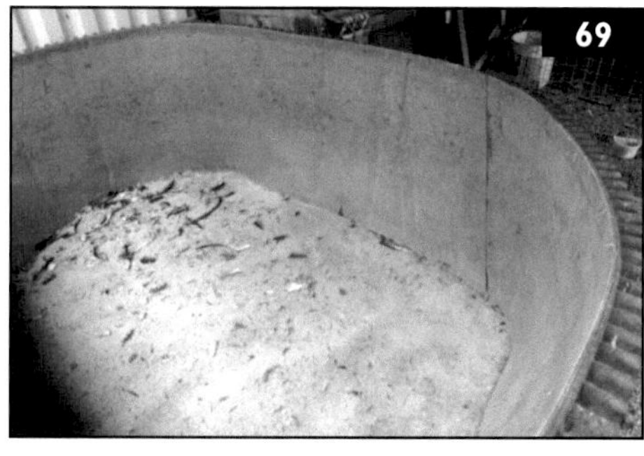

CASE 69 You are in the company of an investigating animal welfare society and have cause to visit a site where it is suspected that illegal cock fighting has taken place. The circular rubber tread from an earth moving vehicle is shown (69). The substrate comprises four layers of carpet. On examination there appear to be blood splatter marks around the wall at about 40–60 cm height. On questioning, the defendant claims that this area has been used as a 'night sleeping accommodation' for his lurcher dog, who had suffered a split tail, the intermittent bleeding from the tail tip being the cause of the blood spots. You are still suspicious that it is a cock fighting pit.

1 What investigations should be carried out to determine if the spots are blood?
2 How can you differentiate between canine and avian blood?
3 How can you determine if the blood is associated with cock fighting?

CASE 70 A 3-year-old male budgerigar (*Melopsittacus undulatus*) presents dead on arrival. You prepare the bird for postmortem examination. What you see once you pluck the feathers is shown (**70a**). You feel a mass over the keel as well as over the ventral coelomic cavity. Once you have cut into the coelom and removed the coelomic organs, you see the liver with what appears to be a yellow and soft mass (**70b**).

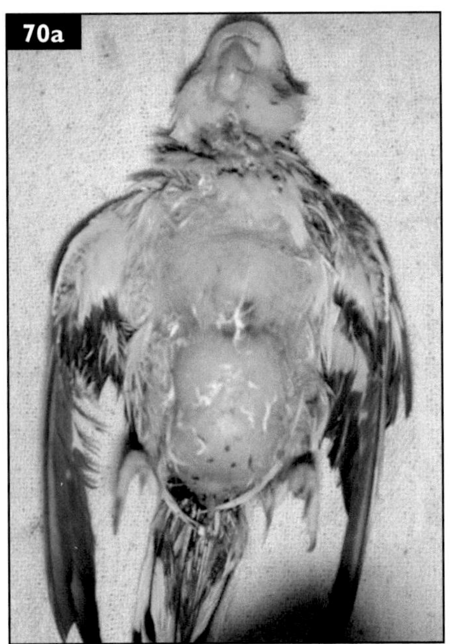
70a

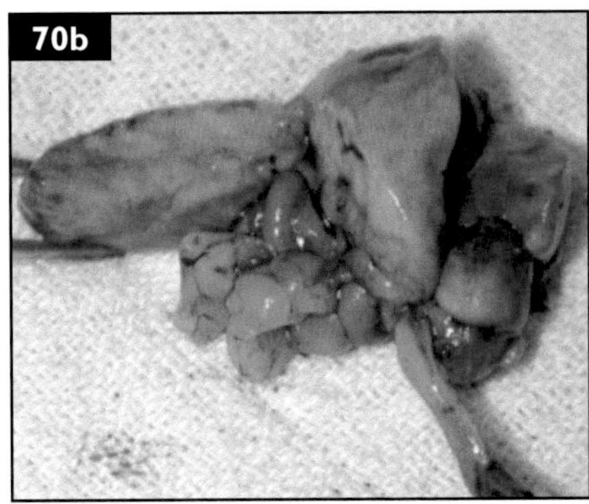
70b

1 Describe your gross findings.
2 What are the main differential diagnoses?
3 Describe a common cause for these lesions.

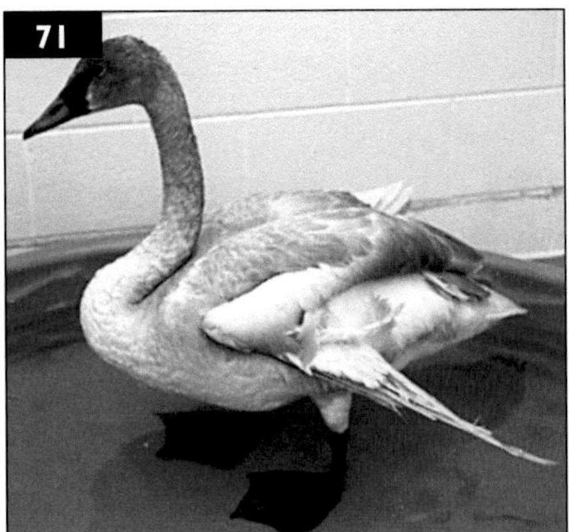
71

CASE 71 A captive-raised juvenile trumpeter swan (*Cygnus buccinators*) is shown with malformation of the left distal wing (**71**).

1 What is this condition called in birds?
2 What is the cause of this condition?
3 How can this condition be treated/managed?

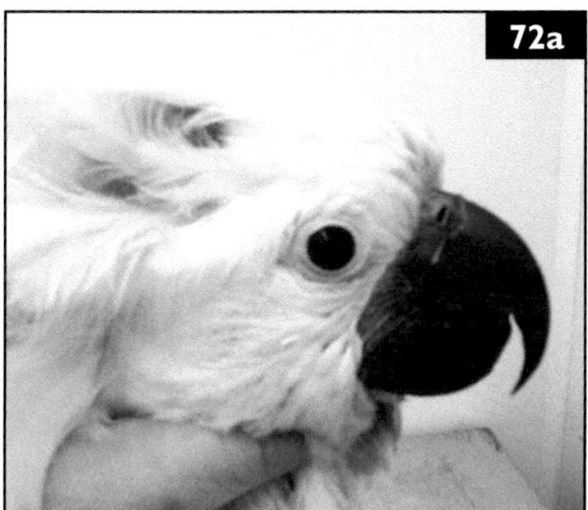
72a

CASE 72 A 24-month-old cockatoo (*Cacatua alba*) is presented by its owner. The bird appears bright, alert, is slightly thin, and its plumage looks somewhat 'tatty'. Examining the head (**72a**), answer the following questions.

1 What is your immediate concern regarding this bird? What disease is likely to be resulting in this abnormality?
2 How would you confirm your diagnosis, and what action can you take to clear infection from the collection?
3 What action must be taken to eliminate the pathogen from the environment and prevent the disease spreading?

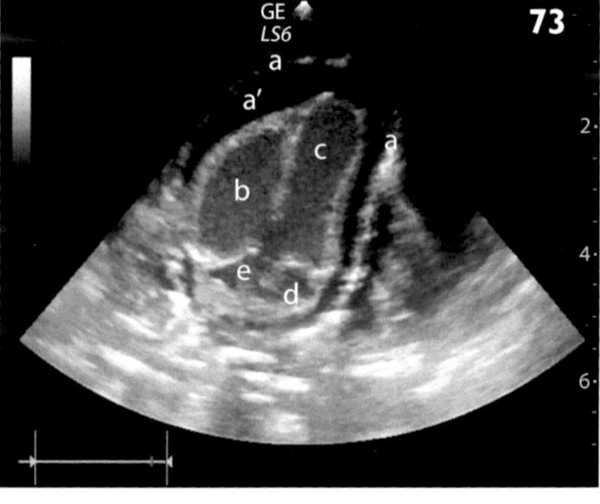

73

CASE 73 A 25-year-old male blue and gold macaw (*Ara ararauna*) is presented with a history of lethargy, anorexia, and increased respiratory effort. Following initial stabilization, a brief physical examination is performed and the bird appears to have a 3–4/6 heart murmur and coelomic distension that appears to be ascites. Radiographs under sedation confirm the suspicion of enlarged cardiac silhouette and ascites. An echocardiogram through a ventromedian approach is performed, which shows severe pericardial effusion and dilatation of the right ventricle (**73**; a = pericardium, b = right ventricle, c = left ventricle, d = left atrium, e = right atrium overlapped by aortic outflow tract).

1 How would you initially stabilize this bird?
2 How would you perform pericardiocentesis in a bird?
3 How would you treat this bird long term?

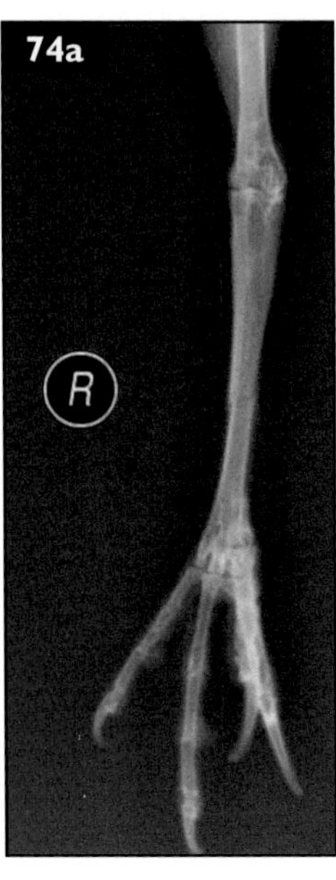

74a

CASE 74 An adult female Cooper's hawk (*Accipiter cooperii*) is admitted to your clinic with a fractured tarsometatarsus (**74a, b**).

1 How would you surgically manage this fracture?
2 What alternative method may be used in smaller avian patients (<150 g)?
3 If this patient was a falcon, what other action would you take during the recovery period?

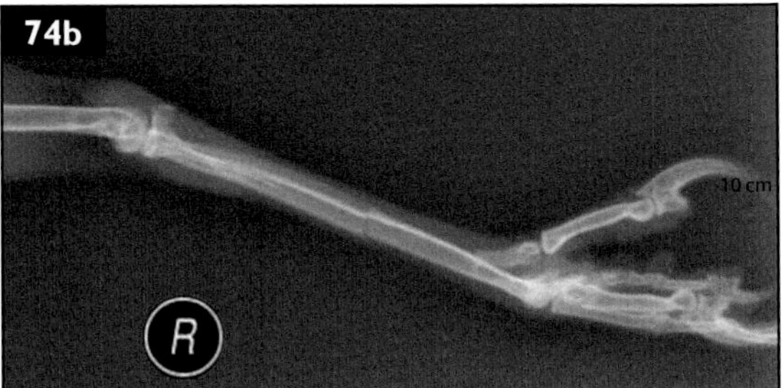

74b

CASE 75 High rates of relinquishment are common for companion parrots. Major reasons for relinquishment include: compatibility factors such as inability of owners to dedicate adequate time to the birds, inadequate space, failure to get along with family members or other parrots in household; personal factors such as owners' financial resources, lifestyle changes, illness, death, divorce, moving, and allergies; and behavioral problems such as feather damaging behavior, aggression, messiness, noisiness, and difficulty to train.

1 True or false? Because many parrot species are long-lived, the majority of parrots are relinquished because of changes in the owner's lifestyle (such as marriage, children, illness, death) after 15–20 years of ownership.
2 In a 2002 survey in the USA, The National Parrot Relinquishment Research Project respondents were asked to indicate the reasons owners gave when relinquishing their parrots. What was the number one reason?
3 What preventive actions might reduce the number of birds relinquished to sanctuaries?

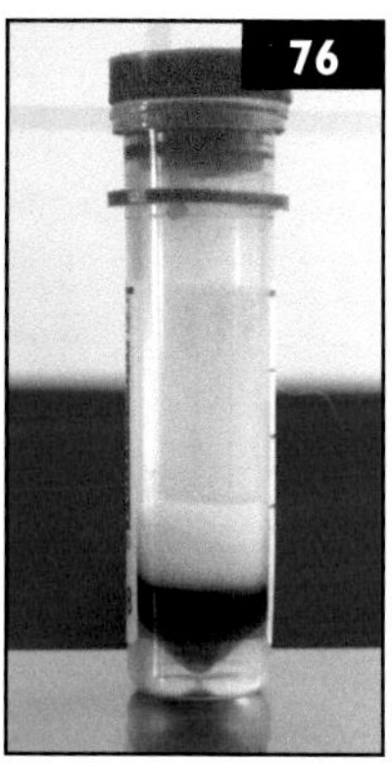
76

CASE 76 Dyslipidemia, in particular hypercholesterolemia (76), is frequently diagnosed in pet psittacine birds and some birds of prey. It is associated with a number of degenerative diseases such as hepatic lipidosis, xanthomatosis, and atherosclerosis.

1 What parameters would you use to evaluate dyslipidemia in birds?
2 What lifestyle and dietary changes would you recommend to correct this disorder?
3 What therapeutic options are available in birds?

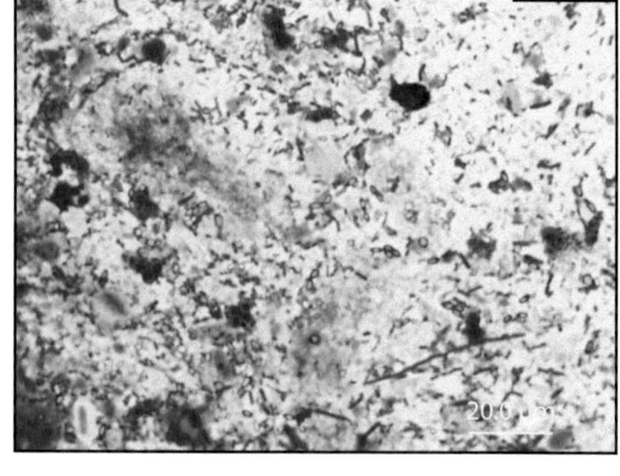
77

CASE 77 A breeding male red lory (*Eos bornea*) died without premonitory signs of disease. Within 10 days, two other lories from the same aviary were found dead. Fecal cytologies with Romanowsky stain from the dead bird and the other live birds were performed (77).

1 What is the most likely cause of such mortality?
2 What is the source of such organisms?
3 What are the recommended treatment options?

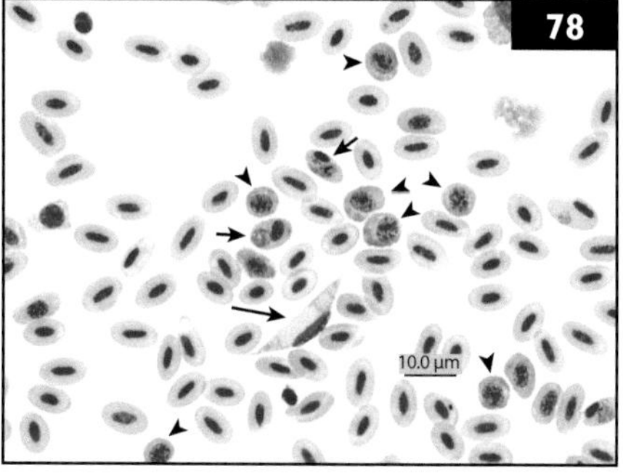

78

CASE 78 An adult female Swainson's hawk (*Buteo swainsoni*) was admitted to a local raptor rehabilitation facility with head trauma and a fractured clavicle. A blood smear obtained from the bird shortly after arrival is shown (78).

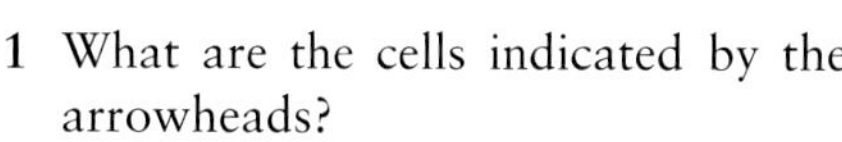
1 What are the cells indicated by the arrowheads?
2 What is the significance of the cells depicted by the short arrows?
3 What is the structure indicated by the long arrow?

CASE 79

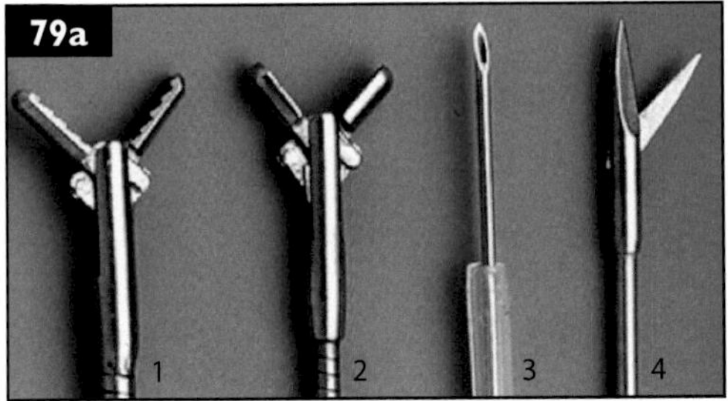

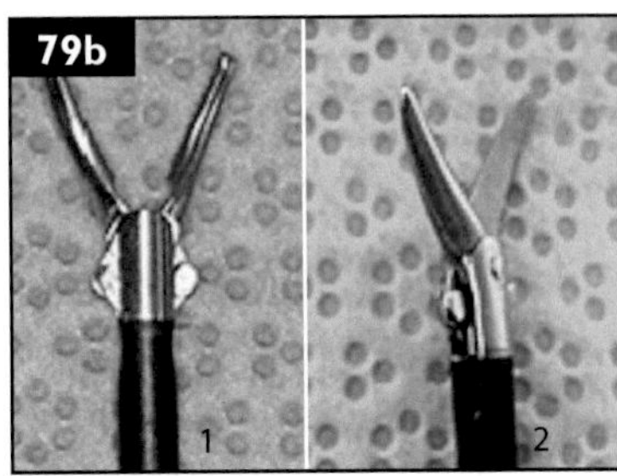

Courtesy of Dr. Stephen Divers, UGA

1 What surgical devices can be used to ensure hemostasis during avian endosurgery?
2 Name the instruments shown (**79a**), which are commonly used in avian diagnostic endoscopy.
3 Name the two instruments shown (**79b**), which are most commonly used in avian endosurgery.

CASE 80 Two lethargic 8-week-old, blue Orpington (*Gallus gallus domesticus*) chicks, crouched sternally with one leg positioned forward and the other leg positioned backward, were euthanized for necropsy. The liver and kidneys from one of the birds with whitish tan masses are shown (**80a, b**).

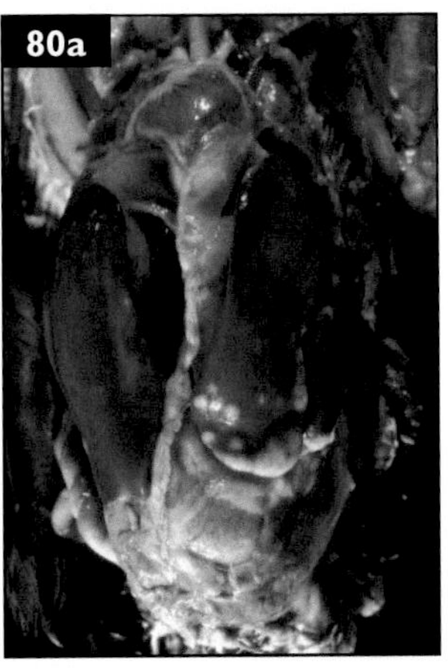

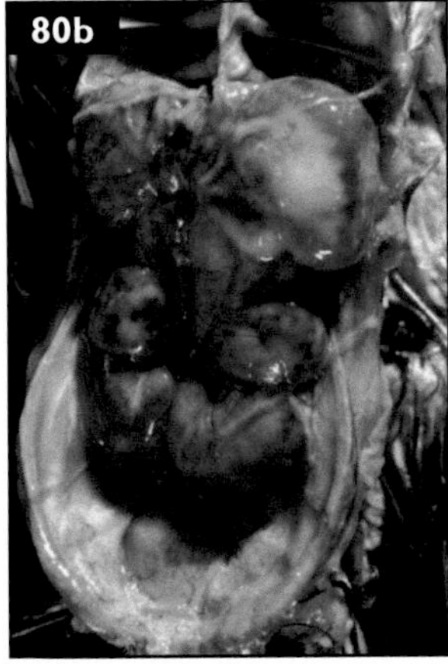

1 What disease is most likely?
2 What gross necropsy findings can be associated with this disease?
3 How do you prevent this disease?

CASE 81 An adult Muscovy duck (*Cairina moschata*) originating from the USA is presented to your clinic in a very lethargic and weak condition. Following blood sampling, obtaining radiographs (**81a, b**), and initial treatment to stabilize the bird, it expires before specific treatment can be started. On gross necropsy you confirm your abnormal radiographic findings: two USA pennies dated from 1990 and 1995 in the ventriculus and a distended proventriculus with what appears to be a stainless steel short chain of a watch.

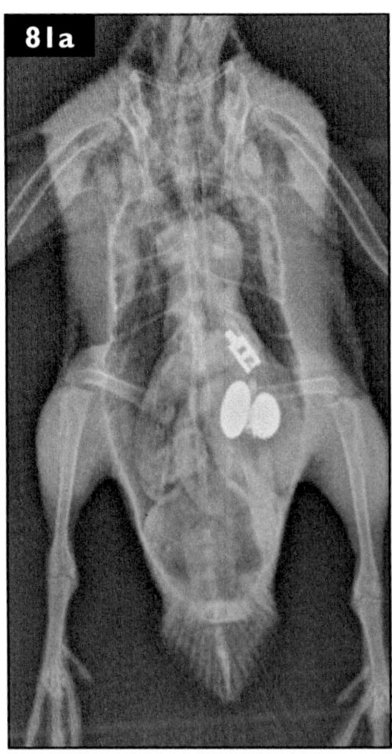
81a

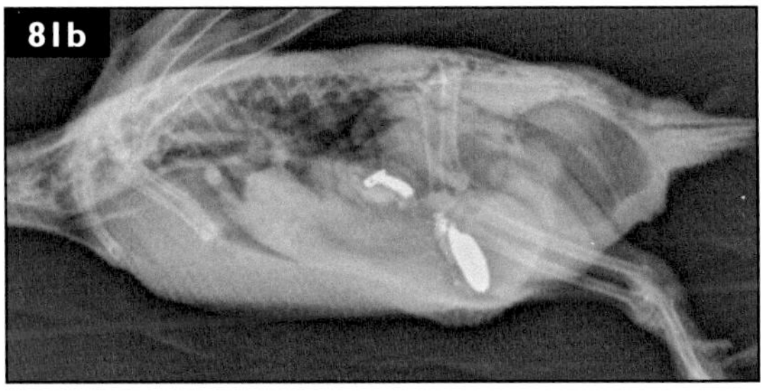
81b

1 What are the most likely differentials in this case?
2 Which organ do you sample in priority for histopathology?

You want to determine whether a conspecific living in the same aviary is affected by the same problem.

3 During what time of the day do you take a blood sample from the remaining bird to improve the specificity of this test? What characteristic of the sampling tube do you check?

CASE 82 Over a period of 3 weeks, a budgerigar (*Melopsittacus undulatus*) flock suffered high mortality. Adult birds, fledglings (more than 14 days), and juveniles were found dead. The owner reported dyspnea, diarrhea, fluffed-up feathers, and lethargy prior to death. One of the owners developed signs similar to flu with night sweats and headaches.

1 What is the most likely causative agent?
2 What diagnostic tests should be performed?
3 What treatment should be implemented?

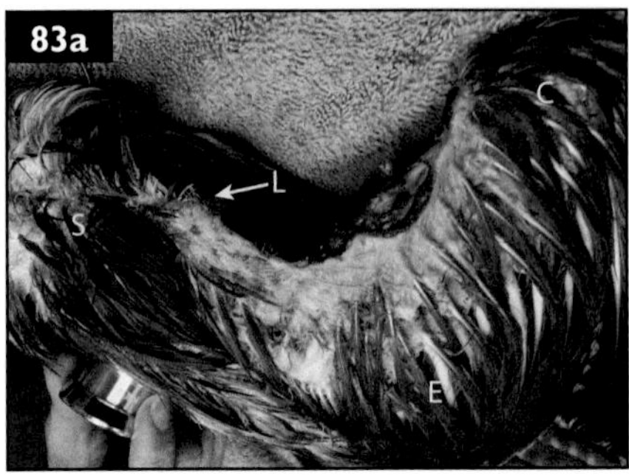

83a

CASE 83 The right wing of a saker falcon (*Falco cherrug*) who has suffered a severe soft tissue injury to the anterior edge of the right wing some 2 weeks previously is shown (**83a**). The skin edges were closed by a local veterinarian, but this has broken down since (S = shoulder, E = elbow, C = carpus).

1 What overall anatomic structure has been damaged, and what structure is arrowed as L?
2 In order for repair of this injury to be possible, what structures need to be repaired and how?
3 What suture technique would be used to repair structure L?

CASE 84 A 7-year-old female cockatiel (*Nymphicus hollandicus*) presents in respiratory arrest and dies during examination. During the postmortem examination you pluck the feathers and see this (**84a**). Once you open the coelom you dissect out this structure from the cranial reproductive tract (**84b**).

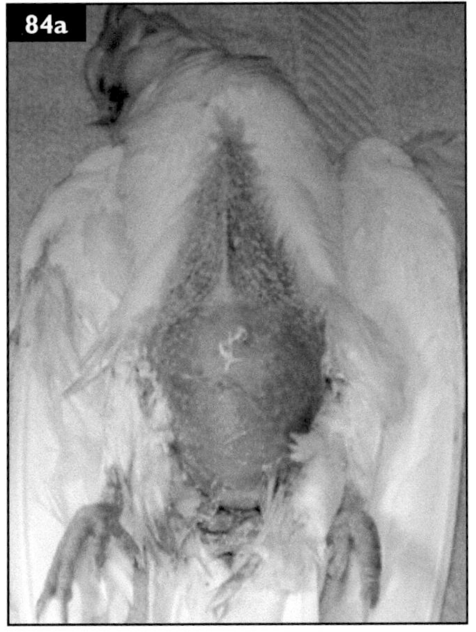
84a

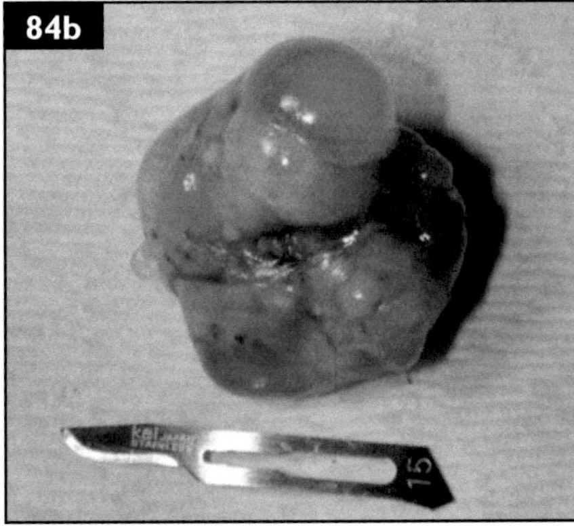

84b

1 Describe your gross findings.
2 What are your primary differentials?
3 What are the treatment options for this condition?

CASE 85 An adult Swainson's hawk (*Buteo swainsoni*) presents after being found at a construction site down on the ground with possible head trauma. On physical examination the bird is bright and responsive. A small amount of blood is noted surrounding the glottis; no lesions or wounds are noticed in the oropharyngeal cavity. Cutaneous sensation is appropriate around the eyelid. Pupillary light reflex is appropiate in both eyes, with symmetrical pupil size. The anterior image (**85a**) shows asymmetry of the crown feathers, with the feathers on the right side more erected. The lateral view (**85b**) shows ptosis with the upper eyelid markedly affected, decreasing the space of the palpebral fissure.

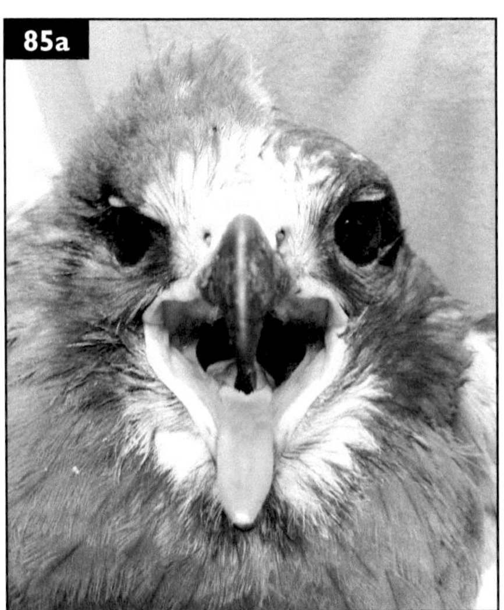
85a

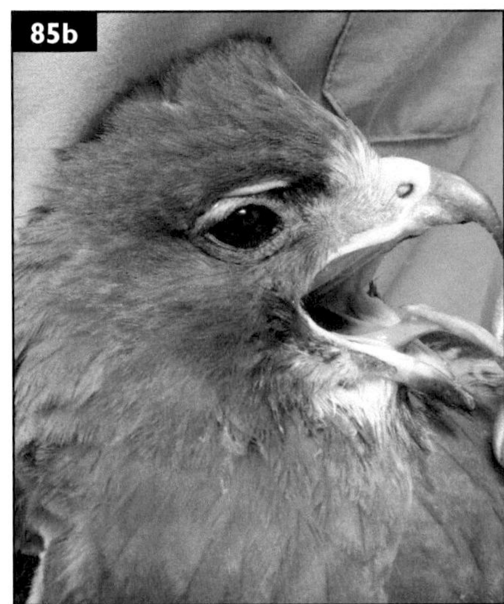
85b

1 What is the most likely diagnosis?
2 How would you confirm your diagnosis?
3 What is the treatment and prognosis for this condition?

CASE 86

1 What are the four parasitic nematode worm species that can inhabit both partridges and pheasants?
2 What are the clinical signs observed in *Capillaria* spp. and *Syngamus trachea* infections?
3 What are the treatments available for game bird species, and how often should these be administered?

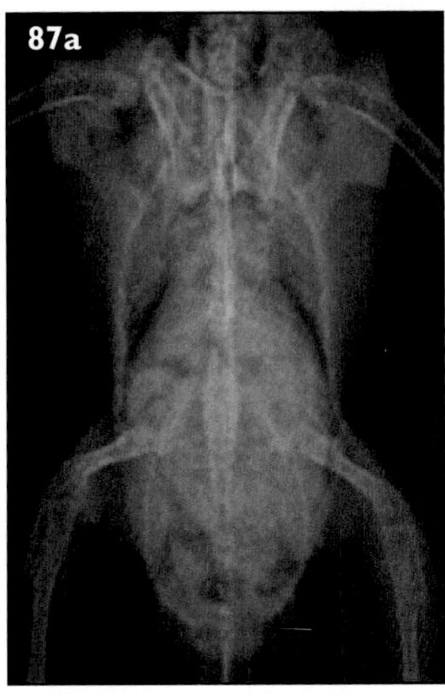

CASE 87 A 13-year-old female cockatiel (*Nymphicus hollandicus*) was presented for evaluation of coelomic distension and biliverdinuria. Ventrodorsal and right lateral whole body radiographs were taken under inhalant general anesthesia as part of the initial evaluation of the patient (**87a, b**).

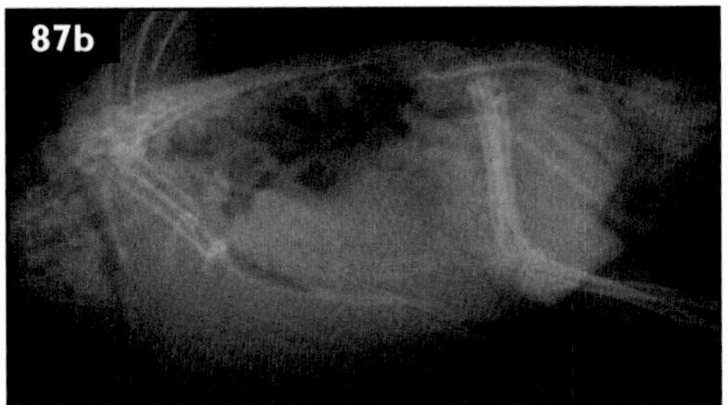

1 What is the cardiohepatic silhouette?
2 What can cause the cardiohepatic silhouette to appear widened with a loss of the 'cardiohepatic waist'?
3 Is the cardiohepatic silhouette widened in this patient and, if so, what diagnostic testing would you recommend to further evaluate this abnormality?

CASE 88 A 7-year-old female budgerigar (*Melopsittacus undulatus*) was presented for a right limb amputation (**88**). A malignant mesenchymatous tumor involving the right distal tibiotarsus circumferentially was diagnosed cytologically. Before anesthetizing the patient, emergency drug dosages were calculated and prepared. Anesthesia was induced using mask delivery of isoflurane, then the patient was intubated. The bird was monitored by ECG and by measuring indirect blood pressure.

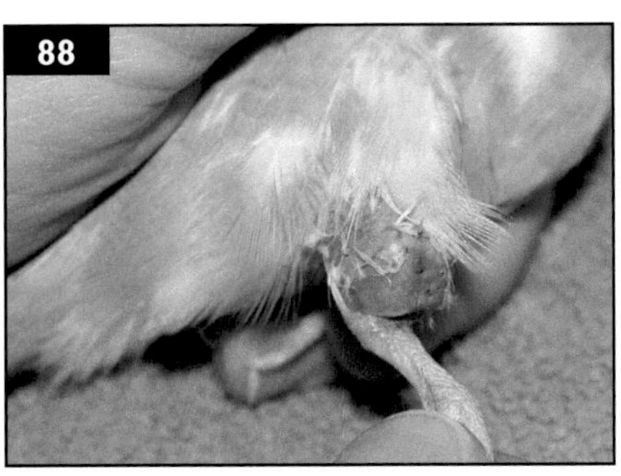

1 How would you correct respiratory arrest if it occurs?
2 How would you address bradycardia and what appears to be hypotension?
3 How would you treat cardiac arrest if it happens?

CASE 89 Intramuscular injections are typically administered into pectoral musculature along either side of the mid-keel region (**89**).

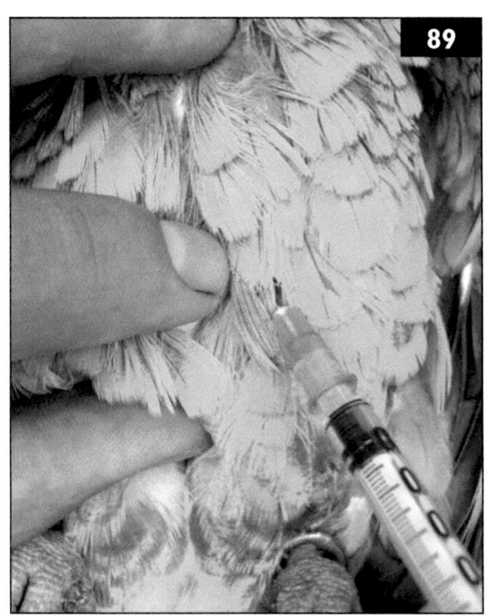
89

1 When giving IM injections, which portion of the pectorals should be avoided, and why?
2 Why are the leg muscles generally not recommended for IM injections in birds?
3 Vascular access can be challenging in small and hypotense patients and in these cases IO access for fluid therapy may be necessary. Where are IO injections most commonly delivered?

CASE 90 A budgerigar (*Melopsittaccus undulatus*) is presented with severe feather loss and feather dystrophy consistent with psittacine beak and feather disease (PBFD) (**90**). You would like to confirm the suspected diagnosis and are considering a number of different laboratory tests for beak and feather disease virus (BFDV) that have been developed.

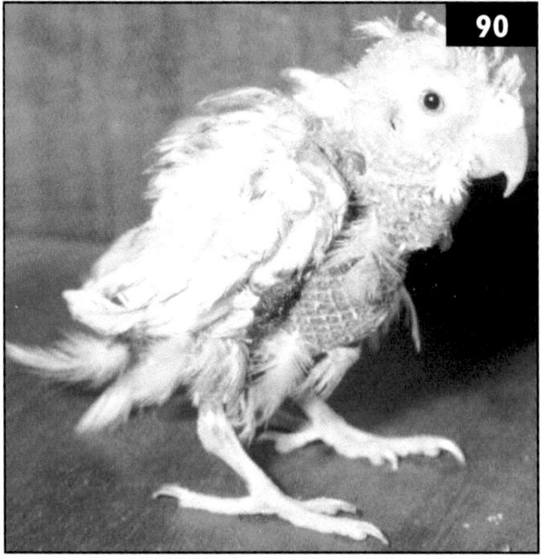
90

1 Which laboratory diagnostic test offers the highest correlation with disease?
2 How many different genotypes of BFDV exist?
3 Would genetic variation in BFDV interfere with diagnostic testing?

CASE 91 Two neonatal ratite chicks are shown (**91a, b**).

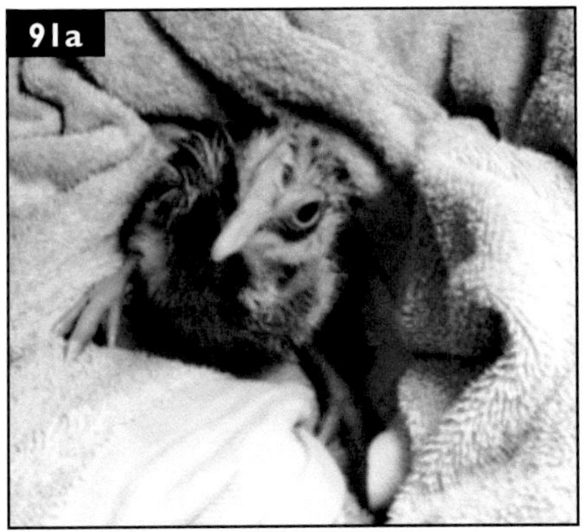
91a

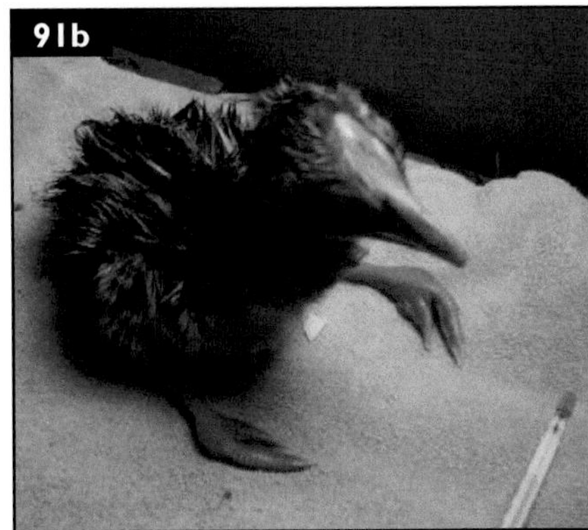
91b

1 What species are these chicks? Are they precocial or altricial?
2 These chicks will be raised by their paternal parent. Why is this?
3 How and what does their paternal parent feed them?

CASE 92 A 3.4 kg juvenile male golden eagle (*Aquila chrysaetos*) presented with a closed, proximal, transverse radial fracture and a closed, proximal, complex oblique ulnar fracture of the left wing (**92a, b**). Surgical repair using an ESF/intramedullary pin (ESF-IM) tie-in was planned.

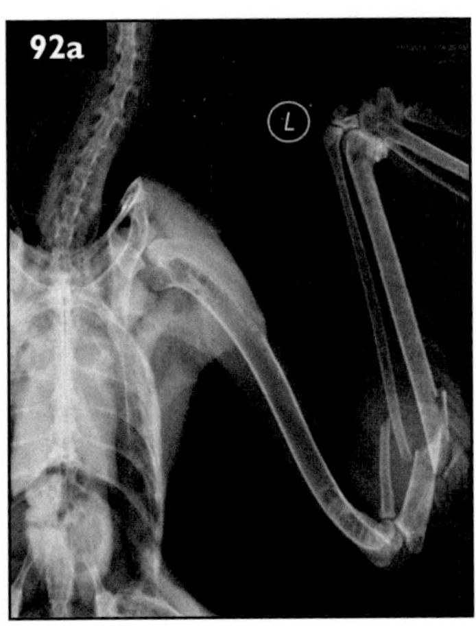

92a

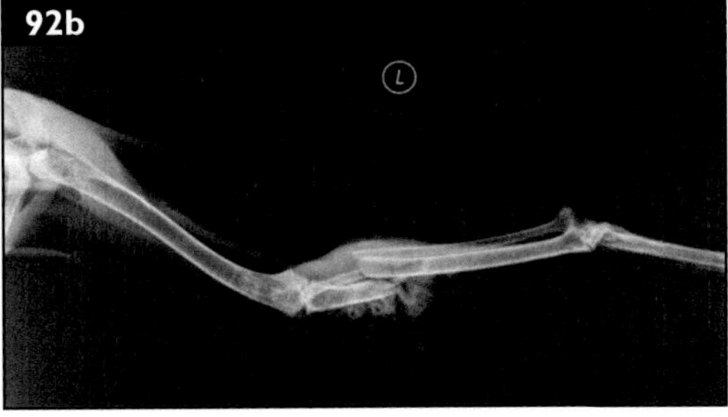

92b

1 Which bone is repaired first?
2 What additional method of surgical stabilization could be added to reduce the oblique ulnar fracture and increase resistance to the distractive force of the triceps muscle?

CASE 93 A 30-year-old female yellow-naped Amazon parrot (*Amazona auropalliata*) was presented for intermittent ataxia. It had been falling off its perch for 2 days. Physical examination was consistent with an overweight bird. Despite supportive care, the bird died in hospital. A necropsy was performed (**93**).

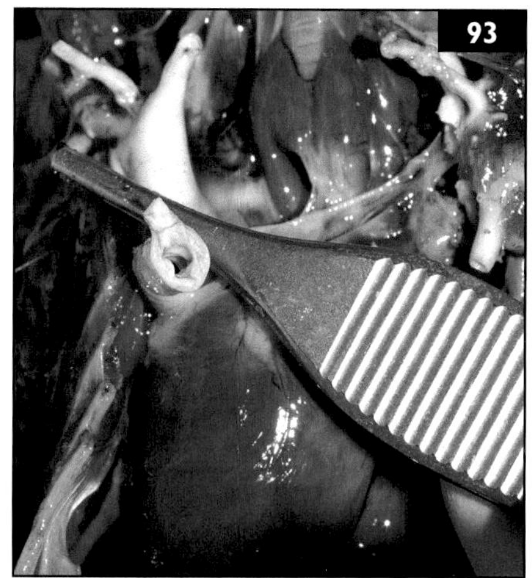
93

1 How would you describe this gross lesion, and what is the most likely cause for it?
2 What are the histopathologic hallmarks of these types of lesions, and what are the different lesion types that have been described?
3 What risk factors associated with the development of these types of lesions were present in this bird?

CASE 94 An adult tawny eagle (*Aquila rapax*) is presented as an emergency. While in flight it had crashed against the wire mesh front of the aviary and was instantly incoordinated and unable to stand normally. It had initially been treated with fluid therapy and NSAIDs on site, but after 3–4 hours had not improved. On physical examination the bird had no obvious cranial nerve deficits. Radiographs were obtained under general anesthesia (**94a**). While there is no apparent spinal misalignment, a fracture has affected the cranioventral aspect of C3.

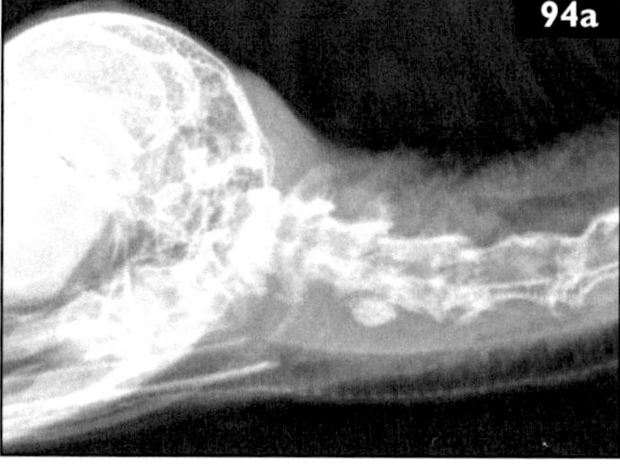
94a

1 What are the treatment options?
2 If external support is to be provided, how can this be achieved?
3 If an external support is provided, how should the bird be fed?

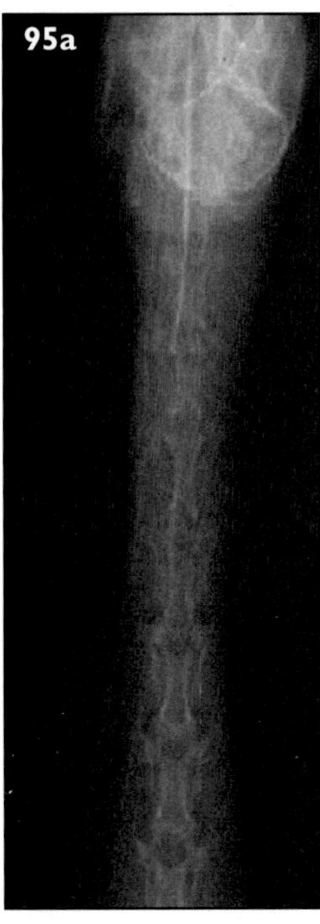

CASE 95 A male mallard duck (*Anas platyrhynchos*) presented for examination for acute respiratory distress and lethargy. The duck had experienced recurrent episodes of respiratory distress since being attacked by a raccoon the previous year, resulting in neck lacerations. Diagnostic tests, including a CBC, plasma biochemical analysis, radiography (**95a, b**), and tracheoscopy, revealed a collapsed trachea (shown in the images at the end of the endotracheal tube), likely resulting from the trauma caused by the raccoon, affecting approximately 12 tracheal rings.

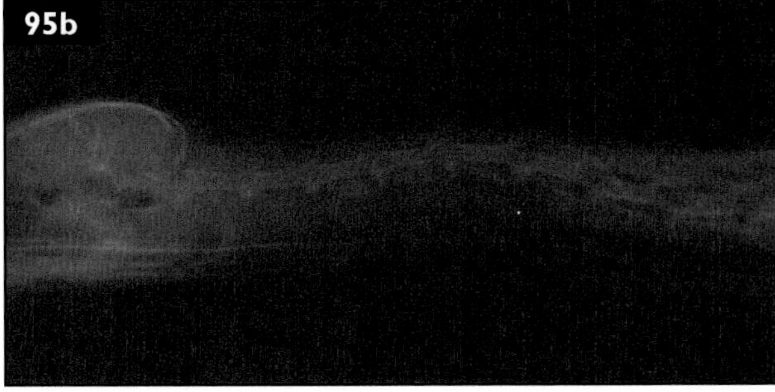

1 What surgical procedure would you perform to resolve this condition?
2 How would you perform this procedure?
3 What postoperative complications might occur?

CASE 96 A 22-year-old blue and gold macaw (*Ara ararauna*) is presented with an abnormal lower beak of a few months' duration (**96**).

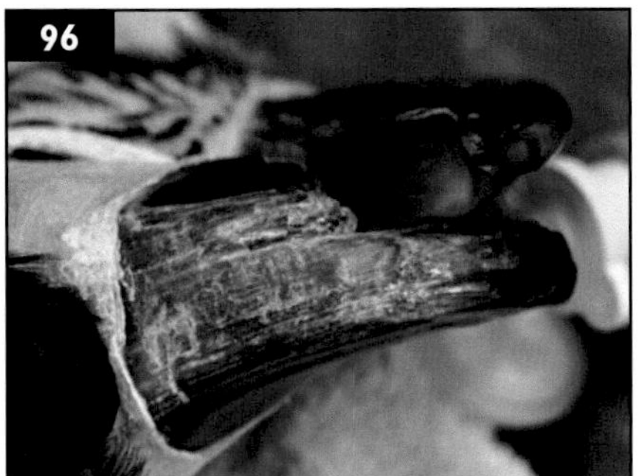

1 What are your differential diagnoses?
2 What diagnostic tests would you carry out to confirm your diagnosis?
3 What treatment would you recommend, and for how long should it be maintained?

CASE 97 A 7-year-old male masked lovebird (*Agapornis personatus*) is presented for surgical excisional biopsy of a supraorbital mass for histopathologic examination. The patient's anesthesia monitoring includes capnography, pulse oximetry, and Doppler flow (97).

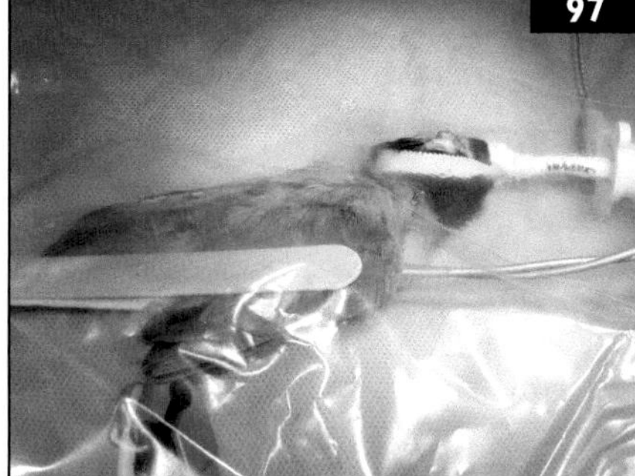

1 How does end-tidal partial pressure of carbon dioxide (PETCO$_2$) correlate with partial arterial pressure of carbon dioxide (PaCO$_2$) in psittacine birds?
2 How do pulse oximetry values correlate with heart rates and arterial oxygen saturation (SaO$_2$)?
3 Doppler has been used in avian anesthesia for indirect blood pressure measurements. What were the conclusions of those studies?

CASE 98 ESF-intramedullary (ESF-IM) tie-ins and ESFs are the most commonly used methods for surgical fixation of long bones (98). Plate fixation has also been reported in birds. It is less commonly used but in some instances might provide an advantage.

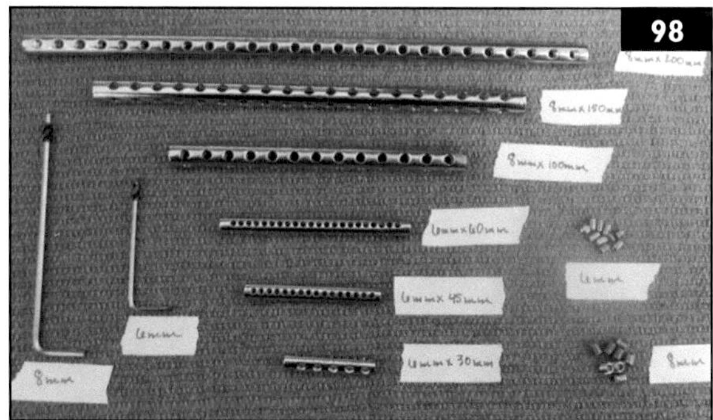

1 What are common options for creating an ESF construct or external connecting bar for birds?
2 What advantages and disadvantages should be considered for each of these constructs?
3 What are the advantages and disadvantages of plate fixation in birds compared with these constructs?

CASE 99 An adult male rainbow lorikeet (*Trichoglossus moluccanus*) presents to you with a history of straining to defecate for several weeks. In the last week, the bird passed a small amount of frank blood in his droppings and has been more lethargic. On physical examination the bird appears healthy but seems to have an approximately 1 cm diameter hard mass in the caudal coelom. Radiographs are obtained under sedation (**99a, b**).

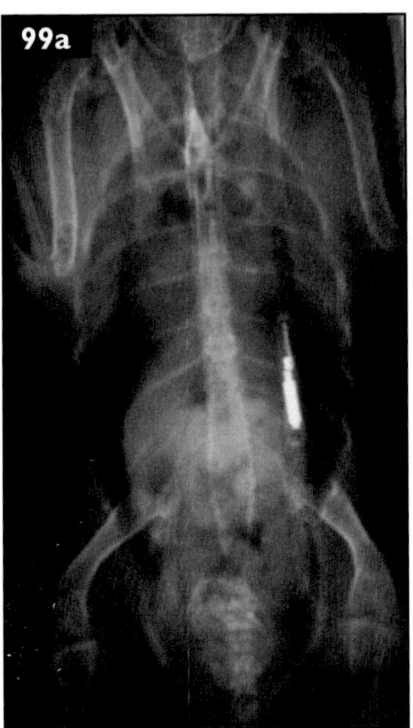

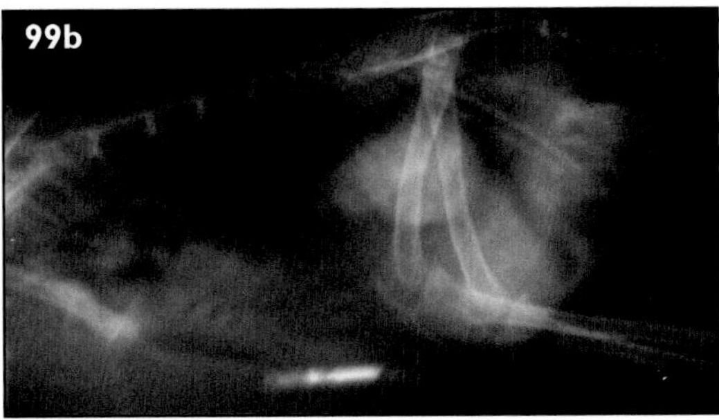

1 What are the abnormal radiographic findings?
2 What is the most likely diagnosis? How would you confirm your diagnosis?
3 How would you treat this condition?

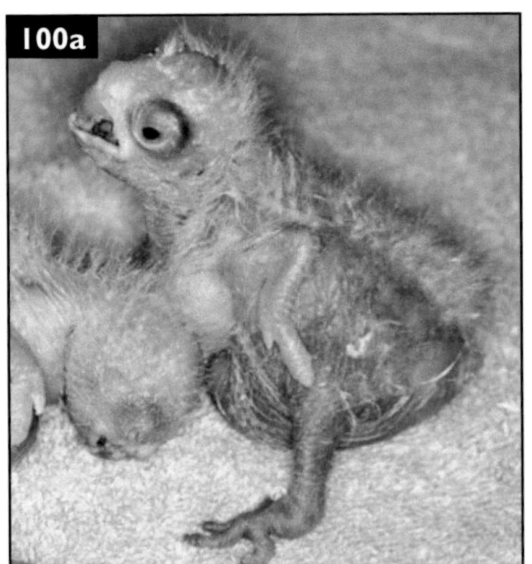

CASE 100 Two neonatal chicks are shown (**100a**).

1 What species are these chicks?
2 Are they precocial or altricial?
3 What is wrong with the beak of the chick that is sitting up?

CASE 101 Thrombocytes are cells that play an important role in the blood clotting mechanism (**101**). These cells are significantly larger than the mammalian counterpart (platelets) and are nucleated. Thrombocytes are produced from mononuclear precursors in the bone marrow. Nonactivated thrombocytes are oval, spindle, or rectangular shaped with a round oval nucleus. Some degree of thrombocyte activation leads to vacuolation of the otherwise pale basophilic cytoplasm. However, vacuolation is exacerbated during fixation and staining with most methods commonly used in hematologic analyses. This makes identification and differentiation from lymphocytes easier.

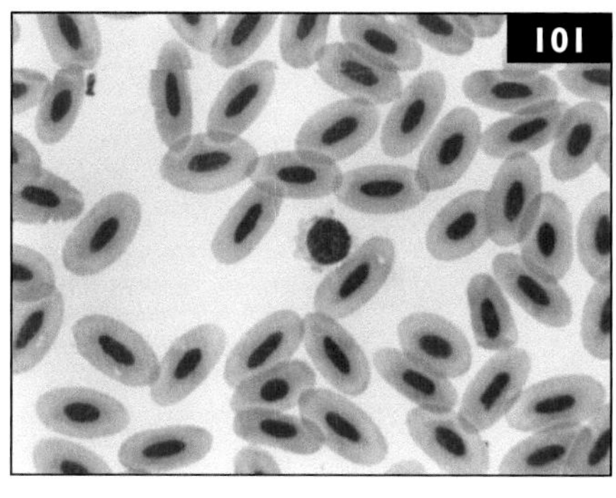
101

1 The presence of megathrombocytes (enlarged thrombocytes) in avian blood films has been associated with which pathologic process?
2 Thrombocyte counts in avian hematology samples are commonly achieved using which quantitative method?
3 What are the main differential morphologic characteristics of thrombocytes in birds?

CASE 102 The macaw skull is a classic example of a prokinetic avian skull (**102a**).

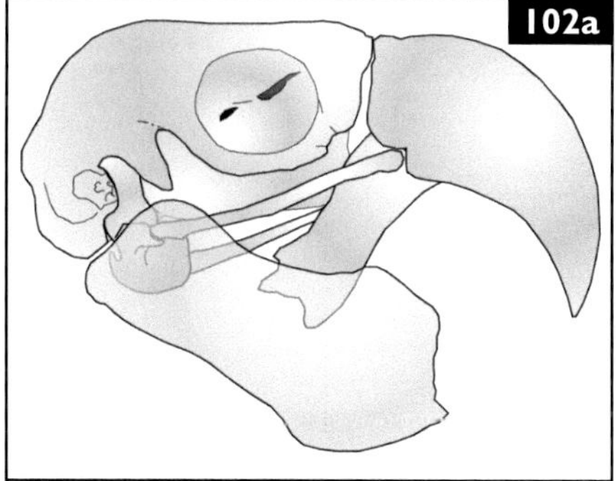
102a

1 What are the four key bones involved in elevating and lowering the upper bill?
2 Explain the role of each of these bones in the kinesis of the psittacine beak.
3 How many synovial joints are involved in prokinetic motion of the upper bill, and what bones are they associated with?

CASE 103 With the banning of the importation of wild-captured parrots, hand-rearing chicks has become the predominant method of producing parrots for the pet trade (**103**). Traditionally, this method has been promoted as the best available option to prepare a parrot chick for its life as a pet, allowing it to be tamed and form a strong emotional and physical 'bond' with its owner. Unfortunately, this process also interferes with the normal behavioral development of the chick and can lead to various medical and behavioral problems.

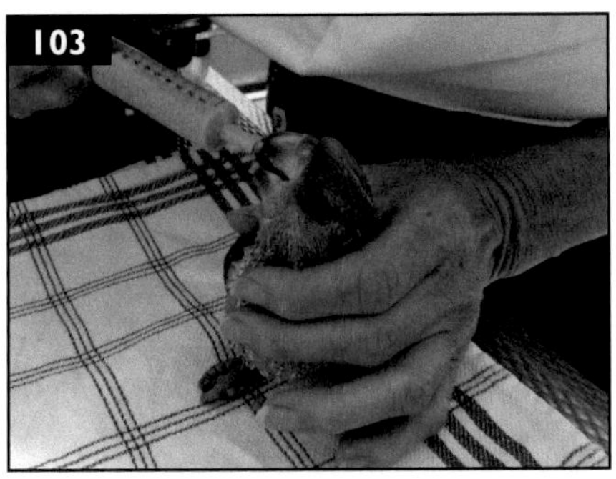
103

1 Which two important behavioral events take place in the life of a juvenile parrot (i.e. in the period from hatching to weaning)?
2 Provide at least three examples of medical issues that may arise following hand-rearing of psittacine chicks.
3 Provide at least three examples of behavioral problems that may arise following hand-rearing.

CASE 104 You examine five birds from a flock of domestic canaries (*Serinus canaria domestica*). The client would like to have the leg bands removed from these birds. They are housed in an outdoor aviary all year round. A few of the birds have visible ectoparasites. You use clear tape to catch a single ectoparasite and view it under the microscope (**104**).

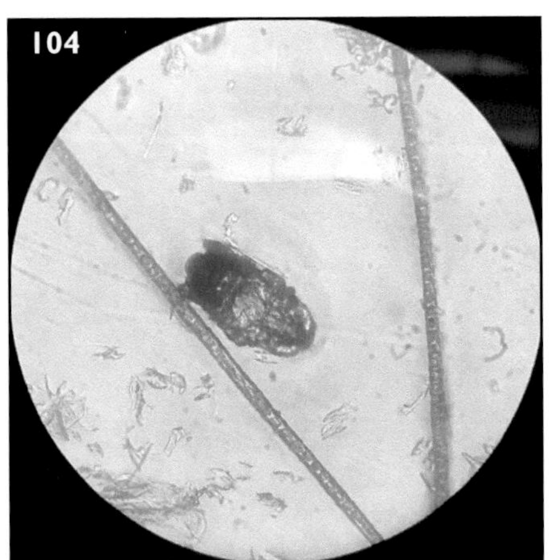
104

1 What type of organism is infesting these canaries?
2 What is the clinical significance of this finding?
3 What treatment options are available for this flock of 60 birds?

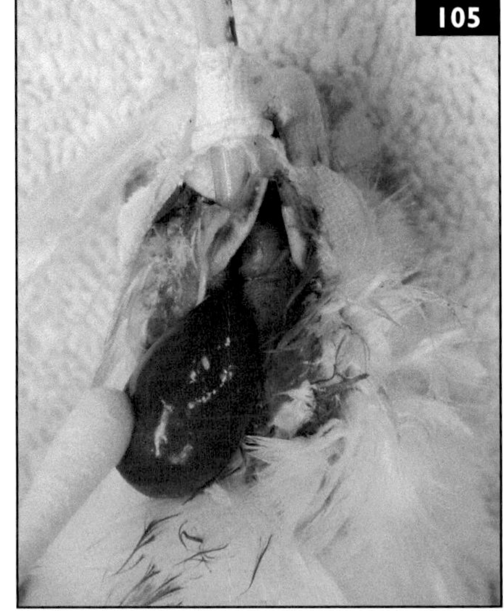

CASE 105 A 16-year-old cockatiel (*Nymphicus hollandicus*) with a split mandible and gnathotheca is presented with a 1 cm diameter red soft pedunculated nonulcerated mass protruding from the oropharyngeal cavity through the split lower beak (**105**). The owner had not noted the mass until today, when the bird appeared to show respiratory distress. The owner reported that otherwise the bird had not been showing any clinical signs. The bird has had a split mandible and gnathotheca for years and has been seen periodically for beak trims.

1 What is the most likely diagnosis for this mass?
2 How would you confirm your diagnosis?
3 What is the prognosis?

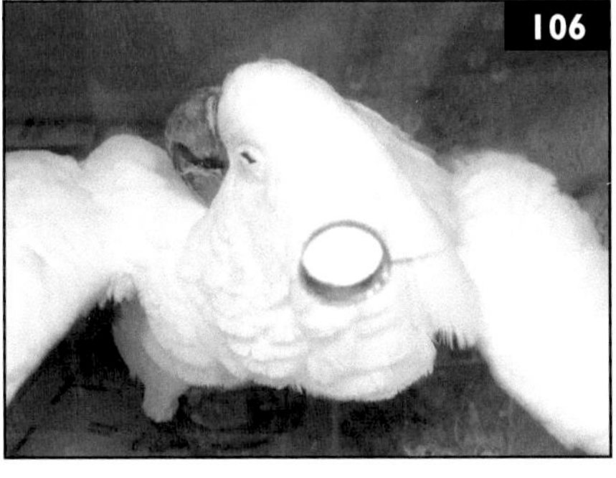

CASE 106 An adult male sulphur-crested cockatoo (*Cacatua galerita*) is presented on emergency for acute onset of lethargy. The bird is stuporous and ataxic. It lives in an outdoor aviary, and the owner has had one other bird dying recently from West Nile virus (WNV) infection. On physical examination, the bird appears in low body condition, and the tips of his rectrices and remiges are unkempt (**106**). Following the examination, the bird has a grand mal seizure lasting about 3 minutes despite emergency administration of anticonvulsant therapy. You suspect that the bird has WNV infection.

1 What diagnostic test can be performed antemortem to confirm the diagnosis?
2 What is the prognosis? What lesions would you expect on postmortem examination?
3 What treatment and preventive measures would you recommend?

CASE 107 The treatment of oiled birds has changed over time. During large spills, arguments have been made to euthanize hundreds of birds because mortalities have historically been over 80% and the cost of rehabilitation is extremely high. Changes in treatment protocols mean survival rates are now above 80%. When and how to wash oiled birds has made a huge difference in the effectiveness of rehabilitation (**107**).

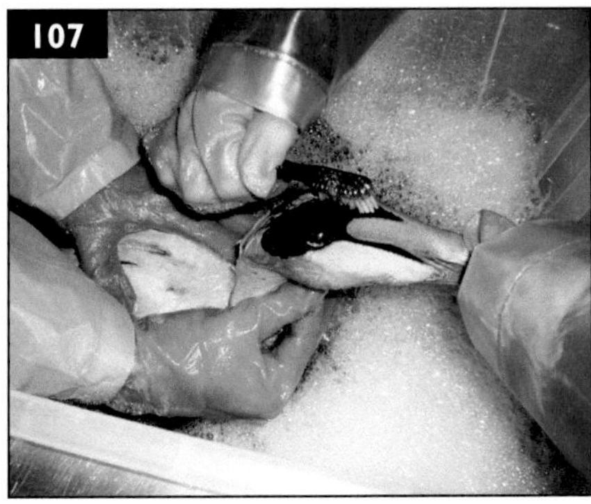

1 What are the effects of oiling on individual birds?
2 What are the different steps in the process of caring for oiled birds?
3 How would you prevent secondary diseases in this process?

CASE 108 An approximately 5-year-old male budgerigar (*Melopsittacus undulatus*) presents for progressive left leg lameness (**108**). There is no history of trauma. On examination, the bird is bright and responsive. There is no voluntary movement distal to the left stifle, but deep pain perception is present and the bird vocalizes when the toes are pinched. No other neurologic deficits are present. There is also mild muscle atrophy in the leg, but no palpable fracture or luxation.

1 What is the most likely diagnosis?
2 What diagnostic test would you perform to confirm your diagnosis?
3 What are the treatment options and prognosis?

CASE 109 A 15-year-old male intact cockatiel (*Nymphicus hollandicus*) presents for decreased ability to grip his perch and swollen toes. On physical examination, several white lesions are noted around the joints (**109**). Blood is collected for a biochemistry panel.

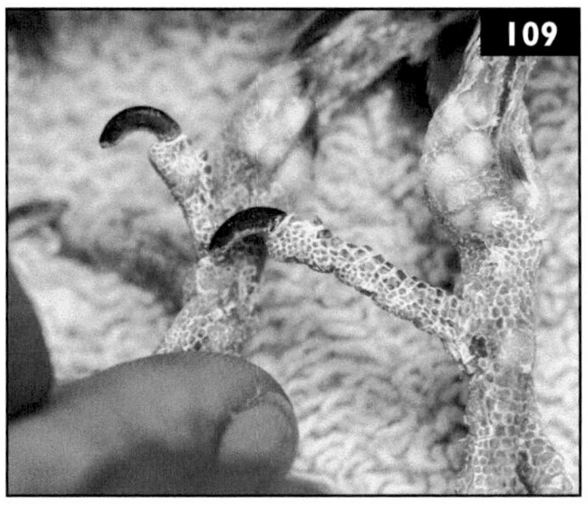

Parameter	Value	Reference interval
AST (U/L)	375	100–396
Calcium (mmol/L) (mg/dL)	2.22 (8.9)	2.12–3.24 (8.5–13)
CK (U/L)	240	30–245
Glucose (mmol/L) (mg/dL)	19.54 (352)	11.1–24.98 (200–450)
Phosphorus (mmol/L) (mg/dL)	1.19 (3.7)	3.2–4.8
Potassium (mEq/L)	4.1	2.5–4.5
Protein, total (g/L) (g/dL)	32 (3.2)	24–41 (2.4–4.1)
Albumin (g/L) (g/dL)	14 (1.4)	7–18 (0.7–1.8)
Globulin (g/L) (g/dL)	18 (1.8)	17–23 (1.7–2.3)
Sodium (mEq/L)	138	132–150
Uric acid (μmol/L) (mg/dL)	1332 (22.4)	208–654 (3.5–11)

1 What is the most likely cause of the lesions noted around the joints?
2 What medications can be used to help this patient?
3 What other systems may be affected by this disease?

CASE 110

1 What are the differential diagnoses for 'swollen head syndrome' in pheasants and/or partridges (**110**)?
2 What are the most appropriate tests available to diagnose the cause of this syndrome?
3 What are the most appropriate treatment methods available for flocks of pheasants and partridges?

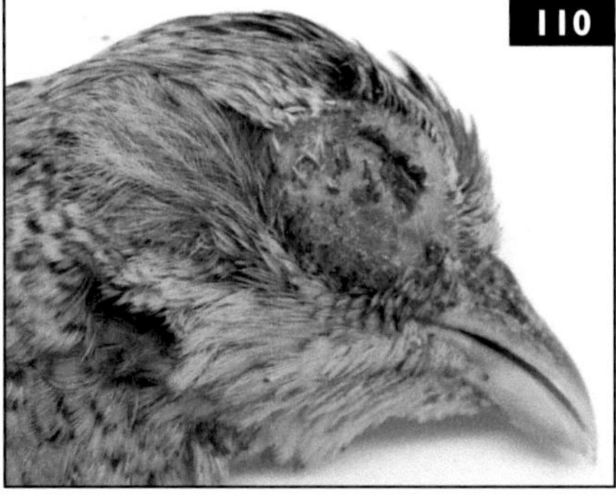

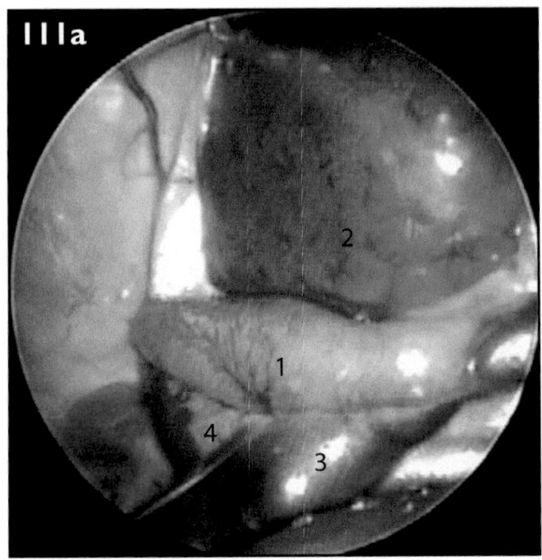

Courtesy of Dr. Stephen Divers, UGA

CASE 111

1 Describe the anatomic entry points for a double-entry orchidectomy.
2 Name the structures labeled (2), (3), and (4) in image **111a** that are closely associated with the left avian testis (1) and need to be avoided during orchidectomy.
3 What are the possible complications of a single-entry vasectomy technique in birds?

CASE 112 A client seeks your assistance after being accused of causing suffering by starvation by a welfare society. The client is accused of having caused suffering between 19th and 28th November 2015. The client had owned a male saker falcon (*Falco cherrug*), which was in mid-flying season at the time. The client was herself in hospital from 27th November until 8th December. An Animal Welfare Inspector visited at 14:00 hours on the 4th December, finding the saker falcon dead (exact date of death unknown). Diarrhea was present under the bird's perch. It was submitted for postmortem examination on the 5th December. The bird was subjected to a postmortem examination by a veterinary pathologist. The pathologist weighed the bird as 645 g; the carcase was somewhat autolyzed and had been dead for an unknown period of time. She measured the bird's 8th primary feathers (P8) as 368–369 mm. She states published data for male saker falcons: P8 average 403 mm, standard deviation (SD) 11.5; weight average 1,105 g, SD 123.6 g. At postmortem examination, no food was found in the gastrointestinal tract, the carcase was markedly dehydrated, the bird was considered to be emaciated, and the gastrointestinal tract findings were consistent with enteritis but hampered by autolysis. A carer had been tasked with feeding the bird each evening while the owner was hospitalized. At the time

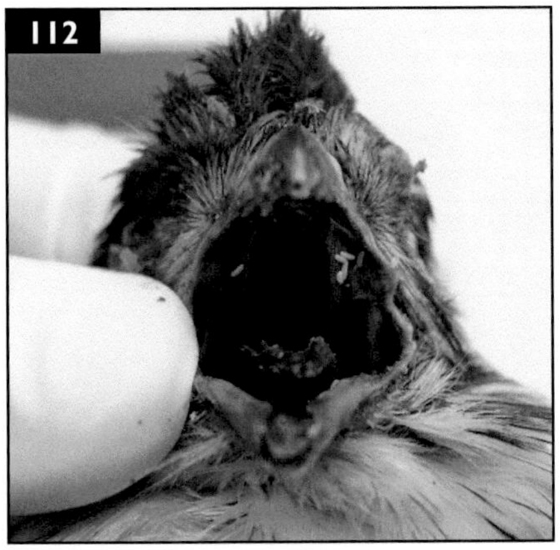

the bird was found dead, the water bowl, which was in reach of the bird's perch, was seen to be knocked over. Maggots are found in the oropharyngeal cavity and cloaca (**112**). The maggots are speciated and instar stage determined, indicating an estimated time of death 1.8–2 days prior to the postmortem examination.

1 What is the most likely date of death?
2 What do you believe the bird's normal flying weight would be?
3 How long do you think it could have been starved for?

CASE 113 An adult sparrow hawk (*Accipiter nisus*) is presented for ophthalmologic examination after the owner noticed a sudden change in the color of one eye (**113a, b**).

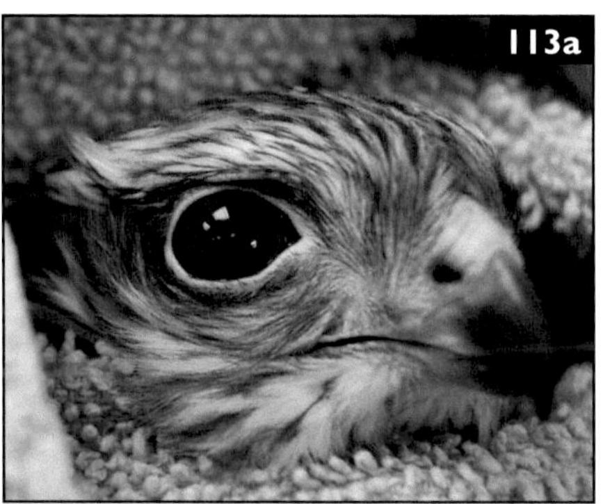
113a

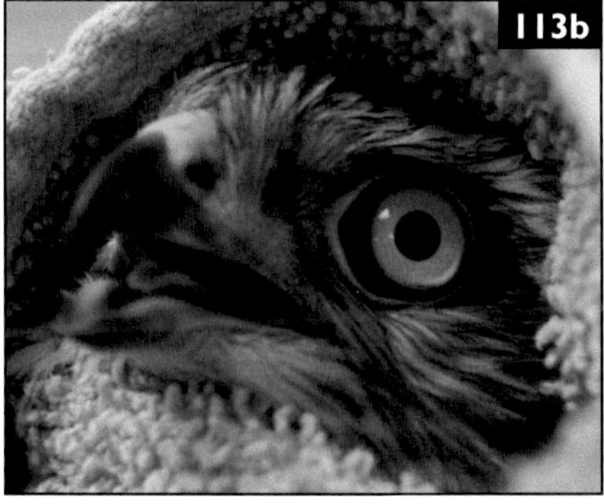
113b

1 What abnormality is seen to be affecting which eye in this sparrow hawk?
2 What is the most common cause for this disorder in birds?
3 What ophthalmologic tests should be conducted?

CASE 114 A local farm is experiencing an acute die-off of almost all their very young mallard ducklings (*Anas platyrhynchos* var. *domesticus*). Clinical disease in these ducklings is rapid. Signs progress from ataxia and lethargy to spasms and opisthotonus to death in as little as 1–2 hours.

1 What is your top differential diagnosis for the cause of death in these ducklings?
2 What pathologic changes do you expect to see on gross necropsy?
3 In addition to necropsy, what diagnostic tests should be performed to confirm the cause of this die-off?

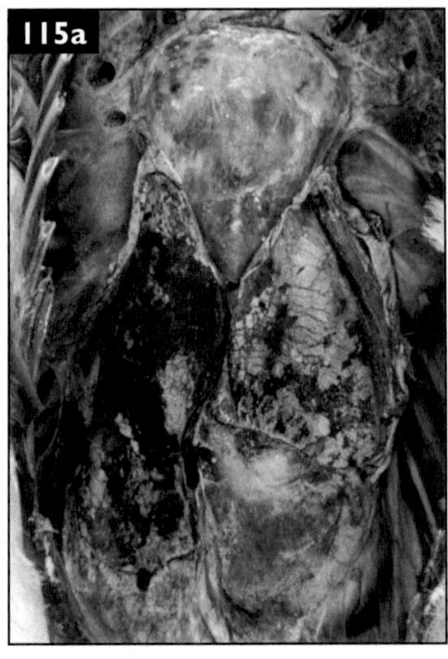

CASE 115 An adult whooper swan (*Cygnus cygnus*) was presented for emergency treatment. The bird was thin (keel score 2/5), severely dehydrated, and weak. Supportive care including intravenous fluids was initiated, but the bird died within 2 hours of admission. At necropsy, serosal changes were observed on the pericardium and liver as well as changes in the kidneys (**115a**).

1. What gross lesions are shown in the image?
2. What is the histologic lesion?
3. What is the pathophysiology of this disease?

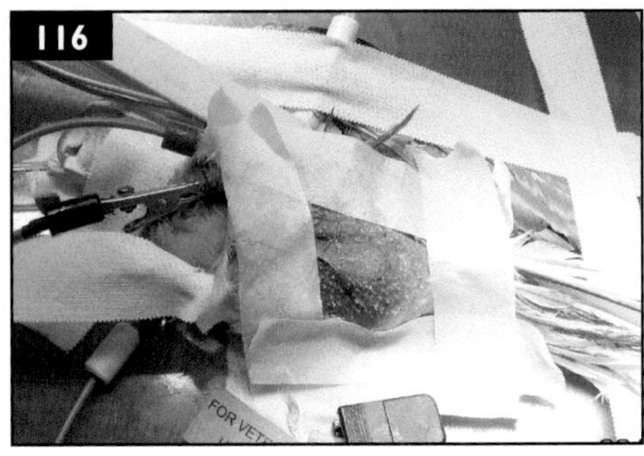

CASE 116 An adult female cockatiel (*Nymphicus hollandicus*) presented with a history of egg binding. The bird first presented 2 months prior for lethargy and increased respiratory effort. Diagnostic tests, including a CBC, plasma chemistry panel, and radiographs, were performed and showed anemia, chronic inflammation, and two well-calcified eggs. The bird was treated medically for egg binding with fluid therapy, calcium, and oxytocin but was not able to lay the eggs. The eggs were collapsed via ovocentesis under general anesthesia through the cloaca (**116**), but the efforts were unsuccessful and the bird was unable to lay the eggs. One week later, the eggs have not been laid.

1. What surgical procedure would you perform to resolve this condition?
2. How would you perform this procedure?
3. What intra- and postoperative complications might occur?

CASE 117 The paired kidneys of birds are divided into three divisions: cranial, middle, and caudal (**117a:** 1 = adrenal gland; 2 = cranial division of the kidney; 3 = common iliac vein; 4 = external iliac vein; 5 = caudal renal vein; 6 = caudal division of the kidney; 7 = urates in the ureter).

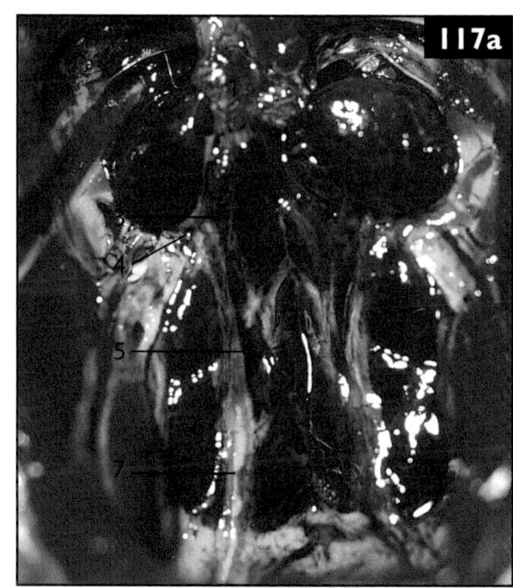

1 What major structure will be revealed if the kidneys of this yellow-crowned Amazon parrot (*Amazona ochrecephala*) are dissected away?
2 How can disease in this area cause paralysis of the legs?

CASE 118 Parrots are commonly reported as species that have a tendency to be neophobic and experience fear when confronted with new or potentially threatening stimuli (e.g. new toys, strangers, other animals such as a cat or dog). Conditioning of a fear response may occur fast, sometimes only requiring a single session, especially in extremely fearful situations (e.g. visits to the clinic or towelling to restrain the bird for a physical examination [**118**]). Undoing this type of conditioning is, however, much more difficult, often requiring repeated favorable experiences to overcome the conditioned fear response.

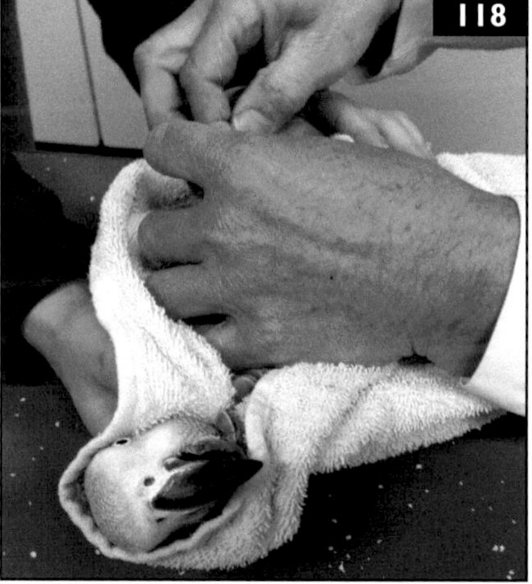

1 What is the correct terminology for the behavior modification techniques that can be used to decrease the conditioned fear response? Also explain briefly how these techniques work.
2 What are the key factors that need to be taken into consideration for the successful implementation of the above mentioned procedure?
3 In case of extreme fear or patients being refractory to behavior modification therapy, pharmacologic intervention may be considered. What drug classes may be used to reduce anxiety?

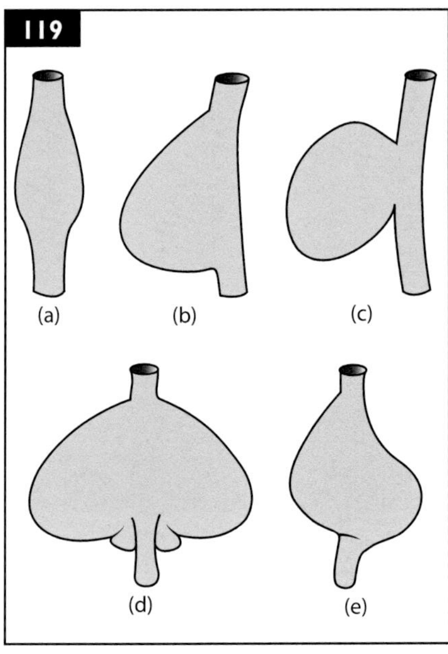

CASE 119 The crop is a diverticulum of the esophagus in birds and is used to store food before it is digested. The degree of development of the crop differs between bird species, and some lack a true crop. Apart from being a food storage organ in adult birds, the crop is also used to store and produce food with which chicks are being fed by the parents. Five crop shapes are shown (**119**).

1 Which crop shape corresponds to the following bird species: budgerigar, cormorant, pigeon, chicken, vulture?
2 Which bird species lack a true crop?
3 Which bird species are known to produce secretions in the crop or esophagus that are used to feed the chicks?

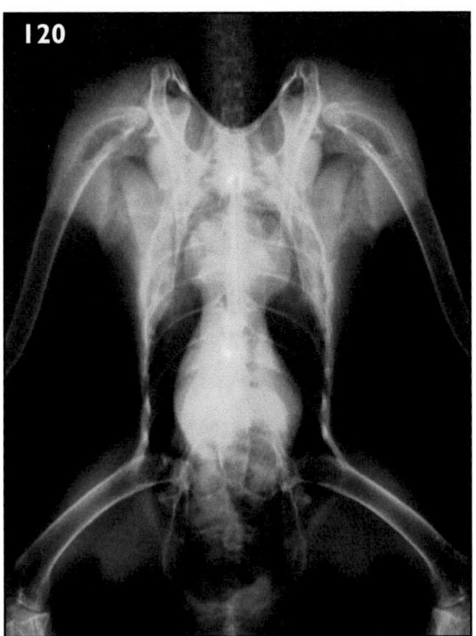

CASE 120 A gyrfalcon (*Falco rusticolus*) was taken to a local avian clinic. On examination the bird had a body condition score of 3/5, was unable to stand or maintain its balance, refused to eat when food was offered, and was passing green colored urates. A radiograph was obtained (**120**).

1 Based on the history and physical examination findings, what are your differential diagnoses?
2 What diagnostic test would you perform to confirm the diagnosis?
3 The falcon appeared to be suffering from lead toxicosis. How is it possible to have such a high lead level? Which is the ideal therapeutic agent for treatment?

CASE 121 You are presented with a 12-year-old blue and gold macaw (*Ara ararauna*) for evaluation of 'abnormally thickened feathers' on the tail (**121**). The macaw was recently adopted and the client is a new bird owner.

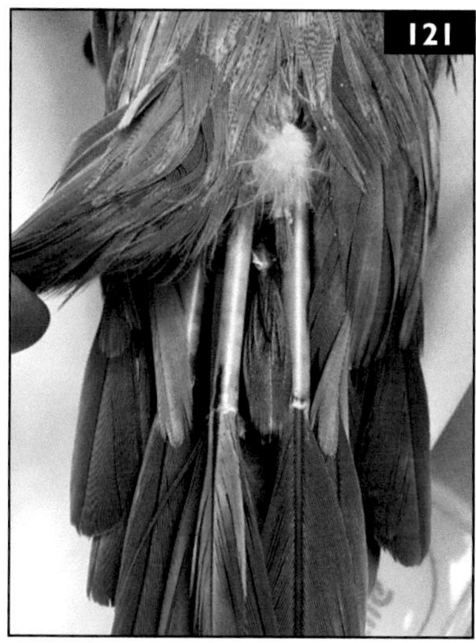

1 What are the 'abnormal feathers' noted by the client and seen in this image?
2 What process is occurring in this bird, and how would you explain this process to a client?
3 The client would like to know how frequently this process will occur, and asks what physiologic factors control this process?

CASE 122 A Harris' hawk (*Parabuteo unicinctus*) is presented with skin lesions on the precrural fold (**122a**). It has been progressively getting worse, and now the bird is self-mutilating. This condition is reported to be particularly common in this species as well as in peregrine falcons (*Falco peregrinus*). Similar skin lesions have been reported also on the ventral aspect of the wing and axillary region of psittacine birds.

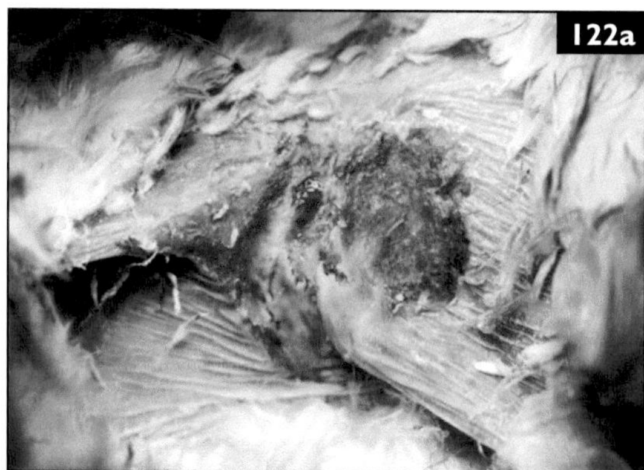

1 What is the most likely diagnosis?
2 How is the disease best managed?
3 How might it progress if left untreated?

CASE 123 A 30-year-old double yellow-headed Amazon parrot (*Amazona ochrocephala oratrix*) of unknown sex was presented for evaluation of lethargy, weight loss, and reduced appetite. The bird had been treated by the referring veterinarian with ciprofloxacin and meloxicam. On physical examination the bird appeared in low body condition and had blunted choanal papillae. A CBC was consistent with moderate nonregenerative anemia and heterophilic leukocytosis. Survey radiographs showed mild proventricular dilatation and loss of serosal intestinal detail. A Gram stain of the feces showed a relative amount of small, normal gram-positive and gram-negative bacteria. Coelomic ultrasound was nondiagnostic and a contrast gastrointestinal study with barium was performed, which showed an irregular and marginated intestinal mucosa (**123a, b**). A fine needle aspirate of the intestines was nondiagnostic. A full-thickness intestinal biopsy was performed under general anesthesia and confirmed the diagnosis of intestinal lymphoma (T-cell).

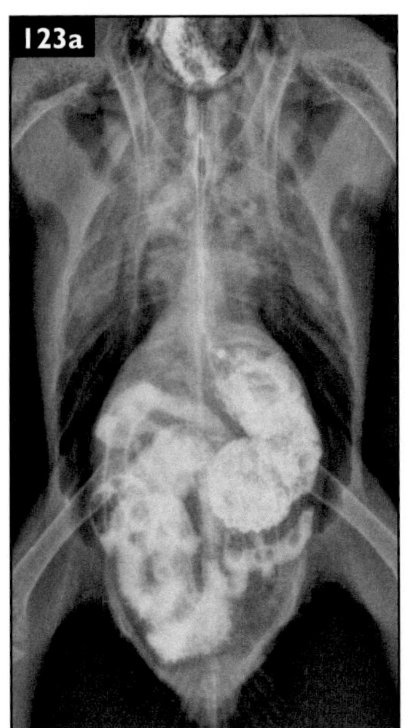
123a

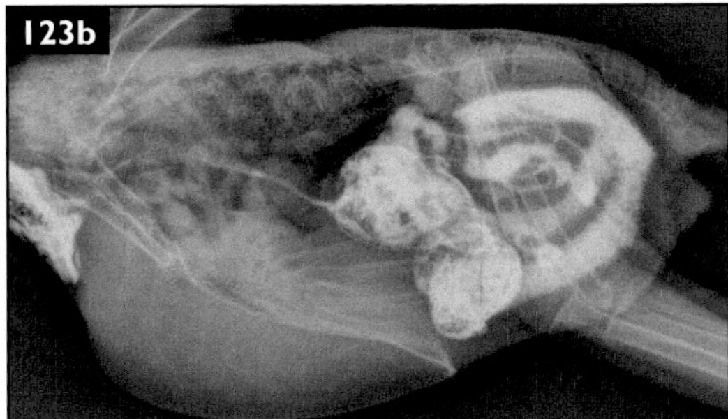
123b

1 What are your differential diagnoses for the radiographic intestinal findings?
2 What are the intra- and postoperative risks associated with this procedure?
3 How would you treat lymphoma in this bird? What is the prognosis?

CASE 124

1 At what age is septicemia usually seen in game bird chicks?
2 What are the main causes of septicemia in chicks?
3 What is the recommended course of action when birds show clinical signs suggestive of septicemia?

CASE 125 An adult female blue and gold macaw (*Ara ararauna*) with a history of straining to defecate and hematochezia is undergoing a cloacoscopy in dorsal recumbency. An abnormal finding was encountered (**125**).

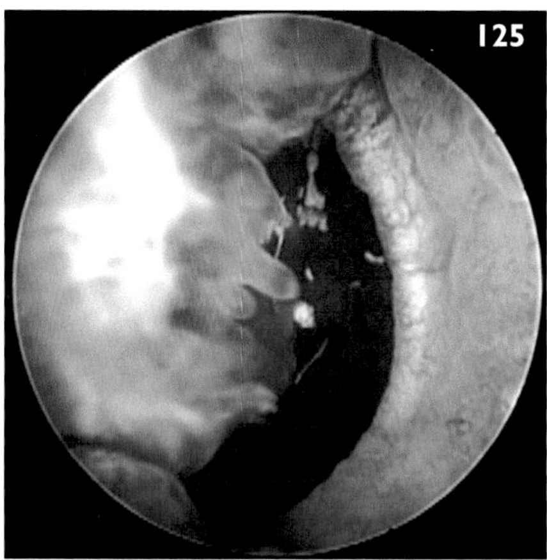

Courtesy of Dr. Stephen Divers, UGA

1 Describe the abnormality and list the most common differential diagnoses for this finding.
2 Describe the technique for obtaining a biopsy of this structure in order to confirm a diagnosis. What is a possible complication of this procedure?
3 What treatment modalities are possible, using the 2.7-mm endoscope system, that may be applicable to this case?

CASE 126 Long bone developmental problems are particularly common in long-legged birds (e.g. flamingos, storks, cranes) (**126**), but can also be seen in birds with short legs (e.g. raptors, psittacines) in some instances.

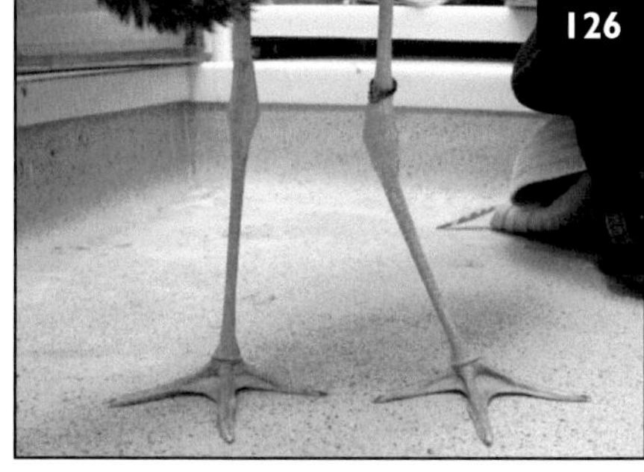

1 What common factors are considered to be involved?
2 How is bone growth different in birds compared with mammals? What are the implications when evaluating birds radiographically?
3 Why might young raptors changing from whole day-old chicks to quartered rabbit or pigeon carcases develop metabolic bone disease?

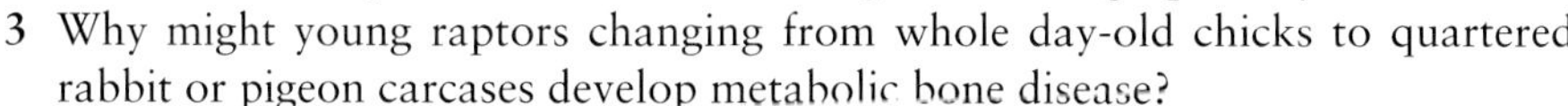

CASE 127

1 What factors cause the death of eggs in each of the first, second, and third trimesters?
2 What levels of fertility and hatchability should be strived for?
3 How often should eggs be turned during incubation?

CASE 128 A type-I ESF and intramedullary pin (ESF-IM) tie-in fixator was used to repair a humeral fracture in this 1.2 kg red-tailed hawk (*Buteo jamaicensis*). The fixator has been in place for 2 weeks and the IM pin has already been removed as part of dynamic destabilization of the fracture.

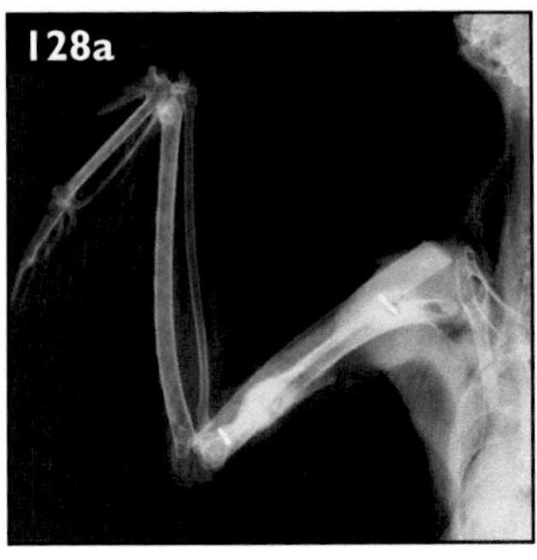
128a

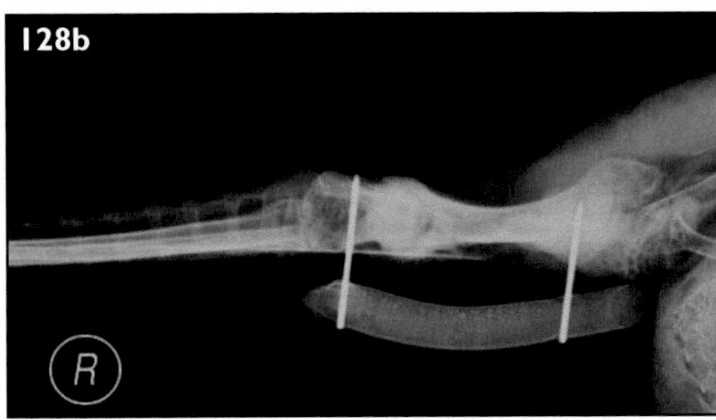

128b

1 What abnormal radiographic findings are seen in the radiographs at this point (**128a, b**)?
2 What is the clinical significance?
3 What is the recommended course of action?

CASE 129 A pigeon, presented to you in July, is one of 80 pigeons from a loft of a renowned pigeon fancier. More than 10% of the pigeons in his loft are showing a range of clinical signs, varying from head tilt (as seen in this pigeon, **129**) to diarrhea and/or swollen elbow joints. In the past week, three pigeons were found dead without having shown previous clinical signs.

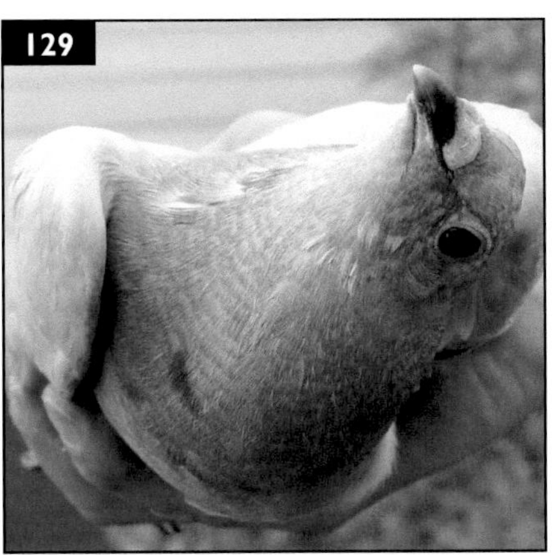
129

1 What is the most likely diagnosis, and how can this diagnosis be confirmed?
2 What treatment and preventive options are available?
3 Does the disease pose a health risk for the pigeon fancier? Explain how and why.

CASE 130 A chestnut-mandibled toucan (*Ramphastos ambiguus swainsonii*) is presented for sinus trephination to further evaluate the soft-tissue opacities found on the radiographic study of the beak (**130**). There was a past history of *Pseudomonas aeruginosa* infection that had been previously treated, although there remained clear nasal discharge afterwards. Rigid endoscopy is used in conjunction with endosurgical forceps to sample and débride these lesions through two separate trephinations. The samples obtained were histologically characterized as sterile granulomas and there were no aerobic isolates detected on culture.

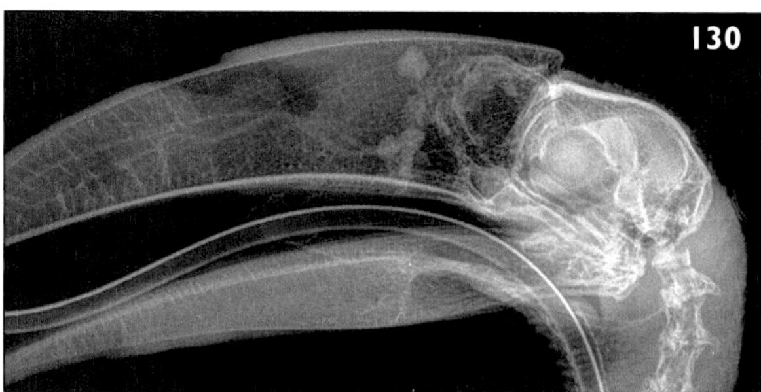
130

1 What structures were entered as the trephination procedure was performed?
2 How would you manage the trephination site postoperatively?
3 How would the trephination affect the growth of the rhinotheca?

CASE 131 Certain aspects of the avian anatomy and physiology, in particular the respiratory system, are markedly different to mammals (**131**). Consider each of the following statements relating to avian anesthesia and state whether they are true or false, and why.

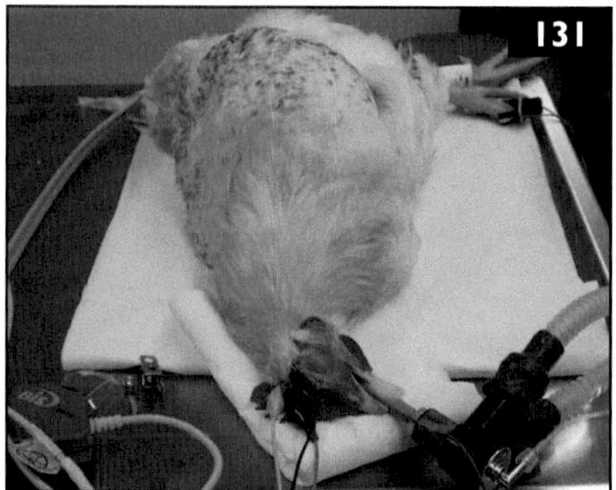
131

1 Birds have a small functional residual capacity (FRC).
2 Oxygen absorption in avian lungs is more efficient compared with mammalian lungs.
3 Birds are more sensitive to hypercapnia.

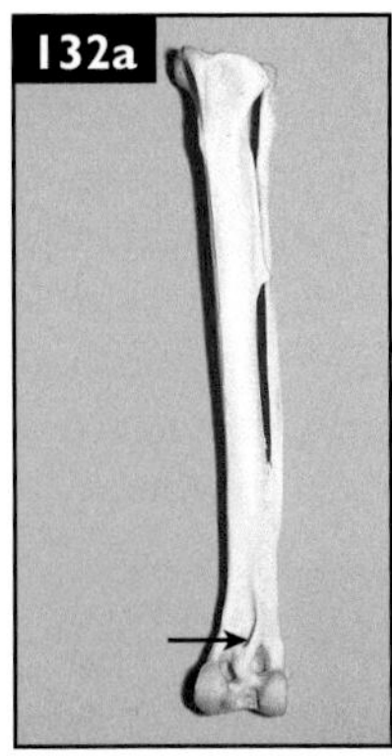

CASE 132 A cranial view of the tibiotarsus of a typical Falconiforme bird (peregrine [*Falco peregrinus*]) is shown (**132a**).

1 What is the structure and function of the tunnel arrowed?
2 What difference is there in this region in Psittaciformes?
3 What complications might occur with distal tibiotarsus fracture repair?

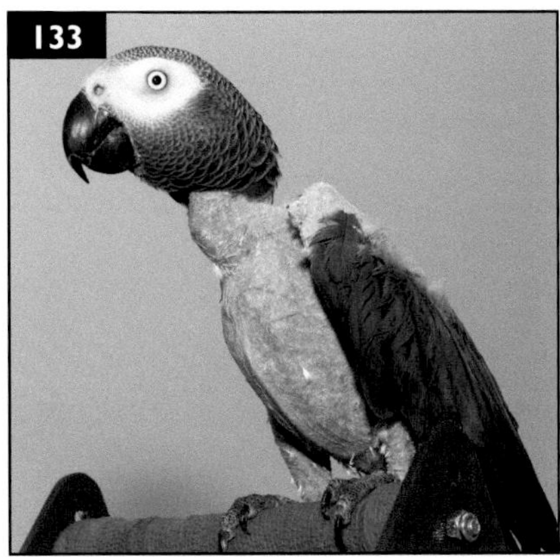

CASE 133 Feather damaging behavior, also referred to as feather destructive behavior, feather plucking, feather picking, or pterotillomania, is a condition that affects many captive Psittaciformes. In particular, African grey parrots (*Psittacus erithacus*) and cockatoos (*Cacatua* spp.) appear predisposed to developing this behavior, which is characterized by self-inflicted damage to the feathers in areas that are accessible to the bird's beak (**133**).

1 What are the medical and nonmedical differential diagnoses that should be considered in parrots presented with this behavior?
2 Describe the different aspects that need to be considered when designing an initial treatment plan for a parrot with feather damaging behavior.
3 In birds that do not respond to the initial treatment plan, pharmacologic intervention may be considered. What categories of pharmacologic agents may be considered for treatment of refractory feather damaging behavior?

CASE 134

1 At what age does coccidiosis typically affect partridges?
2 How is coccidiosis commonly diagnosed in partridges?
3 What are the treatment options for coccidiosis in partridges?

CASE 135 A distraught waterfowl keeper presents this carcase to you one spring (**135**). She had a collection of some 60 birds and in the previous 24 hours 24 birds have been found dead.

135

1 What is the most likely etiology? What would be the most likely postmortem findings?
2 How should the disease outbreak be managed?
3 How can future outbreaks of disease be prevented?

CASE 136 An adult free-ranging red-shouldered hawk (*Buteo lineatus*) is presented by a member of the public to a clinic in the USA for inability to fly. On physical examination, a marked hyphema of the left eye is noted (**136**) together with severe hypovolemia, multifocal subcutaneous hematomas, coelomic distension, and increased respiratory effort.

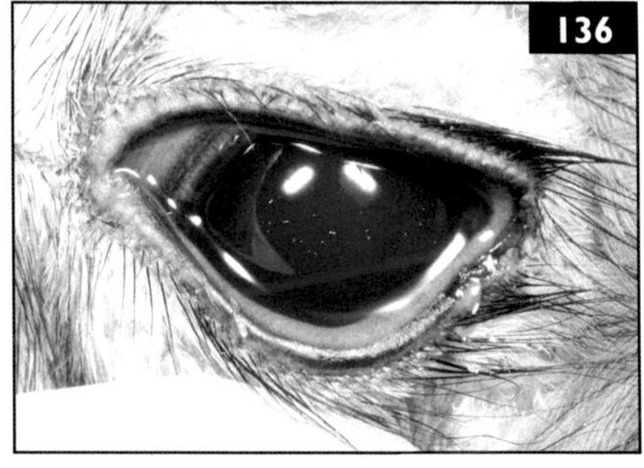
136

1 What is the most likely etiology of the observed clinical signs?
2 How would you confirm your presumptive diagnosis?
3 How would you treat this bird?

CASE 137 The triosseal canal of a bird is shown (**137a**).

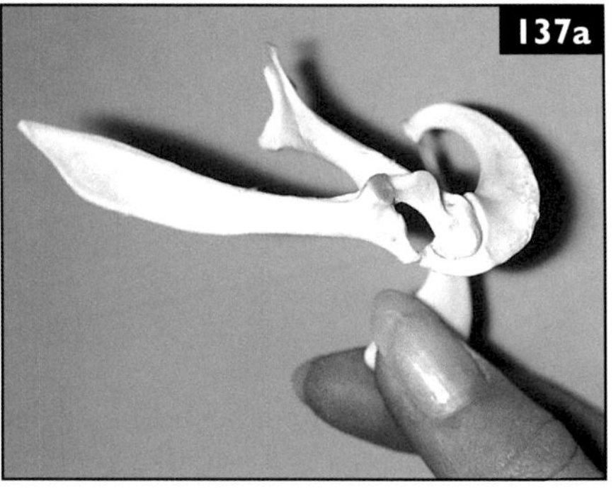
137a

1 What is the function of the foramen formed by the union of the scapula, coracoid, and clavicle? Does it have any clinical significance?

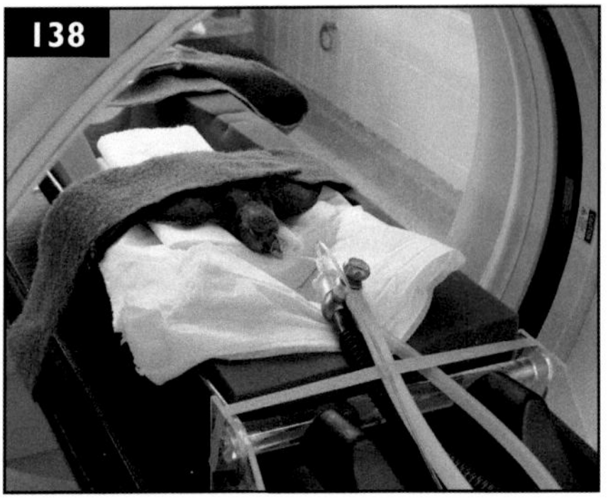
138

CASE 138 Imaging modalities are an important diagnostic tool in avian medicine as they enable noninvasive visualization of the body's anatomy and physiology. Although conventional radiography and ultrasonography are the most commonly used techniques in practice, more advanced imaging modalities such as CT (**138**) and MRI have also made their way into avian medicine.

1 Briefly explain the theory behind the two imaging modalities.
2 What are the main applications for both imaging modalities in birds?
3 What are the main limitations of both techniques with regard to their use in avian medicine?

CASE 139 A photomicrograph of the cerebellum of a euthanized emu (*Dromaius novaehollandiae*) with hematoxylin and eosin staining is shown (**139**). The only abnormalities noted on gross necropsy examination were poor body condition and abrasions on the ventral aspects of the hock joints. This emu comes from a flock of 30 birds.

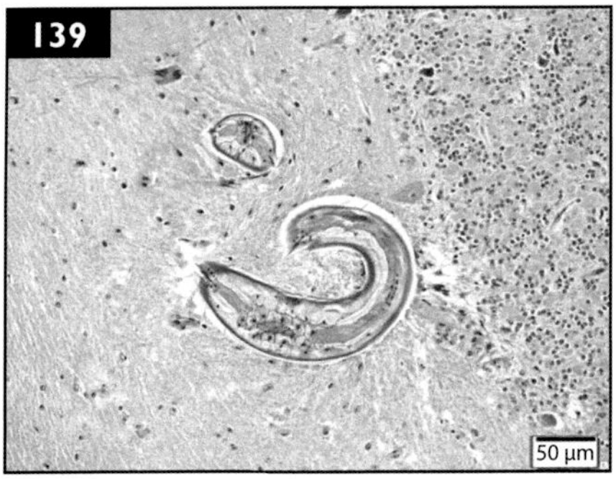

1 What is the most likely etiologic agent?
2 Describe the clinical signs that the affected bird was most likely to have shown.
3 What management steps should be taken to prevent the occurrence of the same disease in other birds in the flock?

CASE 140 Haemosporidians are intracellular protozoan parasites that develop in vertebrate and invertebrate hosts. Blood-sucking dipterans are considered the definitive host as this is where sexual reproduction takes place.

1 Name the three haemosporidian genera known to affect avian species.
2 Name the invertebrate hosts involved in their life cycle.
3 What is the importance of these parasites in captive and wild avian populations?

CASE 141 A neonatal chick is shown (**141a, b**).

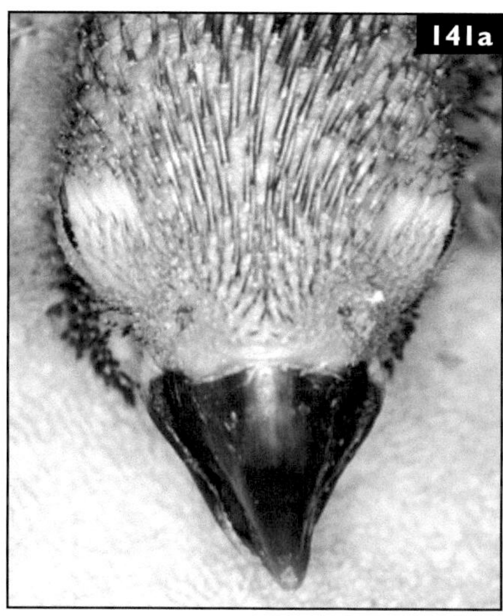

1 What species is this chick?
2 Is it precocial or altricial?
3 What is wrong with its beak?

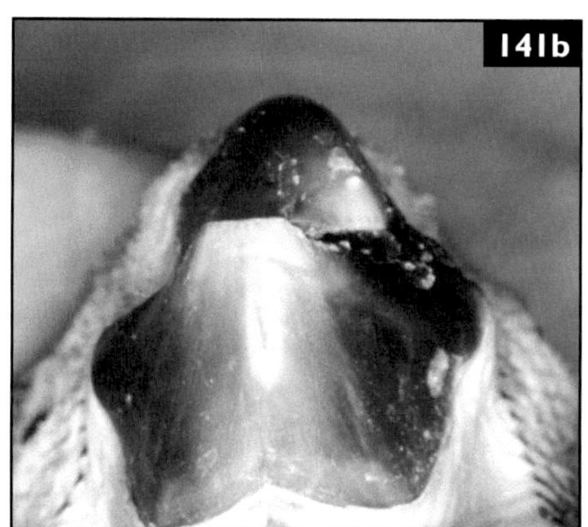

CASE 142 Avian soft tissue surgery imposes many challenges, some of them associated with the size of the patients and others with the fact that the surgeries are performed within the coelomic cavity with limited access to some organs. The choice of surgical instrumentation can facilitate significantly the surgeon's task, and appropriate soft tissue retractors, magnification with surgical loupes, and microsurgical instruments are critical to optimize the exposure, visualization, and handling of the tissues (**142**).

1 List some of the common soft tissue retractors used.
2 What are the ideal characteristics of surgical loupes?
3 What are the key features of microsurgical instruments?

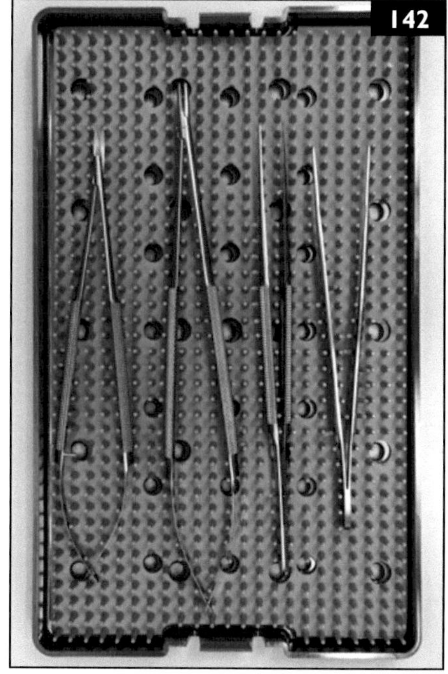

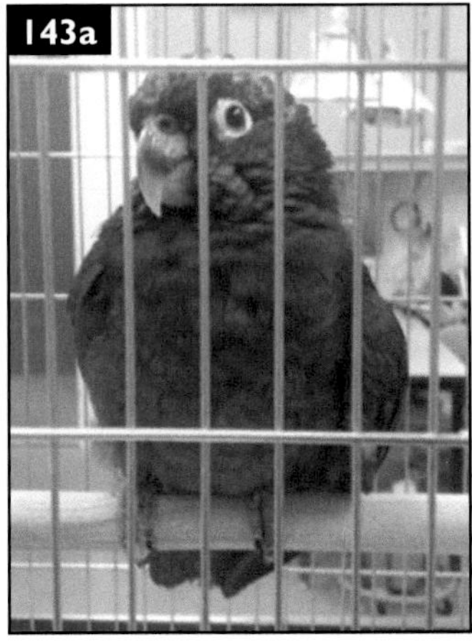
143a

CASE 143 An adult Maximilian parrot (*Pionus maximiliani*) of unknown sex was presented after flying swiftly into a sliding glass door. He was quiet and uncoordinated for 45 minutes following the incident. Both wings were initially drooped, but the left remained drooped (**143a**). On physical examination, there was no evidence of fractures or luxations, and the parrot did not appear to have any neurologic deficits.

1 What is the most likely diagnosis?
2 What are the expected physical examination findings with this type of injury?
3 What diagnostic test would you perform to confirm your diagnosis?

CASE 144 Over a course of 2 weeks during September (autumn), approximately 100 adult and juvenile mallards (*Anas platyrhynchos*), Eurasian teals (*Anas crecca*), gadwalls (*Anas strepera*), and Eurasian coots (*Fulica atra*) were found dead, despite good body condition, in the vicinity of a water treatment plant. Live animals were also detected and clinical signs varied from lethargy, green diarrhea, and ataxia to hind limb weakness/paralysis and an inability to hold the head and neck upright (**144**).

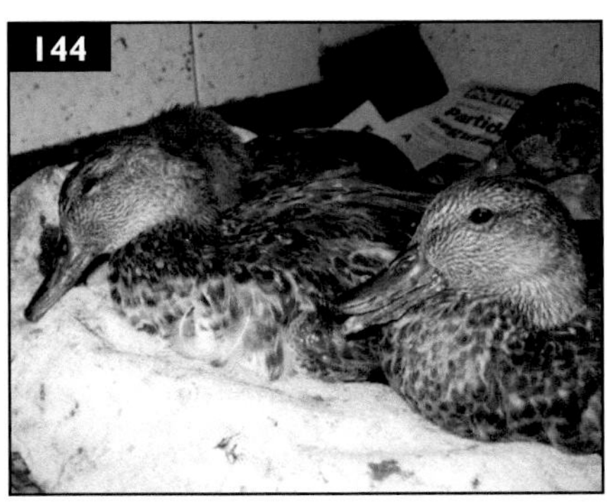
144

1 What is the most likely cause of this disease outbreak?
2 What treatment should be implemented in the live animals?
3 What measures should be implemented to curtail further cases?

CASE 145
1 List the potentially zoonotic diseases that can be encountered in pet birds.
2 For each of the diseases you have listed, give the common clinical signs seen in birds.
3 For each of the diseases you have listed, give the common clinical signs seen in humans.

CASE 146 An umbrella cockatoo (*Cacatua alba*) that presented with regurgitation and radiographic evidence of proventricular dilatation is undergoing gastroscopy for evaluation of the upper gastrointestinal tract using a 2.7 mm × 18 cm rigid endoscope (**146a**).

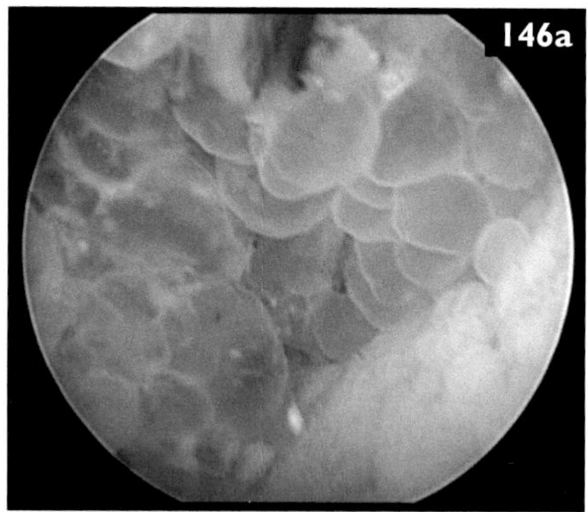

Courtesy of Dr. Stephen Divers, UGA

1 Describe the patient preparation required for this procedure.
2 What are the advantages and disadvantages of using saline irrigation versus air insufflation for a gastroscopy?
3 Describe the abnormalities seen in the proventriculus of this umbrella cockatoo. What is the appropriate next diagnostic step?

CASE 147 Systemic arterial blood pressure in birds is occasionally measured. For convenience, indirect noninvasive blood pressure measured with an oscillometric unit or a sphygmomanometer and a Doppler unit (**147**) are typically performed.

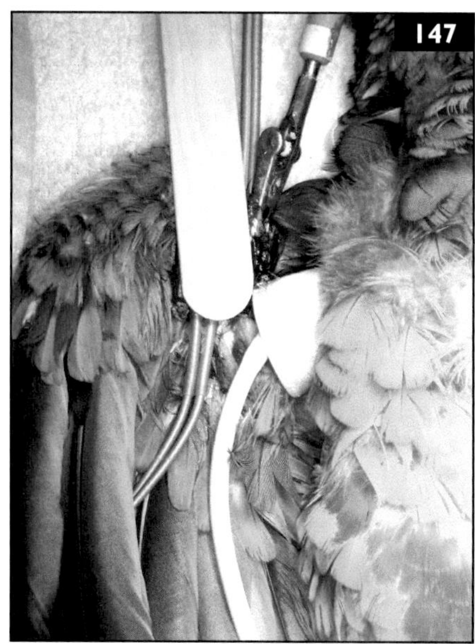

1 What is the reliability of an oscillometric unit or a sphygmomanometer and a Doppler flow unit in birds for the evaluation of blood pressure?
2 What are the main sources of variability in the measurement of indirect blood pressure in parrots using a sphygmomanometer and a Doppler flow unit? What are the clinical implications?
3 Which sites and arteries are used for direct blood pressure measurement in birds?

CASE 148 The avian endocrine glands are considered, in general, similar to those of mammals. However, their anatomic location and histologic appearance can be significantly different from the endocrine organs of some other species (**148**).

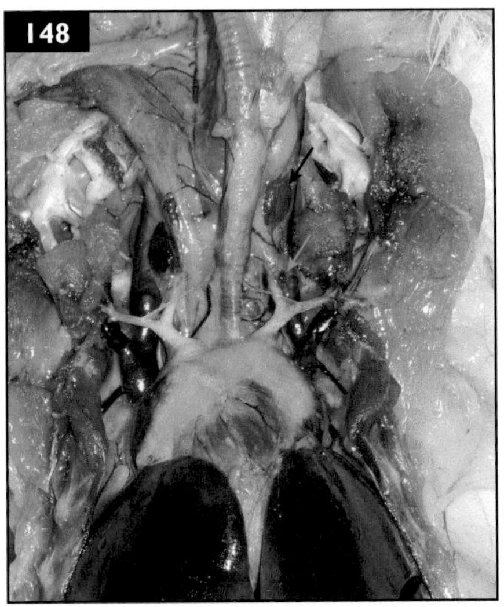
148

1 Review the image shown and name the structures identified with the black and green arrows.
2 List at least two histologic or physiologic features of these structures that are similar and two that are different from those described in mammals.
3 Which disease processes have been described relating to these two structures in avian species?
4 Which specific assays can be used to investigate the function of these structures in birds?

CASE 149 A fledging African grey parrot (*Psittacus erithacus*) is presented with a wet discharge down the front of his neck (**149**). Two other chicks in the group are currently suffering from delayed crop emptying.

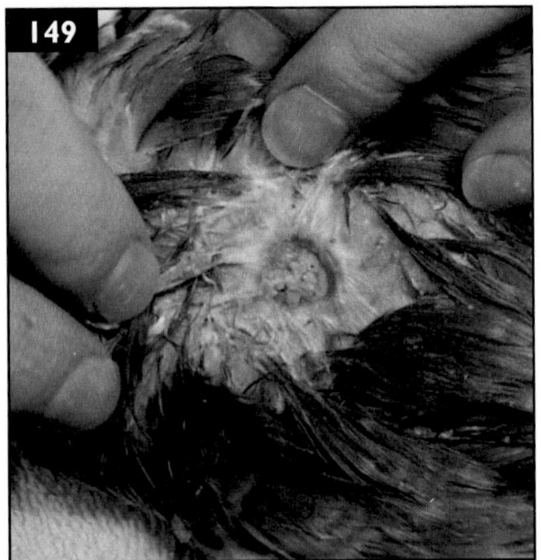
149

1 What condition is the bird suffering from, and what investigations should be carried out on the other youngsters?
2 How should this bird be treated?
3 How can the condition be avoided?

CASE 150 Typical macroscopic findings in a great green macaw (*Ara ambiguus*) with proventricular dilatation disease (PDD) are shown (**150**). Several drugs have been reported to have a beneficial effect on birds affected by this disease.

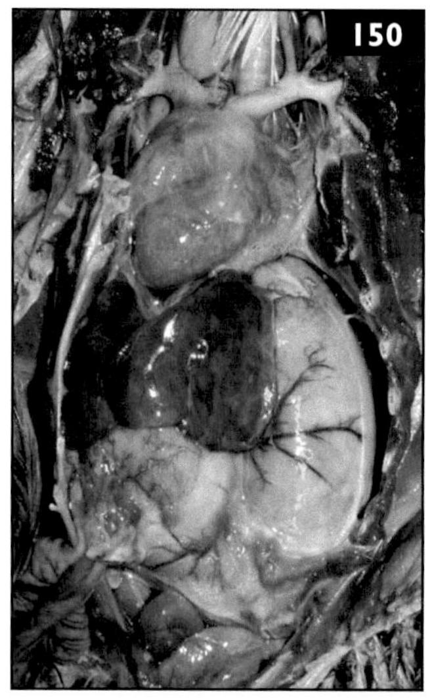

150

1 Name four drugs used to treat PDD and describe their mode of action.
2 Name two groups of drugs commonly used as supportive therapy for patients suffering from PDD.
3 Is PDD a lethal disease?

CASE 151 This 2-year-old cockatiel (*Nymphicus hollandicus*) is presented with acute-onset respiratory distress consistent with upper airway obstructive syndrome (**151**). The owner reports that the bird had not been exposed to any inhalant toxin and there is no recent history of trauma. While collecting the history and visually examining the bird and cage, you note that it is being fed millet seed.

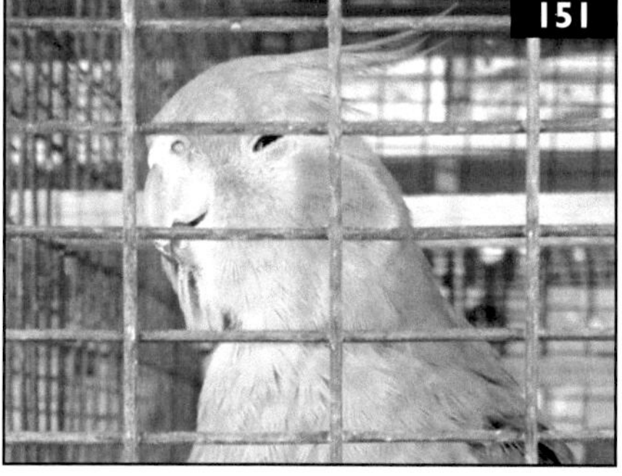

151

1 What would be the most likely differential diagnoses for this case?
2 What initial emergency treatment and diagnostic plan would you pursue?
3 What treatment would be required?

CASE 152

1 List four noninvasive methods of evaluating eggs and avian embryos during incubation.
2 At what stages of incubation are the above noninvasive methods most useful?
3 Which of the above methods may be useful in determining if and when to assist a weak or malpositioned embryo in hatching, and why is each useful?

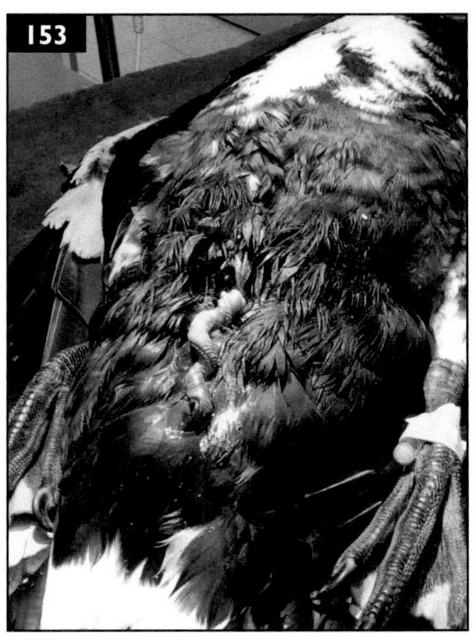

CASE 153 A male Muscovy duck (*Cairina moschata*) is presented with tissue protruding from the vent (**153**), which has been present for at least 48 hours. The bird is well hydrated, in good body condition, and otherwise appears healthy. The drake lives with one other drake and five ducks in a large paddock.

1 What is the organ protruding from the vent?
2 How would you initially treat this condition?
3 How would you treat this condition if it recurs?

CASE 154 A 3.2 kg adult male bald eagle (*Haliaeetus leucocephalus*) was treated for a radius and ulna fracture sustained from a gunshot injury. A solid callus formed at the fracture site, but extension of the wing remained poor during physical therapy. Radiographs of the wing were taken 5 weeks post trauma (**154a**).

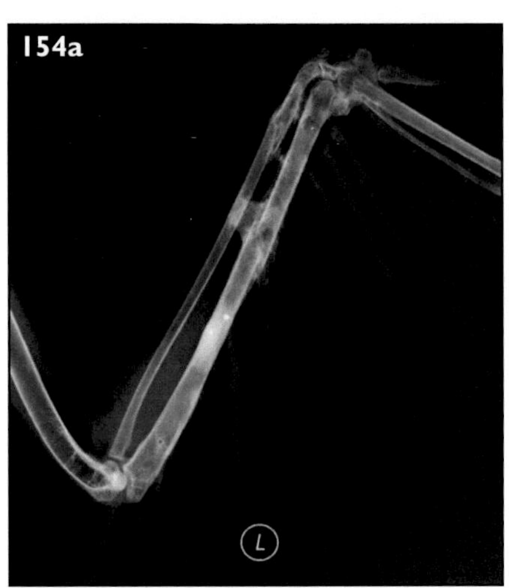

1 Name the condition.
2 How is it prevented?
3 How is it treated?

CASE 155 Erythrocytes in a Major Mitchell's cockatoo (*Lophochroa leadbeateri*) with nonspecific signs of illness including lethargy and anorexia are shown (**155**).

1 What are the main changes present in the erythrocytes?
2 What are the main cytologic features used to assess signs of a regenerative response in avian blood smears?
3 What is the best anticoagulant to use to preserve avian blood for routine hematologic evaluation?

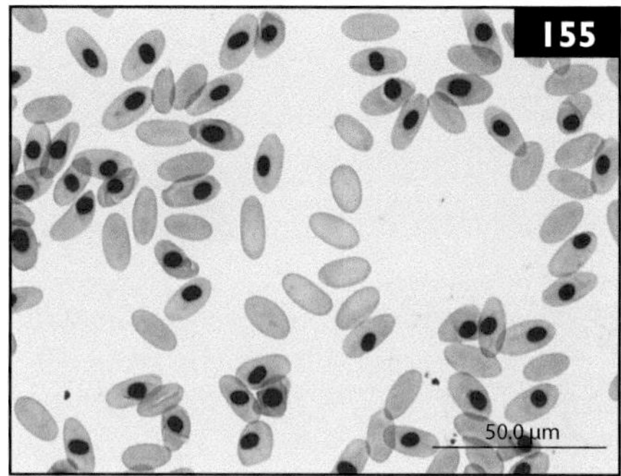

CASE 156 A gyrfalcon (*Falco rusticolus*) is presented with a history of weight loss, regurgitation, and anorexia (**156**). Oropharyngeal cavity examination reveals aggregates of thick, granular yellow exudates.

1 Which nematodes would you consider as the most likely differential diagnoses?
2 How would you confirm the presence of the parasite?
3 What treatment would you suggest in this case?

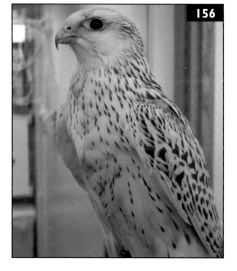

CASE 157
1 What four factors, whether using natural or artificial incubation, are important to the microenvironment surrounding an egg?
2 Why change the air in incubators? Why is the incubator and room ventilation important? Does an egg need ventilation during the entire course of incubation?
3 How much oxygen does a developing embryo (chicken) need in an egg during incubation? How much carbon dioxide does the developing embryo produce during incubation?

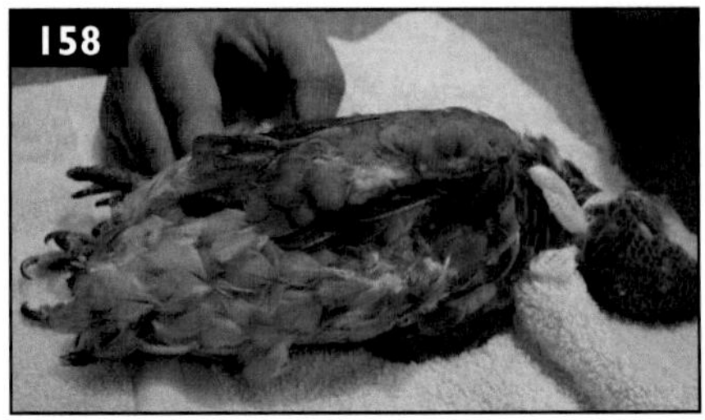

CASE 158 An African grey parrot (*Psittacus erithacus*) is presented for examination. The owner is concerned that the bird may have been feather plucking, as the bird appears to have feather loss (**158**). The owner has three other young birds in the same accommodation.

1 What is the main differential diagnosis?
2 What is your advice to the owner in respect of these birds?
3 What treatment can be provided to these young birds?

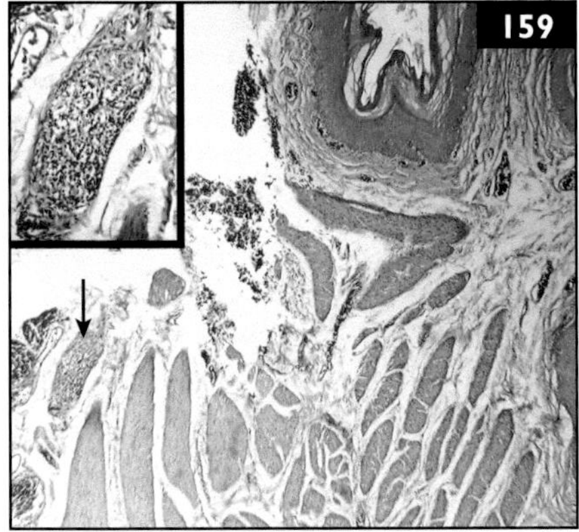

CASE 159 A photomicrograph of a crop biopsy from a yellow-crested cockatoo (*Cacatua sulphurea*) is shown (**159**). The corresponding inset shows the area indicated by the arrow at higher magnification.

1 What is the lesion shown?
2 In what disease is this lesion characteristic?
3 What are the key points for collection and preparation of a crop biopsy?

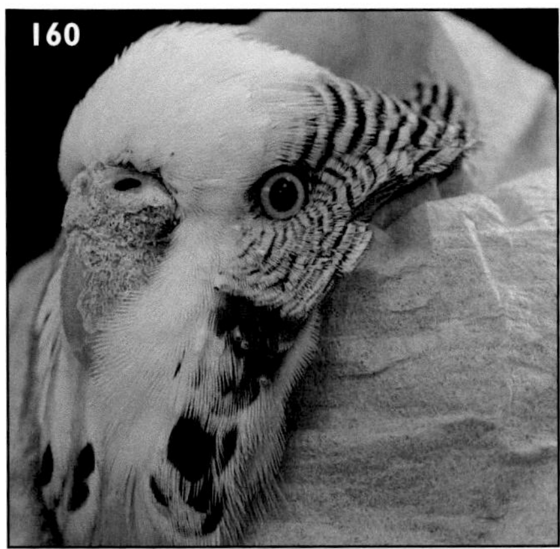

CASE 160 You are presented with a 2-year-old male budgerigar (*Melopsittacus undulatus*) with a 'crusty beak' (**160**).

1 What dermatologic physical examination findings are present?
2 What organism is associated with this finding, and what diagnostic tests would aid in identification?
3 How would you treat this bird?

CASE 161 A 22-year-old female yellow-naped Amazon parrot (*Amazona auropalliata*) is presented for increased appetite, weight loss, and abnormal droppings (**161a**).

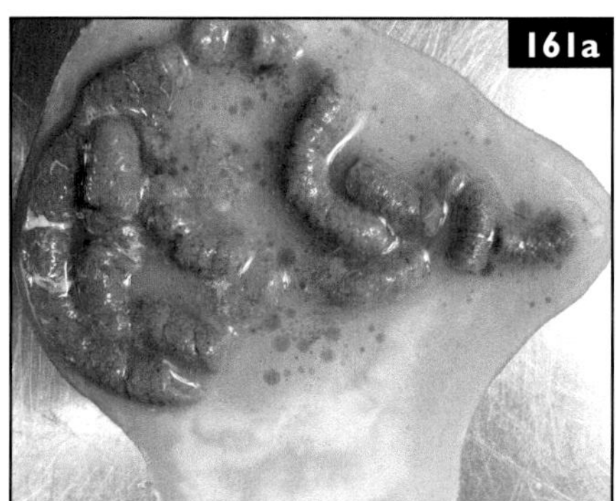
161a

1 What abnormalities of the droppings are present?
2 What is the most likely underlying cause?
3 What simple fecal test can be performed to confirm the diagnosis?

CASE 162

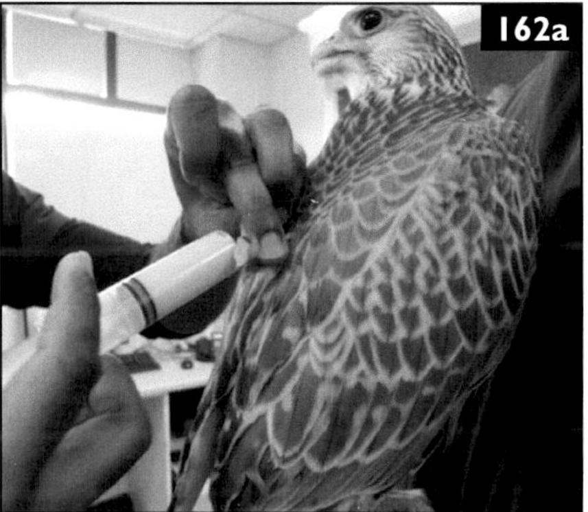
162a

1 What are some of the clinical indications for esophagostomy tube placement in avian patients (**162a**)?
2 Are esophagostomy tubes generally well tolerated in birds?
3 When preparing to place an esophagostomy tube in raptorial species, at what level do you aim to place the distal tube end, and why?

CASE 163 A hematoxylin and eosin-stained section of the ventriculus from a Gouldian finch (*Erythrura gouldiae*) that died acutely with necropsy findings of hepatomegaly and nephromegaly is shown (**163**).

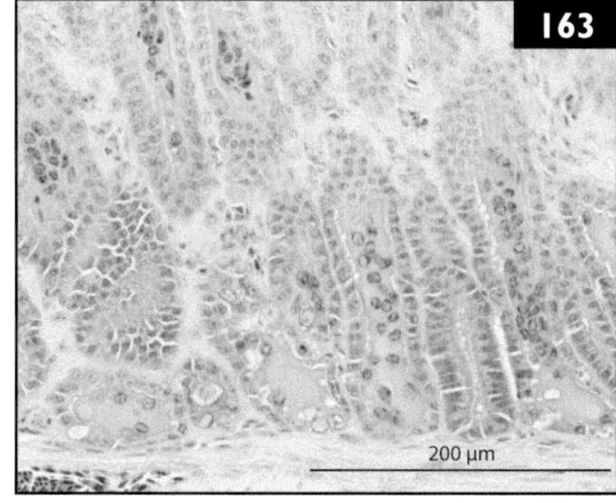

163

1 What abnormalities can be seen in the histologic section?
2 What etiologic agents should be considered?
3 What other diagnostic tests should be performed to confirm a specific etiologic diagnosis?

CASE 164 An adult toco toucan (*Ramphastos toco*) was found dead in its aviary. At gross necropsy an enlarged liver was the most significant finding. Specifically, a firm, caseous mass with irregular edges was occupying an extensive portion of the liver parenchyma (**164a**).

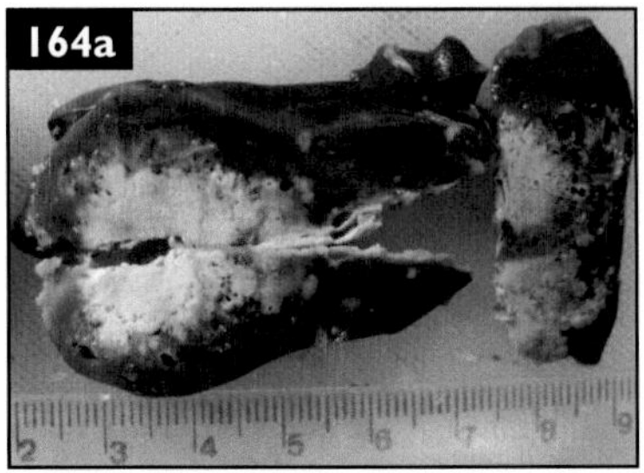

1 What are the main differential diagnoses?
2 What complementary examination would you perform?
3 How would you prevent this disease?

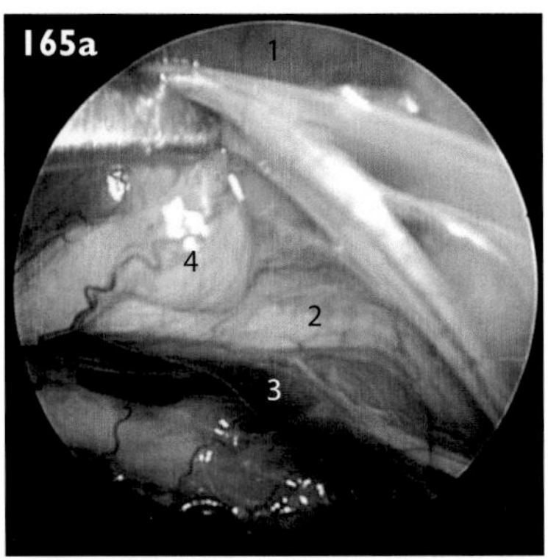

Courtesy of Dr. Stephen Divers, UGA

CASE 165
1 Describe the anatomic entry points for a triple-entry salpingohysterectomy.
2 What structures, labeled (1), (2), and (3) in image **165a**, is the uterus (4) closely associated with and that need to be avoided during salpingohysterectomy?
3 What are the limitations and contraindications of salpingohysterectomy in birds?

CASE 166

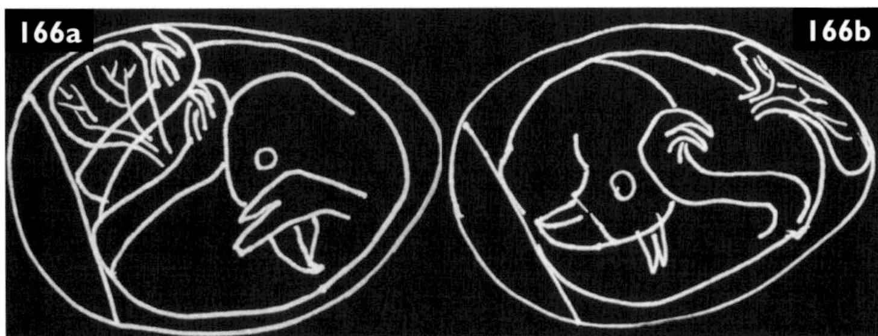

1 What is the normal position for the embryo when hatching?
2 Identify the number of this malposition (**166a**) and the prognosis for the embryo.
3 Describe the effect each of the other types of malpositioning can have on hatching death.

CASE 167 Providing nutritional support by tube feeding, also known as gavage feeding, is an essential part of avian supportive care (**167**). Sick birds are often presented with a history of anorexia, and patient glycogen stores can be depleted within hours in granivorous and omnivorous species, consequent on their relatively high metabolic rates.

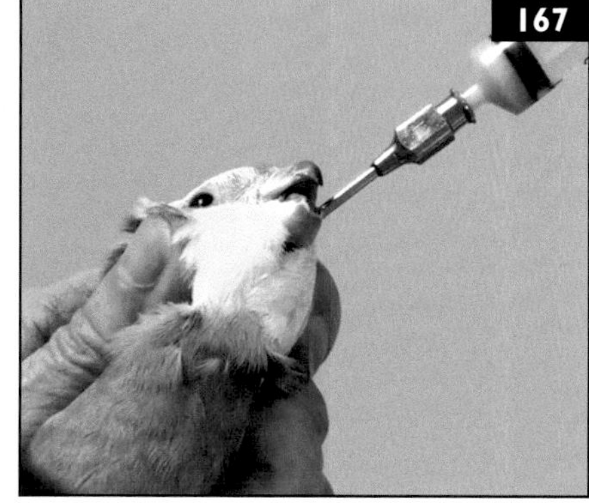

1 What are the contraindications for tube feeding in the avian patient?
2 What is the estimated crop volume?
3 List the potential complications of tube feeding.

CASE 168 One of your clients is incubating various large psittacine eggs. He is concerned that one of the eggs is not fertile. You candle the egg and this is what you see (**168**).

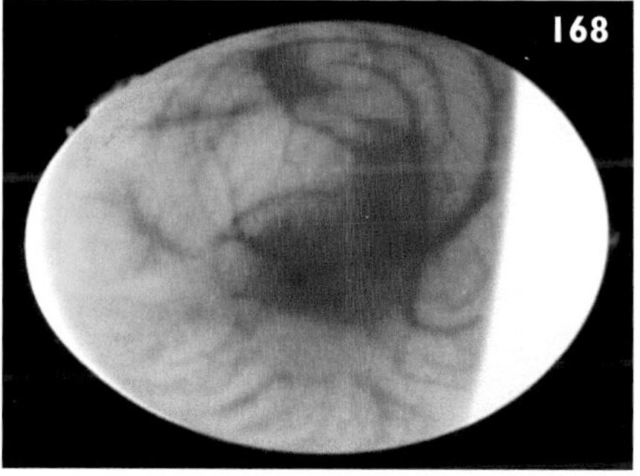

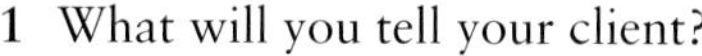

1 What will you tell your client?
2 By what day should you see blood vessels in a candled psittacine egg?
3 What do you see in this egg besides blood vessels?

CASE 169 Part of the ribcage from a juvenile rhea (*Rhea americana*) collected at necropsy is shown (**169**). The farm has had ongoing problems with lameness, poor growth rates, and increased mortality in young birds.

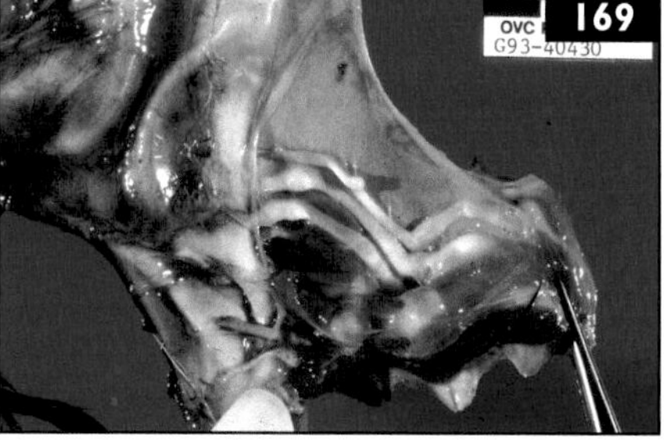

1 What disease condition is affecting this young rhea?
2 Describe the pathogenesis of the lesions shown.
3 What management actions should be taken to reduce disease associated with the condition shown?

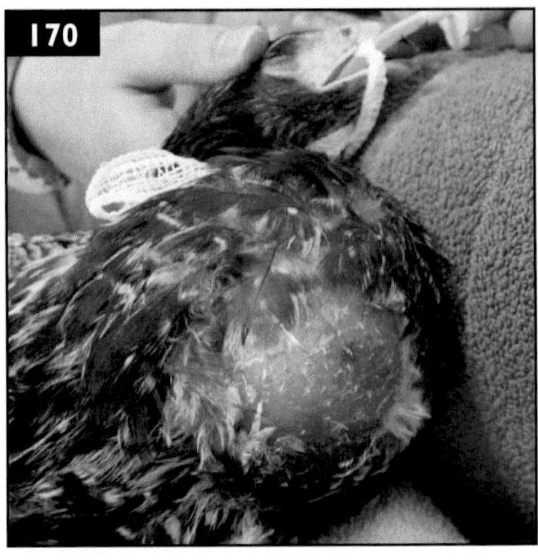

CASE 170 A falconry client calls because he is concerned that his bird has not 'put its crop over' some 18 hours after feeding (**170**).

1 What is the main concern in this bird?
2 When is this clinical presentation most likely to occur?
3 What treatment is recommended?

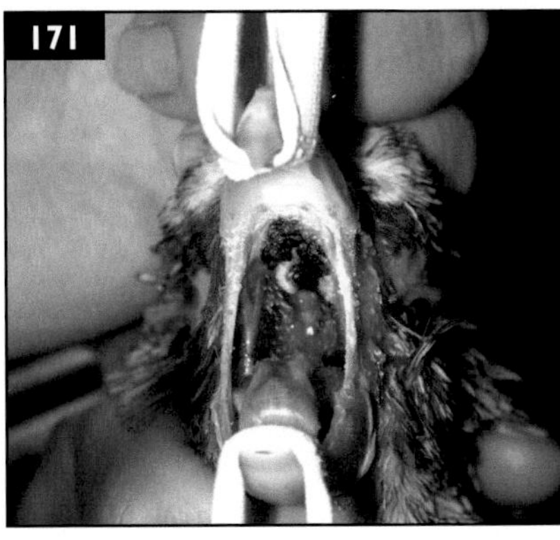

CASE 171 A 33-year-old white-fronted Amazon parrot (*Amazona albifrons*) presented for dysphagia. During the oropharyngeal examination, the lesion shown was found (**171**).

1 List the main differential diagnoses for this lesion.
2 List diagnostic tests that would be appropriate to aid in the diagnosis of this lesion.
3 Discuss the likely progression timeline, treatment options, and prognosis.

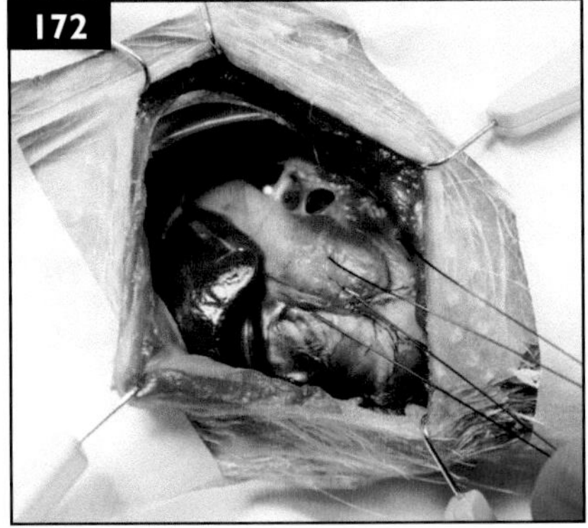

CASE 172 Proventriculotomy and ventriculotomy might be required for removal of foreign bodies (e.g. hook) or toxic material from the proventriculus or ventriculus (**172**).

1 Describe the surgical approach for proventriculotomy and ventriculotomy.
2 What precautions are needed during these procedures?
3 Describe how you would close the surgical incisions in these organs.

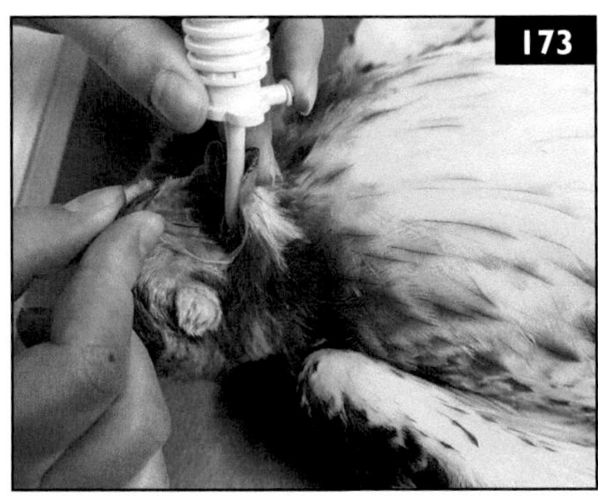
173

CASE 173 An adult red-tailed hawk (*Buteo jamaicensis*) is being anesthetized for whole body radiography (**173**). The bird is unable to fly and was found on the side of a road. On physical examination, no palpable fractures were identified.

1 What is the currently preferred anesthetic gas for avian species, and why?
2 When using isoflurane for raptor anesthesia, what undesirable side-effects may be observed?
3 What are the pros and cons of using sevoflurane?

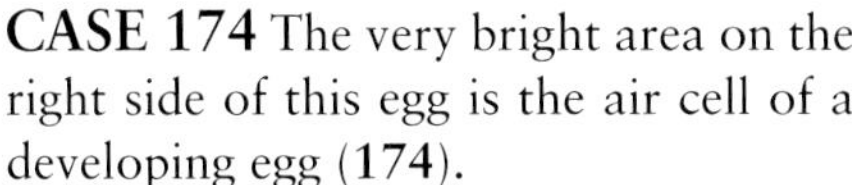

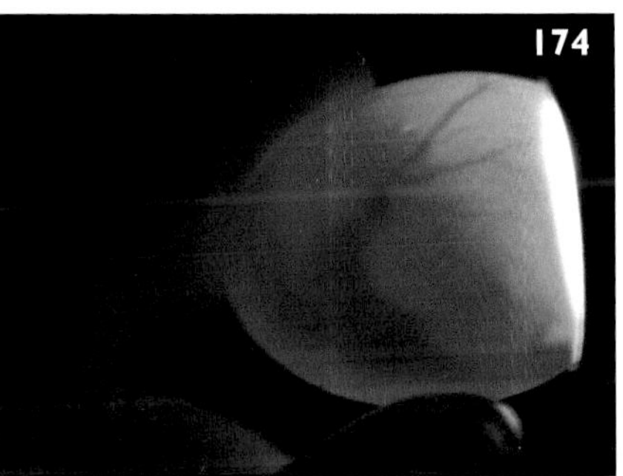
174

CASE 174 The very bright area on the right side of this egg is the air cell of a developing egg (**174**).

1 When is the air cell formed?
2 Where is it located in most eggs, and why is it located there?
3 What function does the air cell perform during the hatching process?

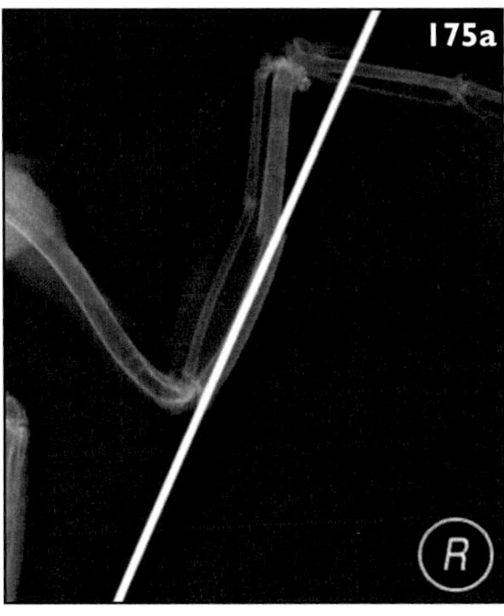

175a

CASE 175 A 230 g juvenile male broad-winged hawk (*Buteo platypterus*) presented with a fractured ulna after being hit by a car. An intraoperative radiograph was taken halfway through placement of an intramedullary (IM) pin (**175a**).

1 What is inappropriate about this initial pin placement?
2 What is the recommended technique for pin placement?
3 What final construct would you use to repair this type of fracture?

CASE 176 A young grey-crowned crane (*Balearica regulorum*) is presented with neck extended, open beak, and increased respiratory effort. Fecal examination reveals the presence of eggs (one shown, **176**).

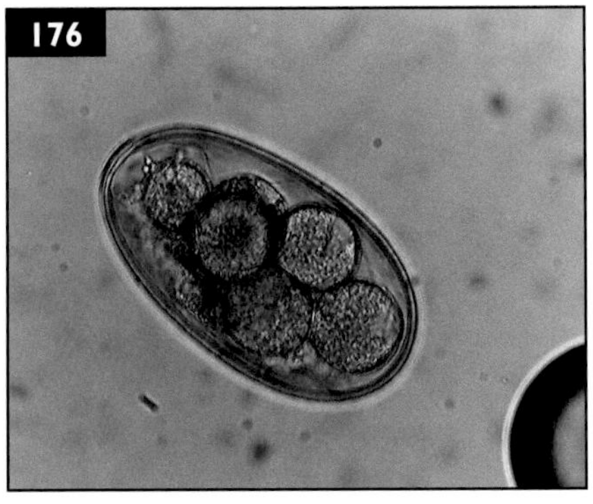

1 Which parasite would you consider as the etiologic agent based on the information provided?
2 If you decide to perform a tracheoscopy, what anatomic considerations should you consider in this species?
3 What treatment and control method would you recommend to the owner to reduce the prevalence in his collection of cranes?

CASE 177 *Sarcocystis* spp. is an apicomplexan protozoon found in wild birds and occasionally in companion or aviary birds. A sporocyst of *Sarcocystis* spp. (15 μm approximately) is shown (**177**). *Sarcocystis chalcasi*, in particular, has been reported in multiple avian species.

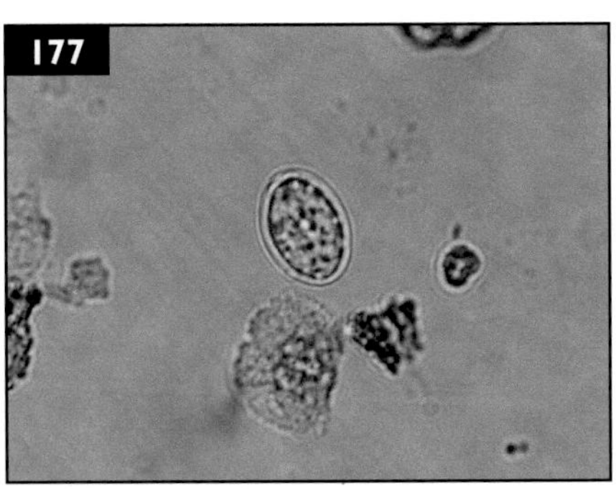

1 Name three avian Orders that may be considered intermediate or definitive hosts for this parasite.
2 What clinical signs have been observed in intermediate hosts?
3 What lesions would you expect during postmortem examination?

CASE 178 A 4-year-old Senegal parrot (*Poicephalus senegalus*) of unknown sex presented for a 2-month history of self-trauma of the feathers and skin at the uropygium area. Most feathers were missing and the uropygial gland was swollen. Uropygial secretion was white to yellow in color and thick in appearance. The owner believed this was a bacterial infection.

1 What diagnostic tests should be performed?
2 Preliminary results from the laboratory are consistent with a *Staphylococcus* spp. infection. What is the significance of this finding?
3 What are the zoonotic concerns?

CASE 179 A dissection of the ventral aspect of the wing of a Harris' hawk (*Parabuteo unicinctus*) is shown (**179**).

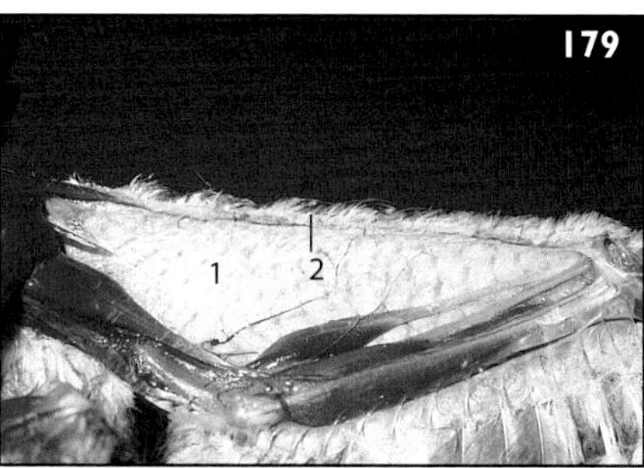

1 What is the structure labeled 1, and what is its function?
2 Name the structure labeled 2.
3 What effect does damage to this structure have on the function of the wing, and how should it be repaired?

CASE 180 Ten 6-week-old pigeons (*Columba livia domestica*) are brought to your clinic. All the pigeons show hunger traces (**180**) at the distal end of all flight feathers. Since all the pigeons show exactly the same signs, a common etiology seems very likely. Based on the development of the feathers it seems likely that the event must have taken place 5 weeks earlier.

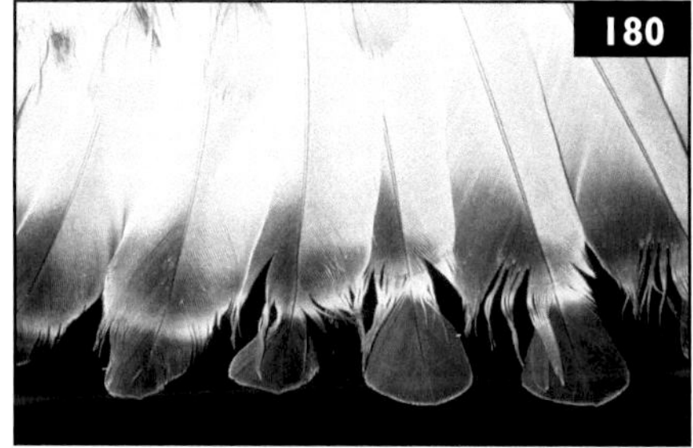

1 What factors may lead to the development of hunger traces?
2 Taking into consideration the time at which these hunger lines were caused, what event took place in these pigeons that may explain the same signs in every one of the 10 pigeons?
3 Provide a possible explanation that could be the reason for these stress lines.

CASE 181 The fundus of an adult tawny owl (*Strix aluco*), found years ago as a roadside casualty and kept since then in a wildlife rehabilitation center, is shown (**181**).

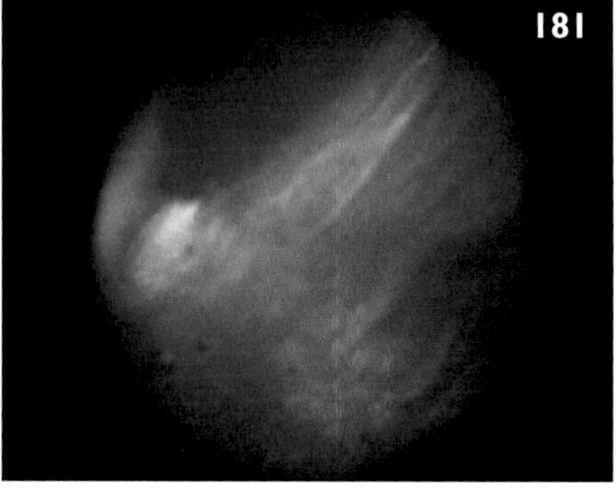

1 Which type of photoreceptor (cone or rod) is more numerous in the nervous layer of a nocturnal bird's retina?
2 What is your diagnosis in this owl?
3 List some potential etiologies.

CASE 182 A newly imported female saker falcon (*Falco cherrug*) from the Middle East was taken to a veterinary clinic for examination. The bird had a history of dyspnea for the past 2 weeks. On examination the falcon had good body condition (4/5) and was bright and alert. There was mild dyspnea, more noticeable during handling. No other abnormality could be detected on physical examination.

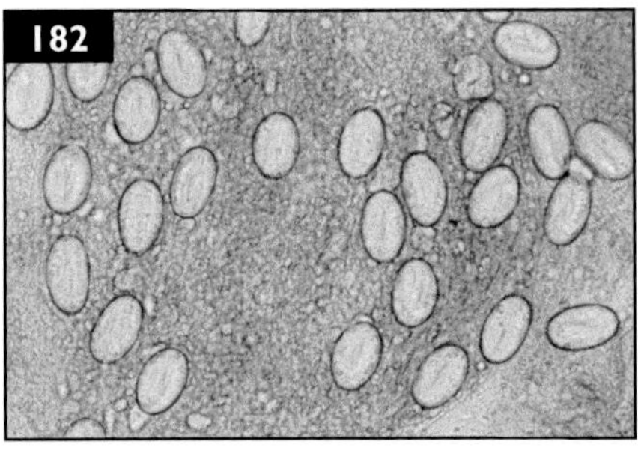

1 Based on the history and clinical presentation, what are the differential diagnoses?
2 What diagnostic tests would you perform to confirm the diagnosis?
3 On direct fecal examination using 0.9% NaCl, numerous thick-shelled embryonated ova could be observed (**182**, ×400). Can you identify the ova in the fecal preparation?

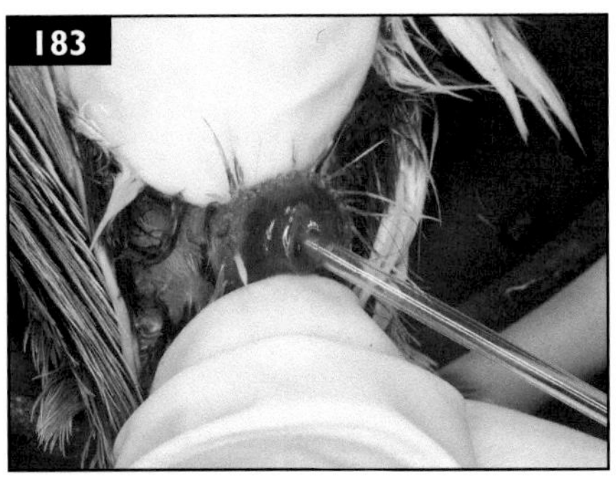

CASE 183 Semen collection and artificial insemination techniques have facilitated important achievements in captive breeding in birds. These techniques have been successfully applied in breeding programs of rare and endangered species, such as geese, cranes, and raptors, and in the production of hybrid falcons for the sport of falconry.

1 What are the most commonly used methods for semen collection in birds? Which method applied in Falconiformes uses males imprinted onto the handlers to collect viable semen samples?
2 What prompted falconers, primarily in the USA, to develop methods for semen collection and artificial insemination in raptors? Which organization was at the forefront in the development of artificial breeding techniques in falcons?
3 What is the preferred method of semen collection in most Passeriformes, as shown in this house sparrow (*Passer domesticus*) (**183**) and similar to that used in budgerigars (*Melopsittacus undulatus*)? What anatomic structure facilitates semen collection in the house sparrow?

CASE 184 This adult Harris' hawk (*Parabuteo unicintus*) is being administered an intracameral injection to induce mydriasis for fundic evaluation during ophthalmic examination (**184**).

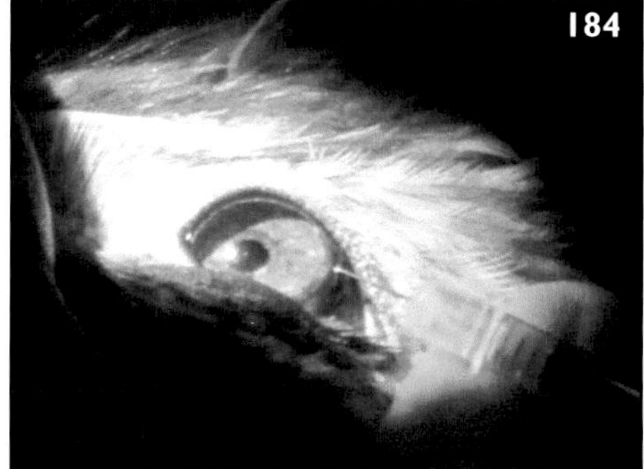
184

1 Which drugs are commonly administered by intracameral injections, and what are the potential complications of this route of administration?
2 When does a clinician induce mydriasis in birds?
3 What alternatives may be used to induce mydriasis in birds?

CASE 185 A mass from a 5-year-old male Pekin duck (*Anas platyrhynchos*) is shown (**185**). He presented with weight loss, increased respiratory rate and effort, lameness, lethargy, and anorexia. On physical examination there was a large palpable firm coelomic mass present dorsally on the right side, displacing the ventriculus ventrally and caudally.

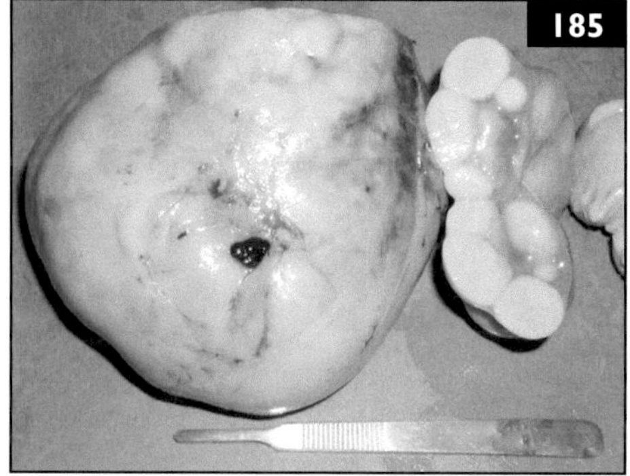
185

1 Based on the gross image, what type of testicular tumor do you suspect?
2 What is the likely cause of the clinical signs?
3 Can you determine malignancy by cytology or even by a small biopsy section?

CASE 186 A cockatiel (*Nymphicus hollandicus*) presented for hepatomegaly and ascites.

1 Why is a lateral coelioscopy contraindicated in this patient for evaluation of the liver?
2 What is the preferred coelioscopic approach in this patient?
3 Describe the technique for obtaining a liver biopsy in this patient. How does this differ from obtaining a biopsy via a lateral approach?

CASE 187 A 2-year-old African grey parrot (*Psittacus erithacus*) is presented with a history of decreased appetite. The bird has a low body condition score on physical examination but a normal body weight. A lateral radiograph of the abdomen is obtained (**187a**).

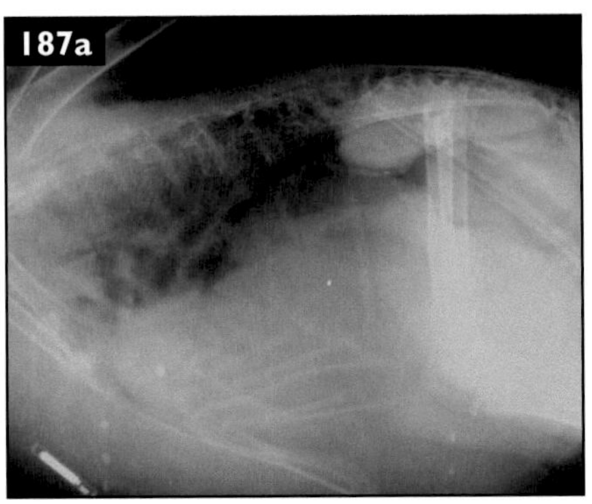

1 How can a bird be losing body condition and yet not be losing weight?
2 What condition is this bird suffering from, and what are the three main etiologies?
3 What steps would you take to further investigate this condition?

CASE 188 Lymphoplasmacytic perivascular cuffing in the brain of a blue and gold macaw (*Ara ararauna*) with proventricular dilatation disease is shown in this photomicrograph (**188**).

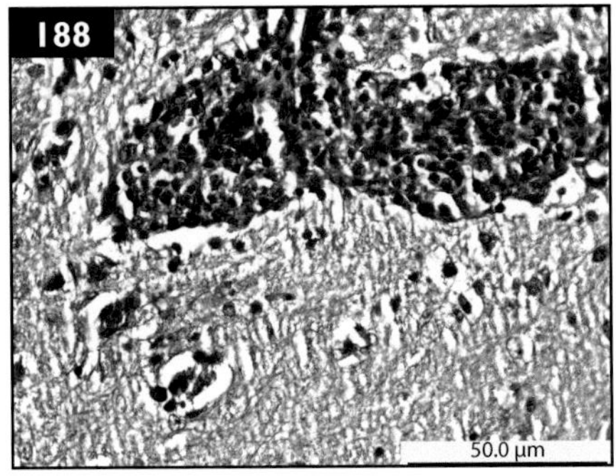

1 In what diseases is this lesion characteristic?
2 Is this lesion always associated with neurologic signs in psittacines?
3 What other histologic lesions would you expect to find in this bird?

CASE 189 A pair of ostriches (*Struthio camelus*) kept in a zoological collection had recently laid eggs from which the keepers had succeeded in hatching three chicks by artificial incubation. Due to space restrictions, these youngsters had to be transferred to another collection. Each bird must have an electronic identification chip inserted.

1 How do you approach and handle an adult ostrich?
2 Where are the microchip implantation sites in adults and chicks in this species?
3 How do you differentiate between male and female ostriches?

CASE 190 You are presented with a 1-year-old male canary (*Serinus canaria domestica*) for evaluation of masses on the wing, which the bird sometimes mutilates and makes bleed (**190**). When pressure is placed on the masses, abundant caseous debris is seen within.

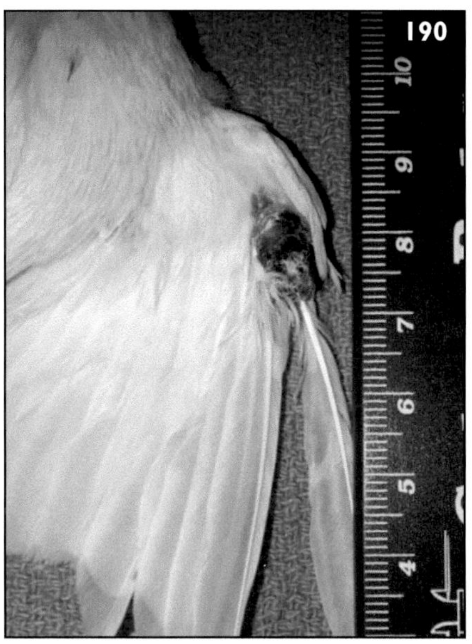

1 What is the most likely cause of the mass in this canary? What is another differential diagnosis for a crusty mass on the skin of a canary?
2 The client would like to know the cause of this abnormality. What information can you share with them?
3 How would you treat this bird?

CASE 191 The American Veterinary Medical Association (AVMA) *Guidelines for the Euthanasia of Animals: 2013 Edition* describes *euthanasia* as "ending the life of an individual animal in a way that minimizes or eliminates pain and distress." Unfortunately, euthanasia technique for companion birds is an area with little scientific evidence, and much of the information for euthanasia of companion birds consists of subjective reports in book chapters, guidelines from various associations, and journal roundtable discussions. The AVMA Guidelines provide acceptable methods of euthanasia for birds, including IV injection of a sodium pentobarbital euthanasia solution with or without the bird being unconscious or under anesthesia.

1 Many veterinarians include sedation prior to IV injection of euthanasia solution. Provide examples of parenteral sedation that can be used when the owner requests to be present for the procedure.
2 Pentobarbital may need to be administered by a route other than IV if the bird is under general anesthesia. What other routes are acceptable for the unconscious bird?
3 IM, SC, intrathoracic, intrapulmonary, intrathecal, and other nonvascular injections are not acceptable routes of administration for injectable euthanasia agents in awake animals. Why?

CASE 192 A hybrid falcon (peregrine cross saker falcon [*Falco peregrinus x F. cherrug*]) is presented bright and alert but the owner complains of poor performance and occasional heavy breathing after exercise. A fecal flotation reveals the presence of multiple ova measuring 50 × 30 µm. Endoscopy shows multiple long filamentous parasites in the air sacs (**192**).

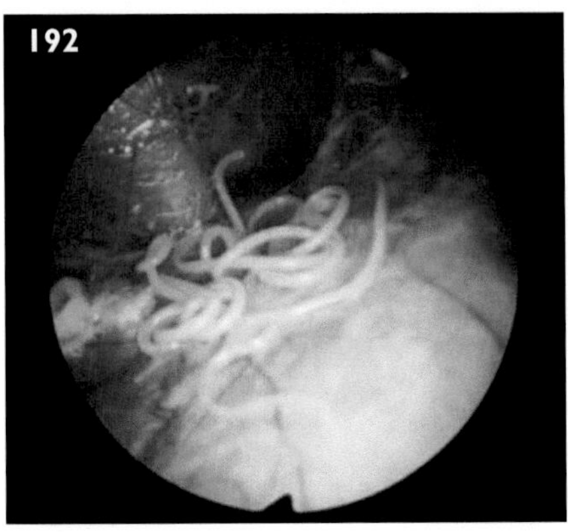

1 What is the most likely diagnosis?
2 Describe the life cycle of this parasite.
3 What treatment options would you consider?

CASE 193 A call duck (*Anas platyrhynchus domesticus*) with a mature cataract in the left eye is presented for ophthalmologic examination (**193**).

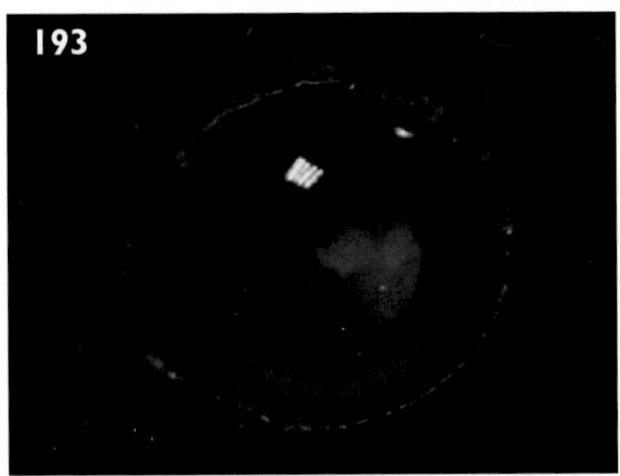

1 What additional diagnostic test would you perform?
2 Which causes have been reported to provoke this condition in birds?
3 How would you treat this condition?

CASE 194

1 The energy cost of maintaining an egg's temperature, whether by natural or artificial incubation, depends on three factors. What are these factors?
2 There are two types of incubation strategies used by different species of birds. Describe each strategy.
3 When using an artificial incubation process, what type of incubation behavior (from the question above) is being duplicated with different types of incubators?

CASE 195 A canary (*Serinus canaria domestica*) breeder client has been experiencing problems with birds losing weight despite showing a good appetite, being fluffed up, and some birds dying. A recent carcase is presented for postmortem examination. Typical gross postmortem findings are shown (**195**).

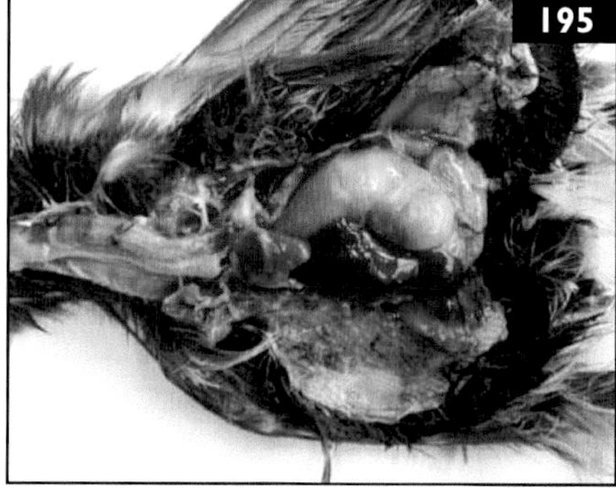

1 What is the most likely cause of the distended proventriculus seen in the image? How could you confirm your presumptive diagnosis?
2 List other differential diagnoses.
3 What would be the treatment plan for a canary breeder confronted with this problem?

CASE 196 A breeder of various species of Passeriformes suffered severe losses of nestling birds aged between 4 days and 6 weeks. They showed signs of diarrhea, no further weight gain, and death within 24–48 hours. No adult birds were affected and there was no drop in the number of eggs produced or in the hatchability. On electron microscopy these virus particles with a diameter of 45 nm were observed (**196**).

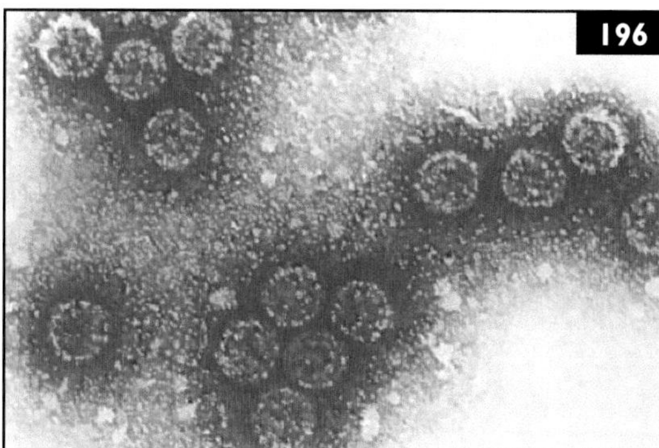

1 What virus would most likely cause these problems in nestling Passeriformes?
2 What findings would you expect on histopathology? How would you confirm your diagnosis?
3 What steps would be necessary to clear the virus from this collection?

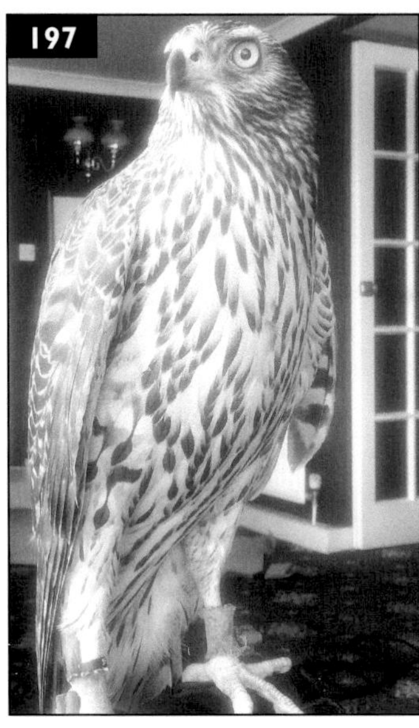

CASE 197 Three juvenile goshawks (*Accipiter gentilis*) are presented with clinical signs that include opisthotonos and circling, which has been progressive over 5 days (**197**). The three were hand-reared by a good Samaritan who found them as chicks and reared them for 35 days on frozen day-old chicks and raw fish.

1 What would be your differential diagnoses for this condition? Which would be your primary differential based on the dietary history?
2 What specific tests would you run to rule out your primary differential? What additional body system could be affected in addition to the central nervous system if your primary suspicion is confirmed?
3 What would be your treatment plan to rectify the nutritional status of these birds?

CASE 198 A 20-year-old female galah (*Eolophus roseicapillus*) is presented with lethargy and diffuse feather loss over the entire body. On examining the bird, you find it to be obese, with excessive fat deposition over the legs and ventral abdomen (**198**). On close examination of the skin you note no regrowth of feathers. A hematologic and biochemical profile reveals mild nonregenerative anemia, mild leukocytosis, and hypercholesterolemia.

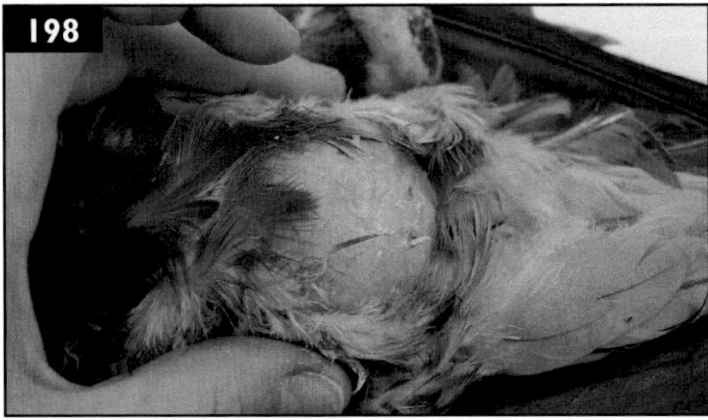

1 What is the tentative diagnosis?
2 What diagnostic tests may be used to confirm the tentative diagnosis?
3 If the tentative diagnosis is confirmed, what would be the recommended treatment for this bird?

CASE 199 Cloacoscopy should be part of a diganostic work up for evaluation of cloacal masses, hematochezia, and straining.

1 Describe how this procedure should be performed.
2 Name the labeled structures in the image shown (**199**), obtained during a cloacoscopy in a pigeon.
3 What difference in cloacal anatomy can be observed during cloacoscopy between a pigeon and a psittacine?

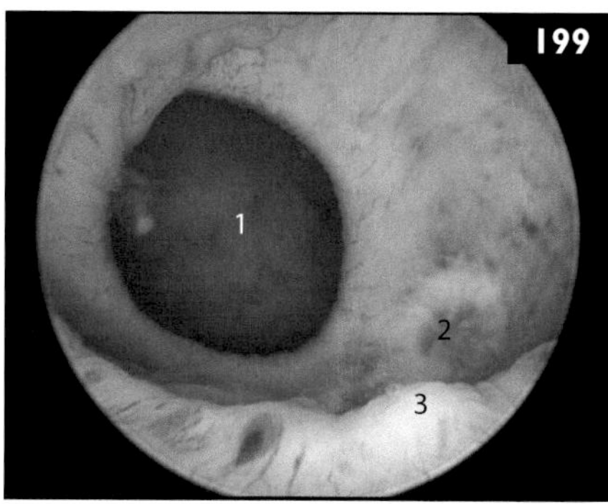

Courtesy of Dr. Stephen Divers, UGA

CASE 200 A falconer presents this gyrfalcon (*Falco rusticolus*) to you for a routine annual examination (**200**). The owner asks whether the B vitamin supplement he uses via intramuscular injection could be toxic if given in large quantities. The supplement contains vitamins B_1, B_2, B_3, B_5, B_6, and B_{12}.

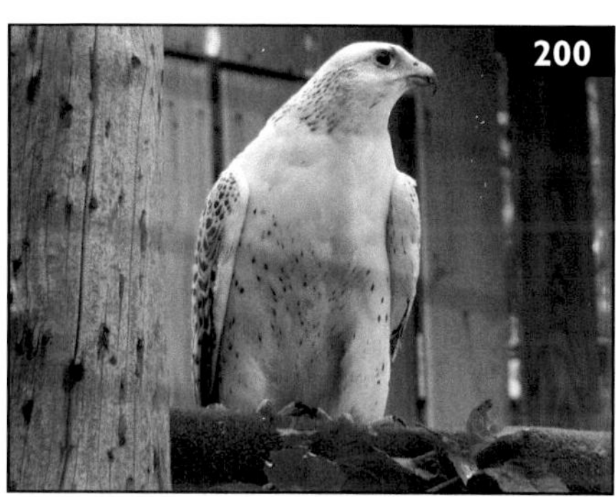

1 Which one of these vitamins has been reported to cause lethal toxicity in gyrfalcons?
2 What are the associated clinical signs?
3 List three food items that naturally contain vitamin B_6.

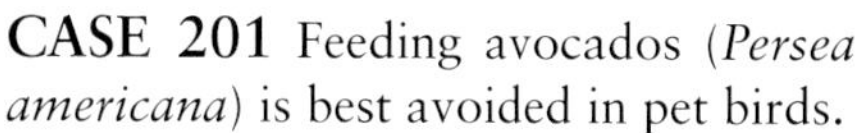

CASE 201 Feeding avocados (*Persea americana*) is best avoided in pet birds.

1 What are the toxic effects of avocados in birds?
2 What is the toxin contained within avocados?
3 What parts of the avocado are toxic?

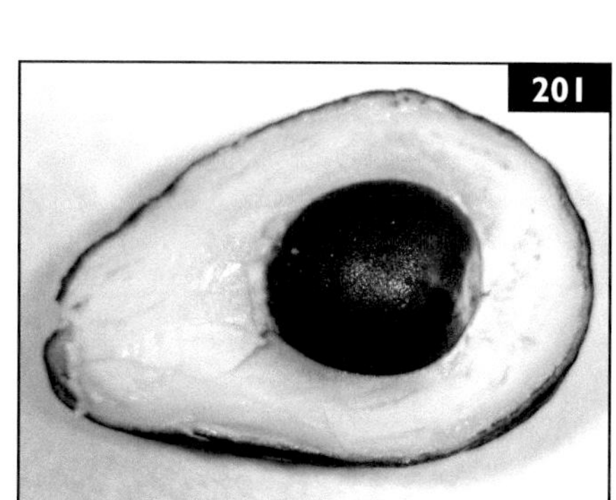

CASE 202 A 2-year-old speckled Sussex hen (*Gallus gallus domesticus*) presented with a history of reluctance to walk over the past 24 hours and not laying an egg for 3 days. The owner suspected a lameness, although there was no history of trauma. On physical examination the hen was reluctant to stand and used her wing for support and balance (**202**). No musculoskeletal abnormalities were detected, but a firm coelomic distension was palpated.

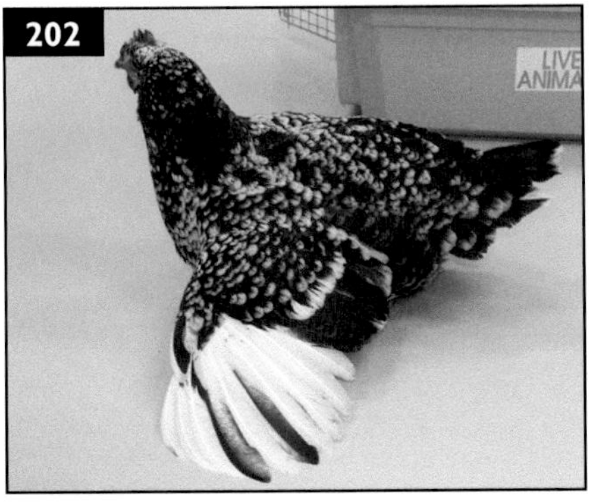

1 What diseases can cause a firm coelomic distension in an adult hen?
2 What would be the possible treatment for each of the diseases listed?

CASE 203 A toco toucan (*Ramphastos toco*) is maintained under isoflurane anesthesia with an air sac breathing tube placed in the caudal thoracic air sac (**203**).

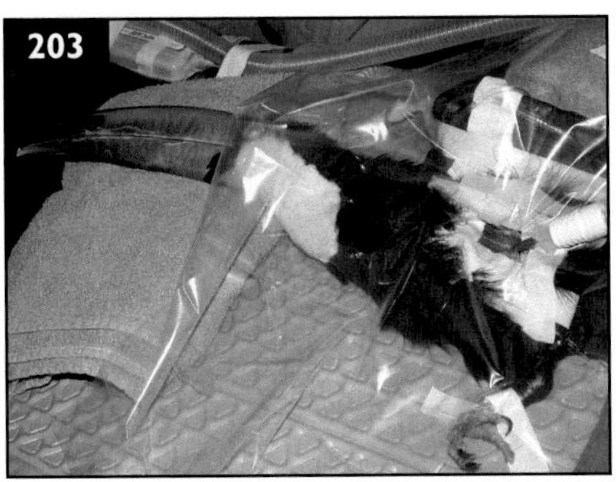

1 What is the methodology for placement of an air sac tube?
2 What are the indications to maintain anesthesia using an air sac tube?
3 How does air sac tube delivery of isoflurane compare with endotracheal administration of isoflurane?

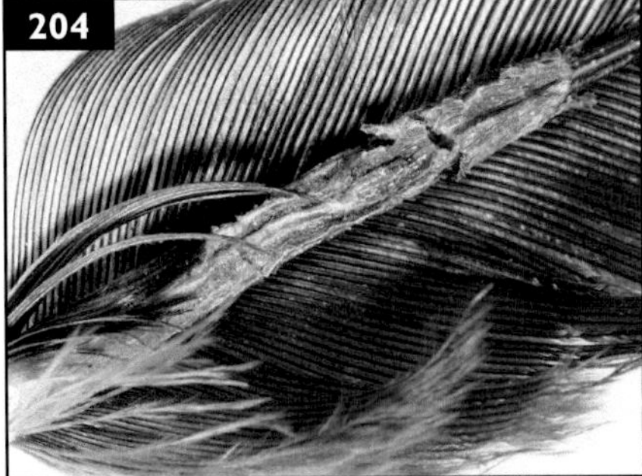

CASE 204 A feather from a young raven (*Corvus coronoides*) that had bilateral feather abnormalities is shown (**204**).

1 What possible differentials should be considered?
2 What diagnostic tests should be performed to investigate the cause?
3 What is the likely prognosis for birds with such lesions?

CASE 205 A canary (*Serinus canaria domestica*) breeder client is suffering losses in his young birds at the time of fledging. He presents a bird from the group, which demonstrates a distended coelom (**205**).

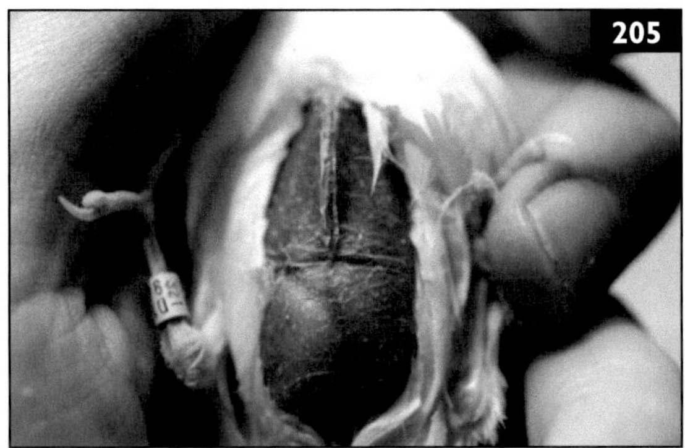

1 What are your differential diagnoses for a distended coelomic cavity in a canary?
2 At what age are canaries most likely to be affected by intestinal coccidiosis, and why?
3 What is the life cycle of intestinal coccidiosis (*Ispora canaria*) in canaries?

CASE 206 An adult male northern goshawk (*Accipiter gentilis*) is presented with mild and short duration seizures (**206**). The bird is currently undergoing retraining, subsequent to a period of being free lofted in an aviary while molting.

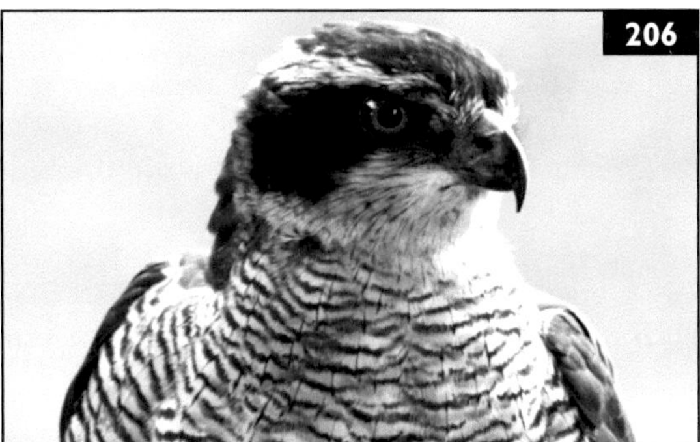

1 What are the differential diagnoses? What is the most likely diagnosis?
2 What is your diagnostic plan? How would you treat this bird if you confirm your suspicion?
3 What action can be taken to avoid this situation?

CASE 207 A 17-year-old peach-fronted conure (*Aratinga aureaconure*) presented for lethargy and weight loss. Physical examination revealed a suspected papilloma on cloacal examination. Gastrointestinal survey radiographs are taken and a barium sulfate contrast study is performed for further evaluation (**207**).

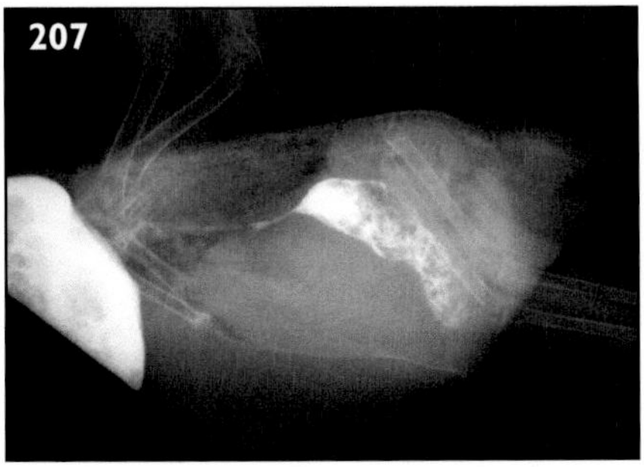

207

1 Describe the abnormal radiographic findings.
2 List the differential diagnoses for this radiographic finding.
3 Based on the suspected concurrent papillomatous lesion, what is your top differential diagnosis?

CASE 208 A Swainson's hawk (*Buteo swainsoni*) is brought to your clinic for evaluation. It has been hit by a car about 30 minutes ago, and there is evidence of head trauma with skin ulceration and feather loss over the head (**208**). The bird appears depressed-to-obtunded and is in sternal recumbency. There are no obvious cranial nerve deficits on the neurologic examination.

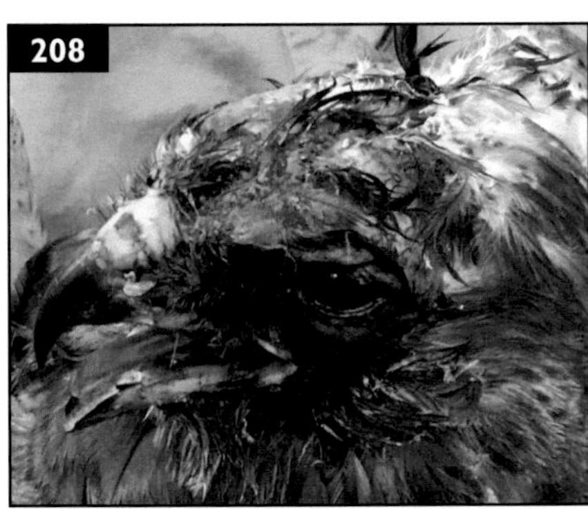
208

1 What are the goals of traumatic brain injury treatment?
2 How would you treat traumatic brain injury in this bird?
3 How would you manage pain?

CASE 209 A 945 g blue and gold macaw (*Ara ararauna*) is presented with a vague history of being unwell. After a physical examination you determine that you will need a hematology and biochemical profile of the bird to better assess its presenting problem.

1 Which blood vessels are suitable for venipuncture?
2 How much blood can be safely collected from this bird?
3 How would you handle the blood sample after collection to maximize the quality of the laboratory results?

CASE 210 This 15-year-old cockatiel (*Nymphicus hollandicus*) presented with a yellow-colored mass on the tip of its wing (**210**). The bird has a history of traumatizing the wing tips.

1 What is your primary differential?
2 What is a unique characteristic of this lesion?
3 What is the recommendation for treatment?

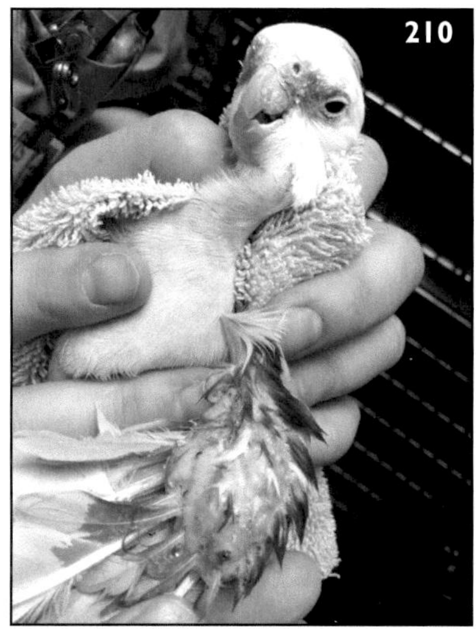
210

CASE 211 A 6-year-old female Gentoo penguin (*Pygoscelis papua*) is presented for swelling of the right elbow joint. Blood collection, whole body radiographs, and fine needle aspirate for cytologic and microbial evaluation under general anesthesia are scheduled in order to investigate the nature of the swelling.

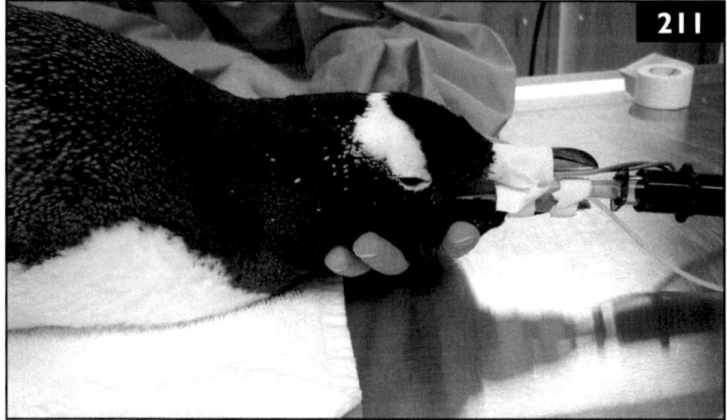
211

1 What anatomic features must be considered for intubation (**211**)?
2 What methods should be considered to maintain body temperature?
3 Which body position is best suited for penguins under general anesthesia?

CASE 212 While the expected rate of fracture healing is dependent on multiple considerations, including type of fracture (open/closed, simple/comminuted, location), patient condition (concurrent health issues, nutritional and exercise status), and method of fixation, there are some general consistencies in bone healing among birds (**212**).

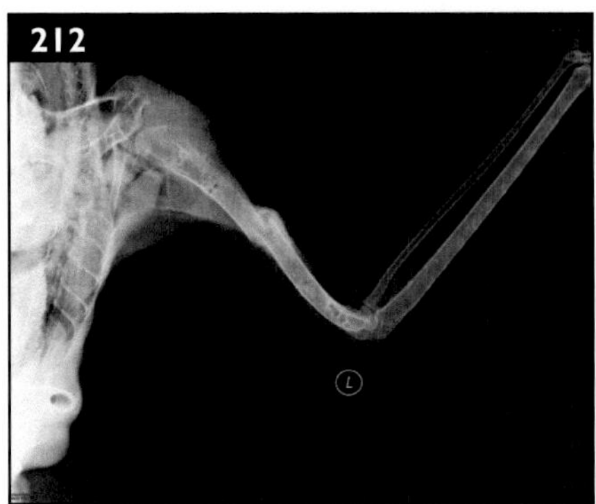

1 How does the healing rate of avian bone differ from mammalian bone?
2 What is the relative healing rate of various long bones in birds?
3 Do bird bones heal by periosteal or endosteal callus formation?

CASE 213 A young wood pigeon (*Columba palumbus*), found on the street, was presented to you by one of your clients. The pigeon was emaciated and had a large lesion on the mucocutaneous junction of the beak and on the eyelid (**213**).

213

1 What is the most likely diagnosis of these lesions, and how could this diagnosis be confirmed?
2 What is the mode of transmission for this disease?
3 What therapeutic and preventive measures can be taken? Include the prognosis in your answer.

CASE 214 Ceca in birds (**214**) aid digestion of plant foods. They are most prominent in fowl and ostriches, in which they functionally resemble the cecum of horses.

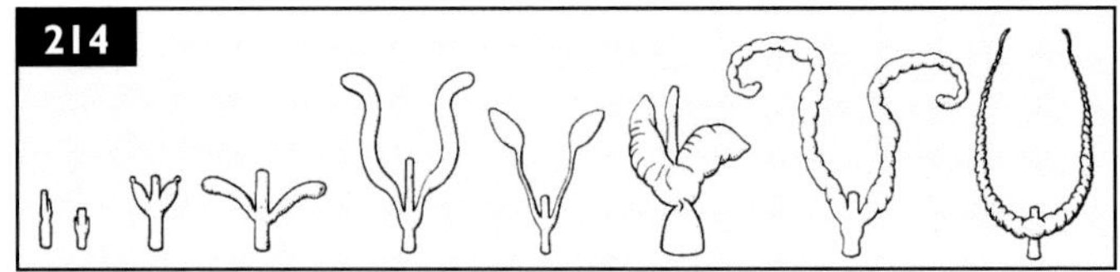

1 What is the most important role of the ceca?
2 Not all birds have functional ceca. Which group of birds lack a functional cecum?

CASE 215 A 1-year-old female cockatiel (*Nymphicus hollandicus*) was presented with a 5-day history of respiratory distress and diarrhea. During general examination, reddening of the oropharyngeal cavity and choanal slit was observed. Following general examination, cytology was performed from an oropharyngeal swab (**215**, ×100).

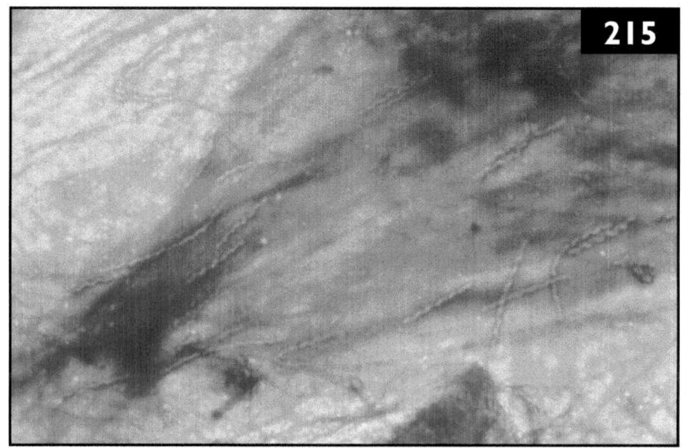
215

1 What is the most probable diagnosis? What other clinical signs are often seen?
2 What is the method of choice for antemortem diagnosis?
3 What is the recommended treatment regimen?

CASE 216 Morphologic gender determination in pigeons is not accurate. However, in the pigeon displayed here (**216**), the gender can be stated with certainty.

1 Name at least four criteria that can be used to determine the gender of a pigeon.
2 The genes for the color of hair in mammals and feathers in birds are in part localized on the sex chromosomes. What is the major difference between sex chromosomes in birds compared with mammals?
3 What is the gender of this pigeon? Based on what criteria can 100% accuracy be given that this is actually the gender?

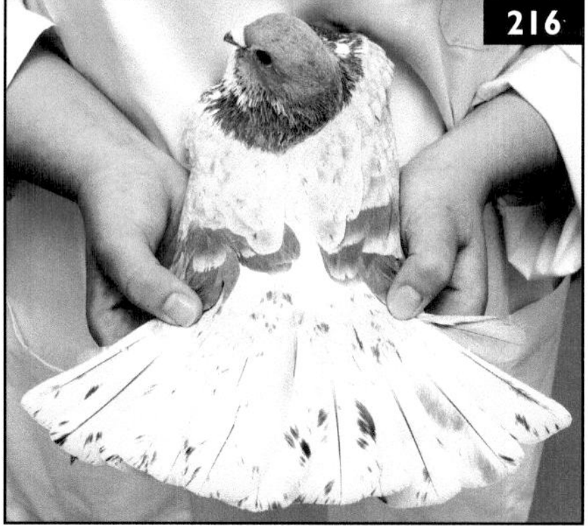
216

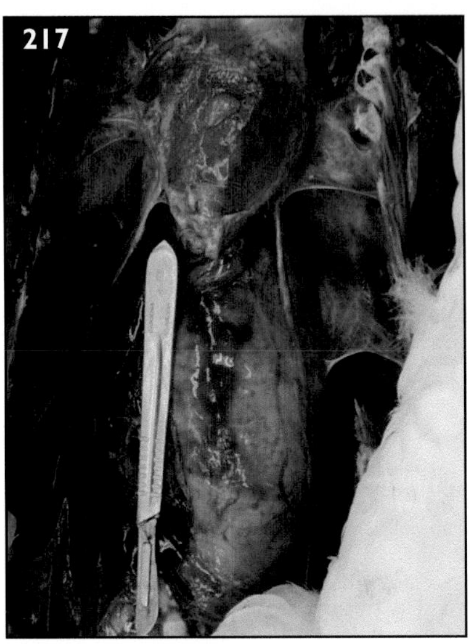

CASE 217 An emaciated adult trumpeter swan (*Cygnus buccinator*) was presented for necropsy and was found to have a severely enlarged proventriculus (**217**; the scalpel handle above the proventriculus provides relative scale). There was no gastrointestinal obstruction in the ventriculus.

1 What is the most likely etiology of this abnormality?
2 What is the most appropriate tissue to submit to confirm your presumptive diagnosis?
3 What are the most common environmental sources for this etiology in waterfowl?

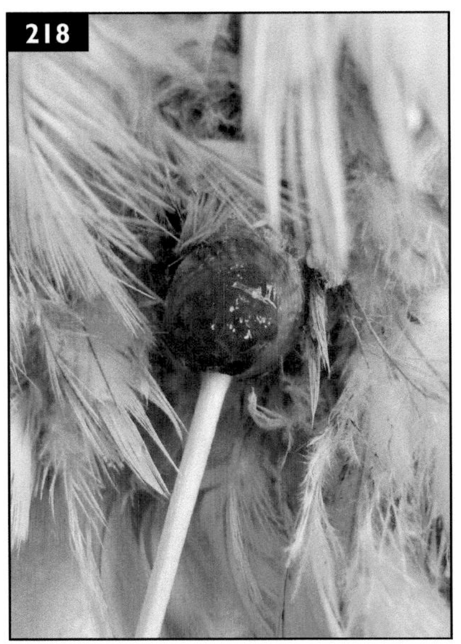

CASE 218 An adult blue-fronted Amazon parrot (*Amazona aestiva*) of unknown age is presented to you for a wellness examination after being recently purchased by a breeder. The client mentions that the bird has been straining to defecate. On physical examination, while trying to gently evert the cloacal mucosa with a cotton-tip applicator, you identify a bright, red, proliferative mass that raises some concerns (**218**).

1 What is the most likely diagnosis? How would you confirm the diagnosis?
2 What surgical treatment would you perform?
3 What are your recommendations to the owner? What is the long-term prognosis for this bird?

CASE 219 An adult great horned owl (*Bubo virginianus*) is presented to a wildlife clinic for evaluation because it is unable to fly. Physical examination reveals a thin body condition and oral lesions (**219**).

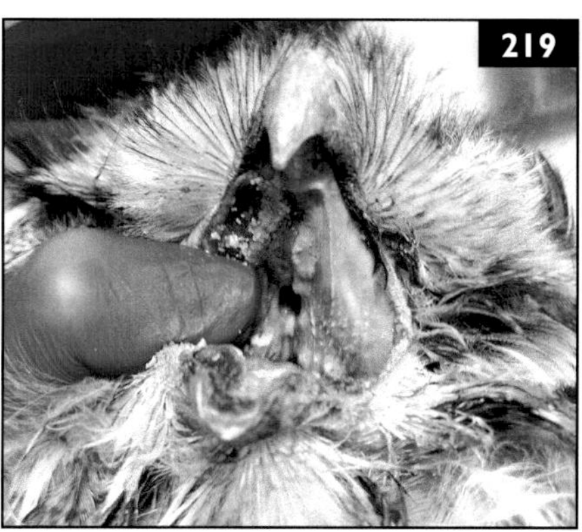

1 What is the most likely underlying cause?
2 What is the most likely source of infection?
3 What is the recommended treatment?

CASE 220 The figure-of-eight bandage or wing wrap is the standard method for stabilizing the wing short term (**220**).

1 What pectoral limb fractures can be adequately stabilized with a wing wrap, and when should a body wrap be incorporated into the wrap?
2 Depending on patient size, what bandaging options can be considered for fractures of the tibiotarsus?

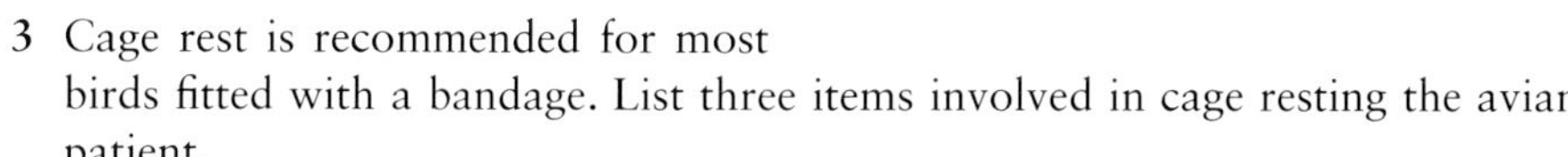
3 Cage rest is recommended for most birds fitted with a bandage. List three items involved in cage resting the avian patient.

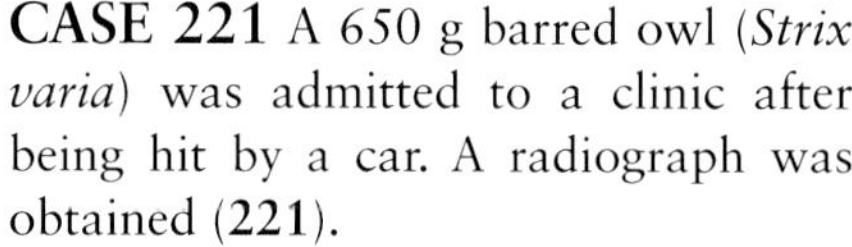
CASE 221 A 650 g barred owl (*Strix varia*) was admitted to a clinic after being hit by a car. A radiograph was obtained (**221**).

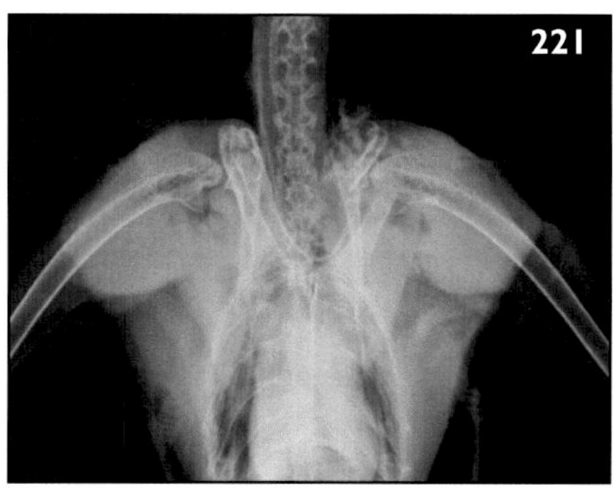

1 What is the main radiographic abnormal finding?
2 Provide a treatment plan for this patient.
3 What is the prognosis for release?

CASE 222 A gyr cross saker hybrid falcon (*Falco rusticolus x F. cherrug*) is presented with respiratory distress, laryngeal stridor, nasal discharge, sneezing, and bilateral conjunctivitis (**222**).

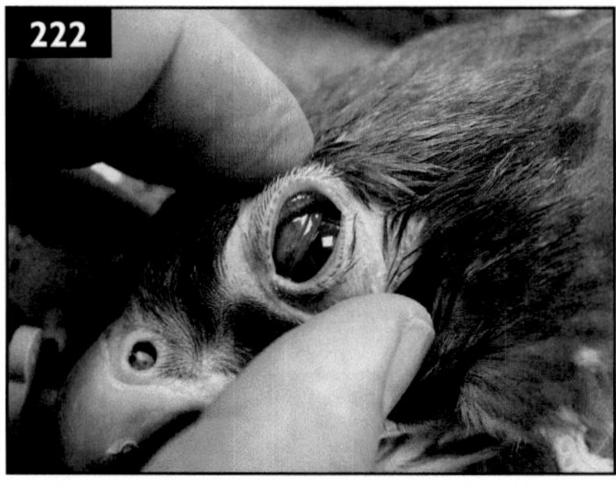

1 Which protozoal parasite would you consider as the most likely etiologic agent?
2 What additional diagnostic procedures would you perform?
3 What therapeutic options would you consider? What prognosis would you offer?

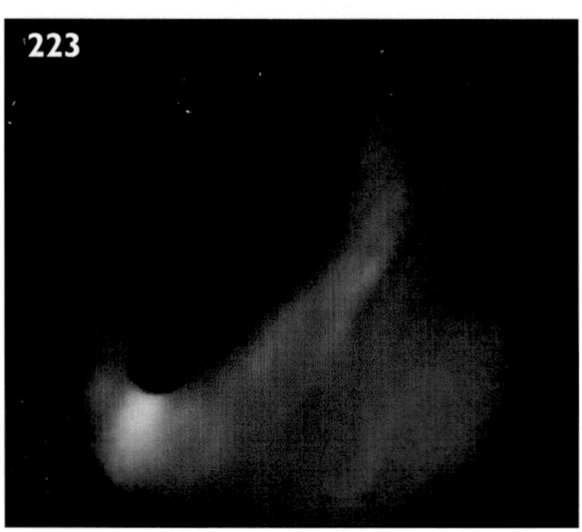

CASE 223 Examination of the posterior chamber of an owl's eye shows a pigmented structure projecting into the vitreous body originating from the point where the optic nerve enters the ocular globe (**223**).

1 What is the black structure observed in the upper left side of the image?
2 List the different types of pecten in birds and the species they belong to.
3 List potential functions of the pecten.

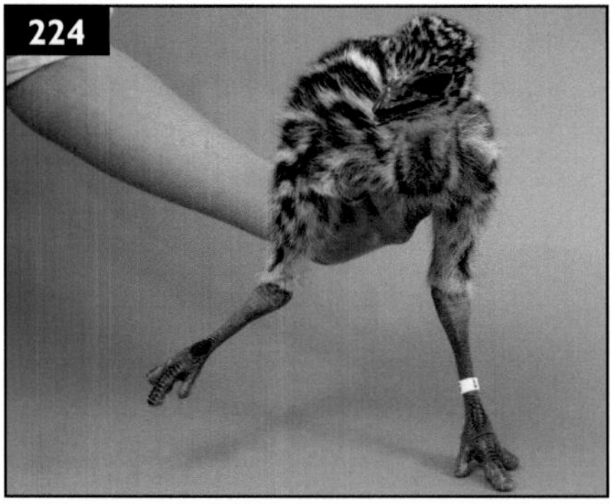

CASE 224 A young, rapidly growing emu (*Dromaius novaehollandiae*) became unable to stand or walk over a period of several days (**224**).

1 What is the problem with its legs?
2 How can this problem be managed?
3 Incidental to the bird's primary issue, what management procedure has been carried out on its feet?

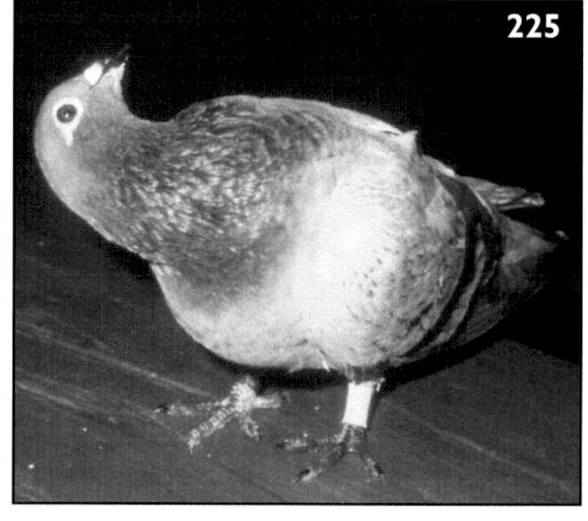

CASE 225 A 2-year-old female pigeon is brought to your practice with a torticollis (**225**). Multiple birds in the flock have similar signs. In addition, the pigeon fancier mentions that the pigeons are producing loose stools. You suspect the disease is caused by a paramyxovirus rather than *Salmonella typhimurium* var. Copenhagen.

1 How can the two diseases be differentiated from each other based on clinical signs?
2 What paramyxovirus serotype is most likely to be responsible? What other serotypes of this virus have been associated with disease in birds?
3 What therapeutic and preventive measures can be taken for the viral disease responsible for the clinical signs observed in these pigeons?

CASE 226 A breeder of lady Gouldian finches (*Erythrura gouldiae*) presents a recent carcase for postmortem examination. The finch had shown signs of dyspnea, clicking breathing noises, and head shaking. Various birds within the collection show similar clinical signs.

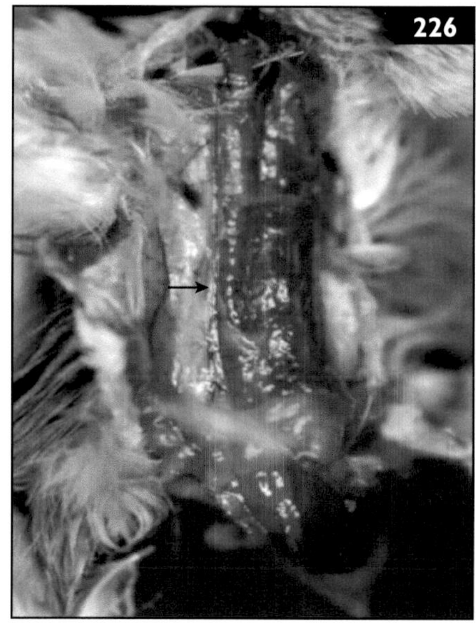

1 What is the name of the parasite shown in the image (**226**), which is responsible for these clinical signs?
2 What are your differential diagnoses for these clinical signs in finches and canaries?
3 How can you evaluate for the presence of this parasite antemortem? What treatment regimens would you recommend?

CASE 227 Several toxins may be inhaled by birds (**227**), causing severe irritation and damage to the respiratory tract and other organ systems in the patient's body.

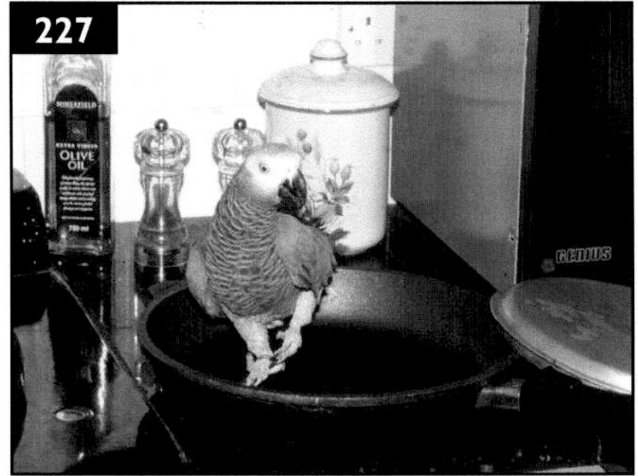

1 What toxins may cause inhalation toxicity in birds?
2 List the commonly reported clinical signs seen in birds suffering from inhalation toxicity.
3 What is the advised treatment regimen in cases of inhalation toxicity in birds?

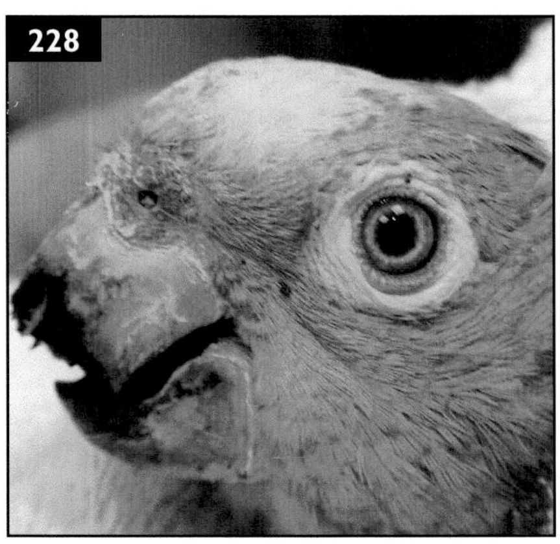

CASE 228 An adult yellow-crowned Amazon parrot (*Amazona ochrocephala*) is presented to you for treatment immediately following a traumatic injury to the upper beak (**228**). You evaluate the bird and confirm traumatic amputation of the upper beak or bill.

1 What anatomic parts of the beak seem to be affected?
2 How can this injury be treated?
3 What is the prognosis for a traumatic amputation of the bill?

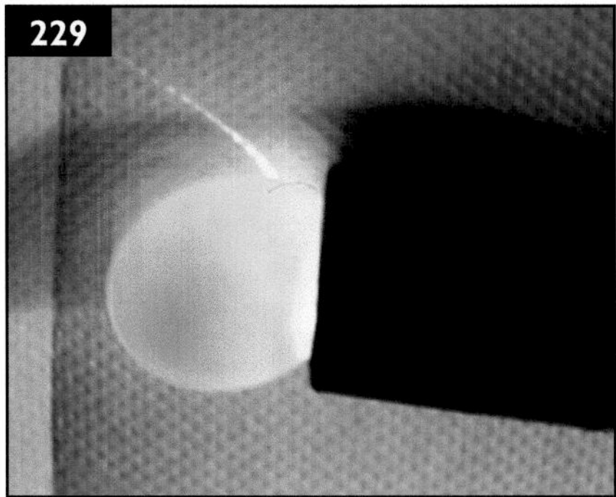

CASE 229 Your client is incubating various large psittacine eggs. He is concerned that one of the eggs is not fertile. You candle the egg and this is what you see (**229**).

1 What will you tell your client?
2 Should you remove the egg from the incubator? If so, by what day?
3 What is missing from this egg?

CASE 230 A 6-year-old female lovebird is being surgically prepared for exploratory coelomic surgery in order to remove and débride yolk material resulting in effusive yolk coelomitis, presumably secondary to ectopic ovulation (**230**).

230

1 What procedure may be considered to stabilize this patient prior to anesthesia?
2 When performing coelomic surgery in patients with coelomic effusion, what measures should be implemented to avert possible respiratory complications?
3 If an air sac is inadvertently perforated during surgery, how will this affect the anesthesia?

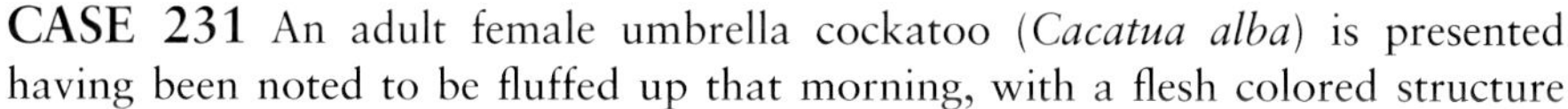

CASE 231 An adult female umbrella cockatoo (*Cacatua alba*) is presented having been noted to be fluffed up that morning, with a flesh colored structure protruding from the cloaca (**231a**). On physical examination, the bird appears dehydrated and in a low condition. The tissue prolapsed is found to be the oviduct and appears swollen but viable.

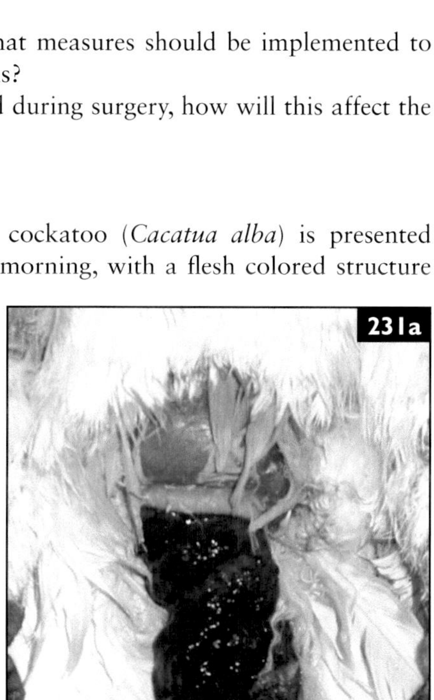
231a

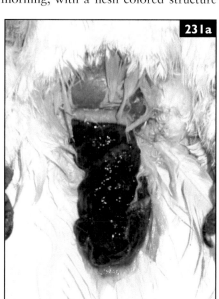

1 How would you stabilize this bird prior to performing additional diagnostic tests?
2 What diagnostic tests would you perform?
3 How would you surgically manage this condition? What are the possible complications?

CASE 232 A red-breasted toucan (*Ramphastos dicolorus*) was presented to the clinic suffering from general weakness, fluffed feathers, and loss of body condition. It had soft, mucous stools. A direct parasitologic fecal examination was performed (**232**, ×400).

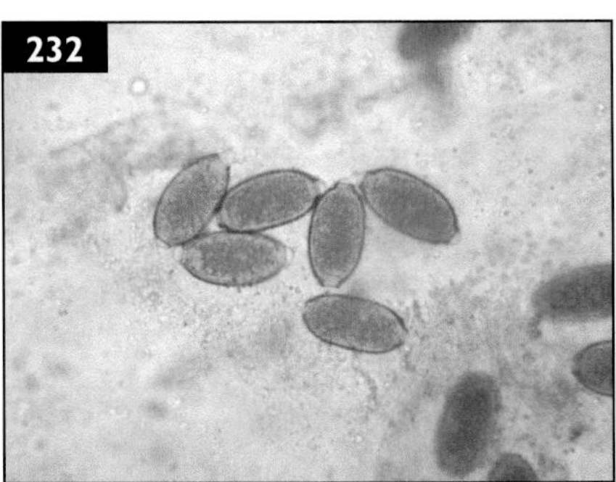

1 What is your diagnosis?
2 How would you treat this condition?
3 What sanitary measures should be undertaken to prevent this condition?

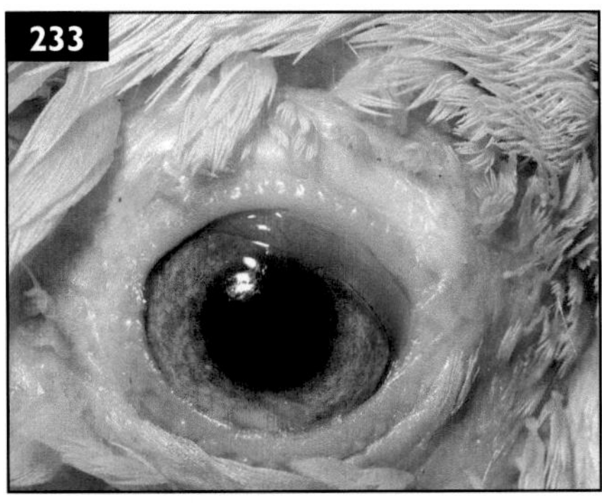

CASE 233 This adult double yellow-headed Amazon parrot (*Amazona ochrocephala oratrix*) is presented in emergency after his owner found him playing with a product containing trichlorphon used to treat fish lice (**233**).

1 What clinical signs do you anticipate after ingestion of this product?
2 How can you confirm ingestion?
3 How would you treat this bird?

CASE 234 A 5-week-old African grey parrot (*Psittacus erithacus*) is presented following ingestion of a foreign body (**234**). On radiographs, the proventriculus is mildly distended and a foreign body is visible. Endoscopic removal of the foreign body under general anesthesia is scheduled.

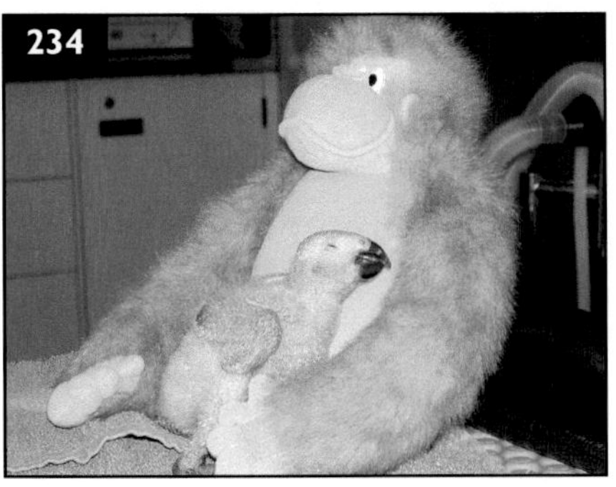

1 Would you consider fasting such a patient prior to general anesthesia?
2 How do you minimize hypoglycemia?
3 How do you prevent hypothermia in this patient?

CASE 235 A swan goose (*Anser cygnoides*) in a large waterfowl collection is presented with difficulty swallowing. A foul smell is noted while examining the oropharyngeal cavity, and endoscopy reveals caseous lesions in the esophagus and proventriculus (**235**).

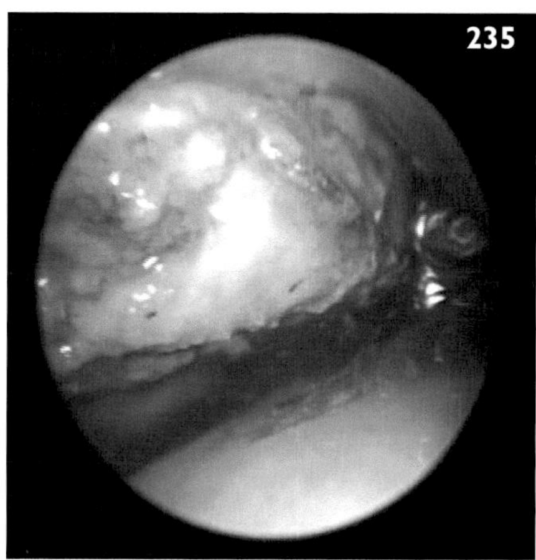

1 Which nematodes would you consider as etiologic agents?
2 What additional diagnostic test would you perform?
3 What treatment and control methods would you implement in the collection?

CASE 236 A group of six juvenile, 2–3-month-old peregrine falcons (*Falco peregrinus*) from a breeding centre in mainland UK were reported ill. The birds showed progressive weight loss, reduced appetite, and mucoid bloody diarrhea.

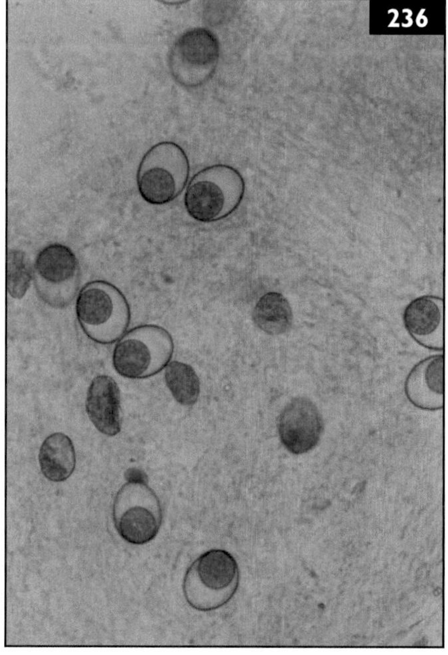

1 Based on the history and clinical findings, what are your differential diagnoses?
2 What diagnostic tests would you perform to confirm the diagnosis?

   Direct and flotation fecal examinations revealed large numbers of protozoan oocysts (**236**, ×400).
3 Which parasitic genera could be implicated? Which one is most likely? What treatment would be recommended?

CASE 237 A canary (*Serinus canaria domestica*) breeder client has recently experienced significant mortalities in his aviary. He presents a recent carcase for postmortem examination.

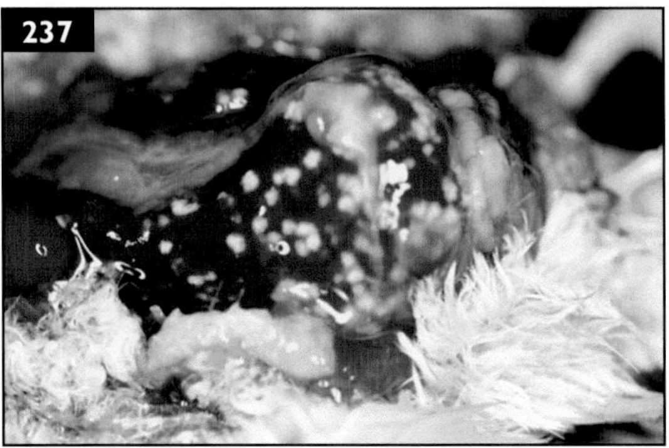

1 What are your differential diagnoses for these liver lesions seen at postmortem examination (**237**)?
2 What clinical signs would you expect to see in canaries with this disease, from this breeder?
3 What diagnostic test would you perform to confirm the diagnosis, and what treatment regimens would you recommend?

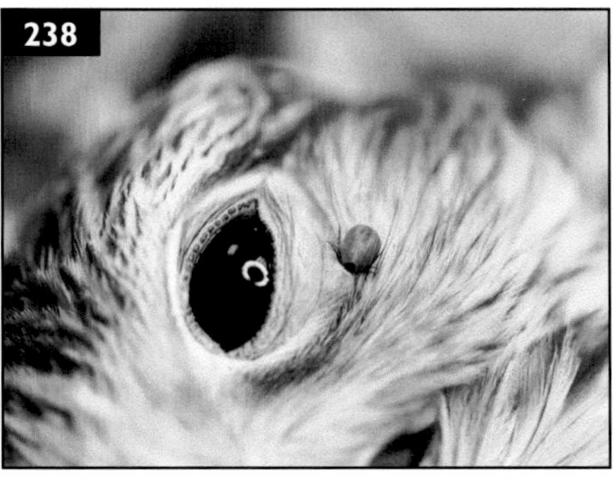

CASE 238 When the owner placed this peregrine falcon (*Falco peregrinus*) in its aviary two days ago, it was clinically normal. Today the bird is noticeably lethargic. A tick is found attached to the lower eyelid (**238**), surrounded by a dark red, subdermal ring (hematoma). No ocular abnormalities are detected on full systematic ophthalmologic examination.

1 What is the most likely diagnosis?
2 What treatment should be provided to the bird?
3 What additional actions should be taken?

CASE 239 A 30-year-old female umbrella cockatoo (*Cacatua alba*) is presented with lethargy, exercise intolerance, and falling off its perch. During the physical examination you note a bradycardia of 120 bpm. You decide to perform an ECG to determine what type of bradycardia is present (**239**).

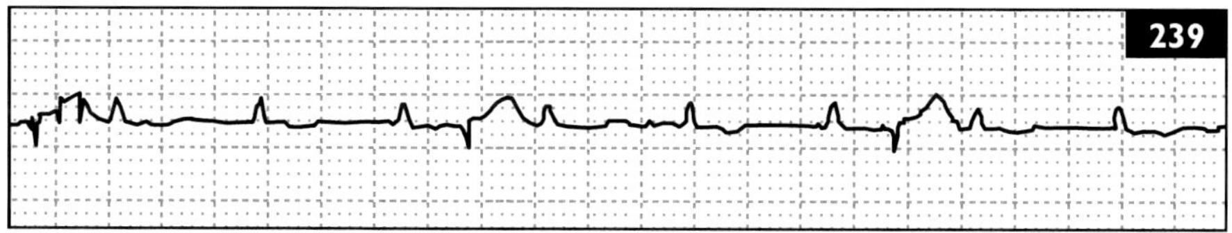

1 How do you perform an ECG in a bird?
2 What is your diagnosis with regard to the bradycardia present in this bird?
3 What test can be performed to diagnose an underlying increase in vagal tone?

CASE 240 Most birds possess a uropygial gland or preen gland (**240**).

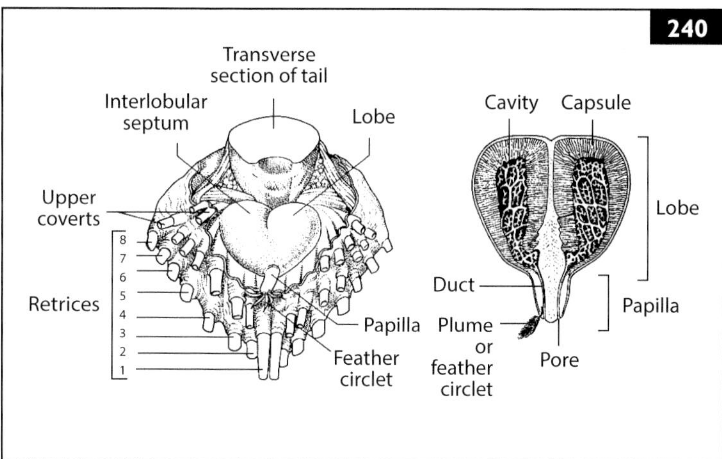

1 Where is it located?
2 What does it produce?
3 What are the main functions of its product?
4 Name some birds that totally lack a preen gland.
5 What clinical abnormalities may affect the preen gland, and how would each be treated?

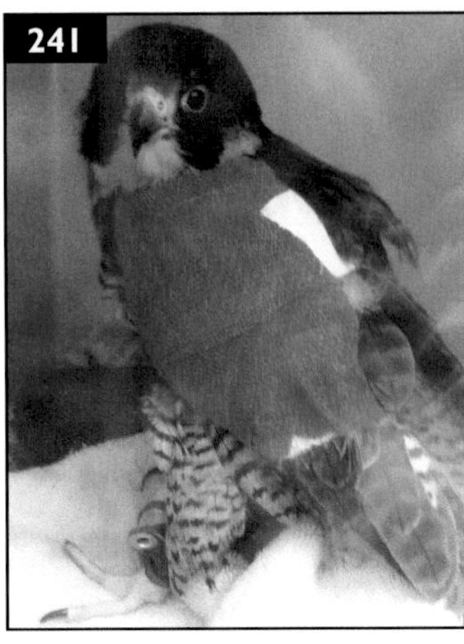

CASE 241 A peregrine falcon (*Falco peregrinus*) is presented with a left humeral fracture. The owner reports that it happened this morning during hunting. The bird appears quiet but responsive, and is carrying the left wing lower. The owner requests that you surgically repair the fracture, keeping the patient hospitalized during the initial postoperative period (**241**).

1 How would you manage pain in this patient (1) during the preoperative period, (2) during the intraoperative period, and (3) during the postoperative period?

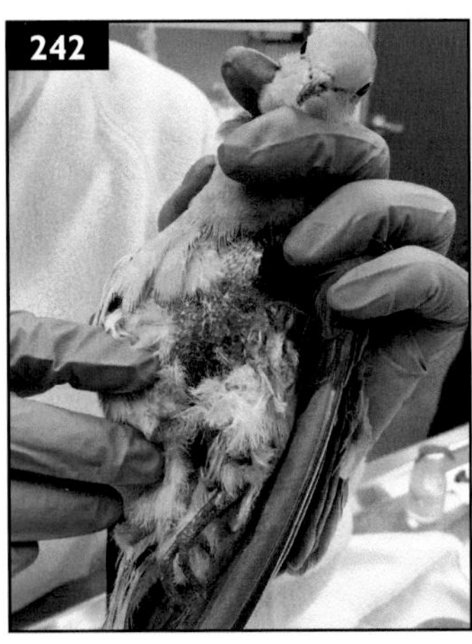

CASE 242 An adult mourning dove (*Zenaida macroura*) of unknown sex was presented after being attacked by a dog (**242**). He had a degloving wound of the pectoral muscles immediately medial to the left humerus. He had diffuse bruising and was missing most of the feathers over the left side of his body.

1 What are your main concerns with a predator bite?
2 What is the normal flora of the oral cavity of the dog and cat?
3 How would you treat birds bitten by dogs or cats?

CASE 243 A 20-year-old male intact blue and gold macaw (*Ara ararauna*) is presented for evaluation of polyuria, polydipsia, and weight loss despite polyphagia. The bird has been seen by another veterinarian, who reported a persistent hyperglycemia (blood glucose >44.41 mmol/L [800 mg/dL]) and the presence of glucose in the urine.

1 What is your most important differential diagnosis for this case? List other differential diagnoses.
2 What other diagnostic tests should be considered for this bird?
3 What treatment options have been used in birds with this condition?

CASE 244 A waterfowl keeper presents a thin Hawaiian goose (Nene, *Branta sandvicensis*) to you for postmortem examination. The liver is mottled with discrete white nodules (**244**). On Ziehl–Neelsen stain microscopic examination, acid-fast organisms are identified.

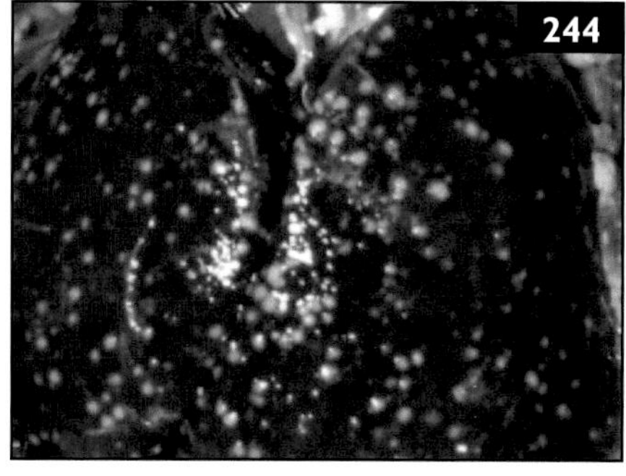

244

1 What is the most likely diagnosis? How often is this seen in waterfowl collections?
2 How can this disease be prevented from entering a collection?
3 What can you do to decrease the risk of spreading the disease in a collection?

CASE 245 A 3-week-old African grey parrot (*Psittacus erithacus*) chick is presented with a strange looking toe (**245**). Other chicks in the clutch show similar changes.

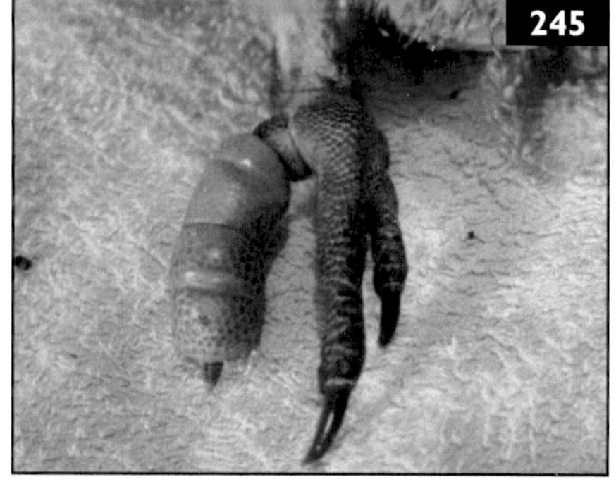

245

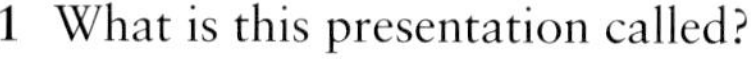

1 What is this presentation called?
2 What is the etiology?
3 What treatment and preventive actions should be taken?

CASE 246 This ventrodorsal radiograph (**246**) shows the cranial portion of the coelomic cavity of a male mallard duck (*Anas platyrhynchos*).

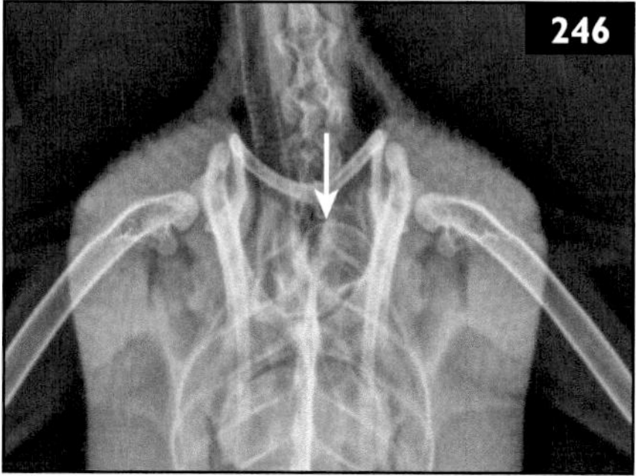

246

1 What is the structure indicated by the white arrow?
2 In what avian family is this structure found?
3 Which cranial nerve innervates this structure?

CASE 247 Domestic geese (*Anser cygnoides*) kept in a backyard are presented with vesicular and necrotic cutaneous lesions on the unfeathered and non-pigmented areas of skin on the feet and head. These lesions seem to develop seasonally between March and September (Northern Hemisphere) and resolve spontaneously. The grass shown (**247**) is found in the backyard. No mortalities have been reported.

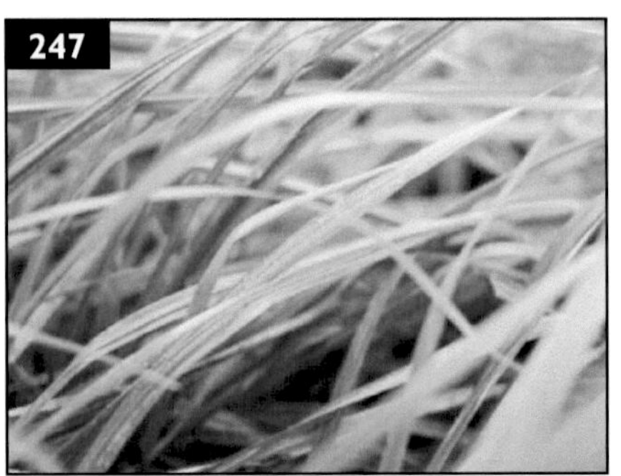

1 Give a possible differential for these lesions.
2 What is the name of this dermatologic disorder?
3 What is the name of the toxin?

CASE 248 A Wright's-stained impression smear of the spleen from a young red-bellied parrot (*Poicephalus rufiventris*) that died acutely, with necropsy findings of splenomegaly and hepatomegaly, is shown (**248**).

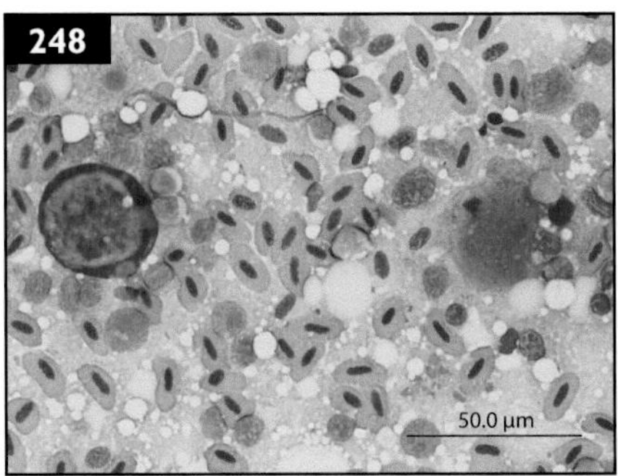

1 What abnormalities can be seen in the impression smear?
2 What etiologic agents should be considered?
3 What other diagnostic tests should be performed to confirm an etiologic diagnosis?

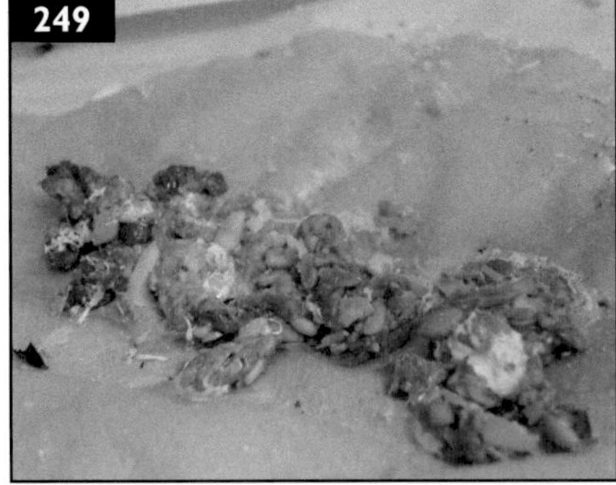

CASE 249 The excrement from a 2-year-old female African grey parrot (*Psittacus erithacus*) is shown (**249**).

1 What abnormality is evident in the excrement?
2 What diseases could result in similar clinical signs?
3 What diagnostic tests would you use to investigate the cause of the clinical signs?

CASE 250 A 32-year-old captive African penguin (*Spheniscus demersus*) with an 8-week history of vomiting, anorexia, and weight loss is evaluated by gastroscopy. Significant findings included a raised partially ulcerated luminal mass at the junction of the proventriculus and ventriculus (**250**).

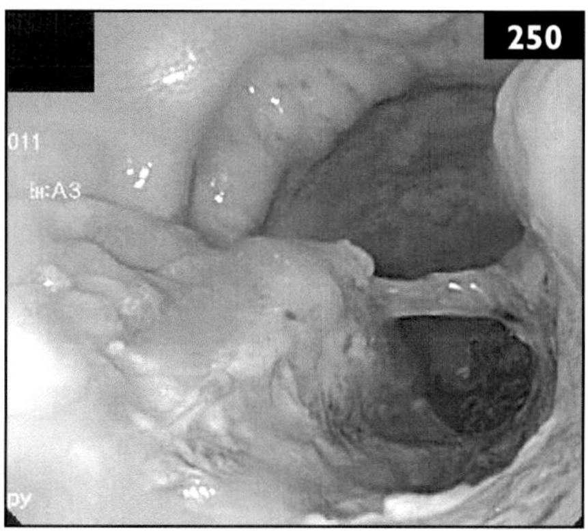

1 What is the most likely diagnosis?
2 What further diagnostics are recommended?
3 What is the prognosis?

CASE 251 A 2-year-old saker falcon (*Falco cherrug*) is presented with a grade 2/5 unilateral bumblefoot of the left foot (**251**).

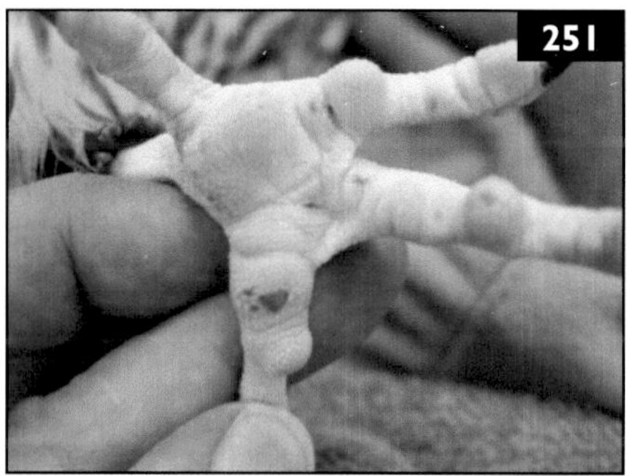

1 Which taxon is most commonly affected by bumblefoot?
2 What are the risk factors most commonly responsible for this disease?
3 Why is that bumblefoot cases are often said not to respond to treatment?

CASE 252 You are presented with an 11-month-old male eclectus parrot (*Eclectus solomonensis*) for post-purchase examination and general wellness (**252**).

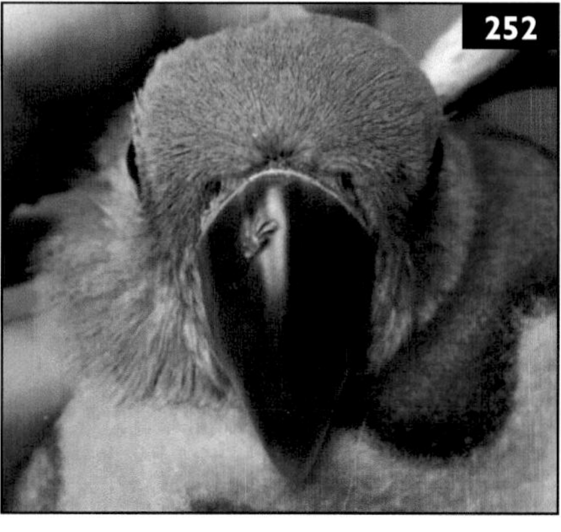

1 What two physical examination findings are present?
2 What can you tell the client about the expected clinical progression of the physical examination findings?

CASE 253 A red-tailed hawk (*Buteo jamaicensis*) was presented after being hit by a car (**253**). The bird had a distal ulnar fracture that was successfully repaired with a IM-ESF tie-in fixator, with the goal of the bird being released back to the wild when deemed fit.

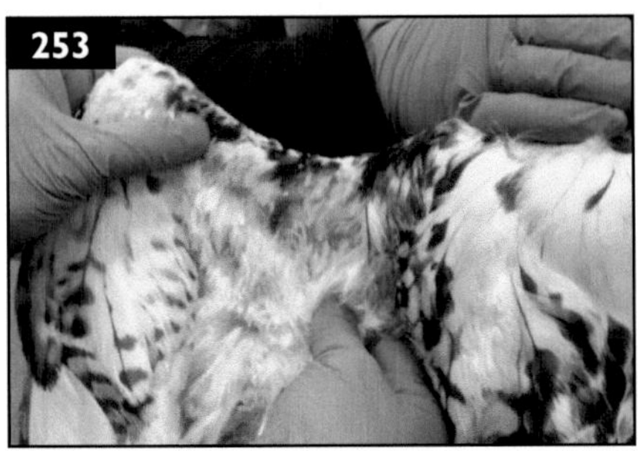

1 When should physical therapy be initiated?
2 Describe the approach to physical therapy.
3 What ancillary therapeutics should be considered during physical therapy?

CASE 254 A common Indian hill mynah (*Gracula religiosa*) is presented after a few weeks of decline in appetite and increasing lethargy (**254**). On physical examination the bird is in a low body condition, with abdominal swelling due to ascites and/or hepatomegaly and increased respiratory effort. An increase in liver enzymes is noted on the biochemistry profile.

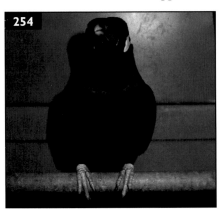

1 What would be the most likely differential diagnosis?
2 What species are most commonly affected by this condition?
3 What would be your nutritional management plan for this patient?

CASE 255 A captive flock of 150 ring-necked doves (*Streptopelia capicola*) suffered mortality rates of 20 animals per month for 4 months. On necropsy, most of the birds had lesions on the spleen and liver and, occasionally, the intestines and lungs. Most of the hepatic lesions were severe, diffuse, pale orange–tan discoloration and enlargement, but in some animals hepatomegaly was detected and contained single or multiple white–yellow foci of variable size.

1 What is the most likely causative agent, and which special stain should be used for initial postmortem diagnosis?
2 What diagnostic tests have the highest sensitivity?
3 What are the treatment options?

CASE 256

1 What are the anatomic landmarks for a left lateral coelioscopy – where exactly is the telescope inserted?

2 On entering the coelomic cavity via the landmarks described above, which air sac is most commonly entered in a psittacine?

On entering the left abdominal air sac, an enlarged structure is encountered cranial and ventral to the gonad and adjacent to the proventriculus (256).

3 Name the structure. What are the differential diagnoses for enlargement of this organ? Can this organ be biopsied?

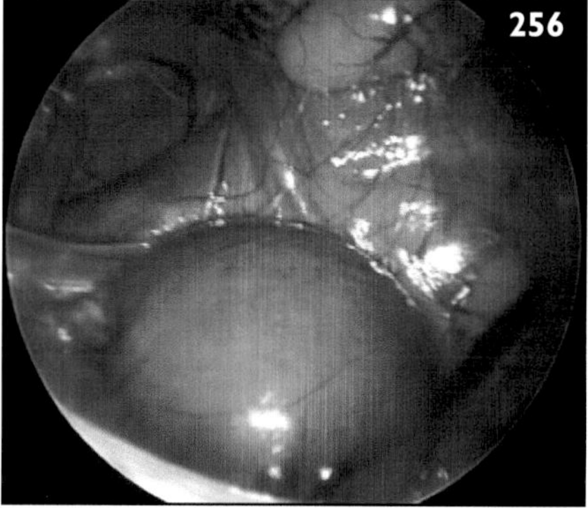
256

Courtesy of Dr. Stephen Divers, UGA

CASE 257 Most avian species have four toes. The arrangement of the toes depends entirely on function. Parrots have two toes directed forward and two toes directed backwards when they perch (257).

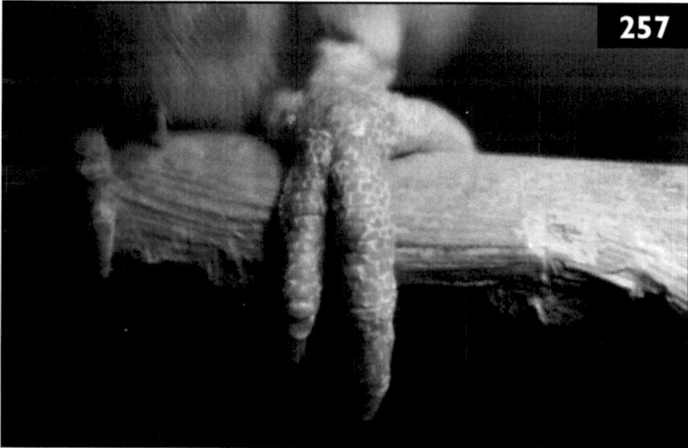
257

1 Name this foot arrangement.
2 This foot arrangement is particularly useful to a group of small parrots from South East Asia that hang upside down from branches. Provide the name and the genus of this group.
3 The foot arrangement also allows parrots to perform what particular everyday task efficiently, which proves so useful during feeding?

CASE 258 The gastrointestinal tract of a young emu (*Dromaius novaehollandiae)* during necropsy is shown (**258**). This bird is from a group of 16 recently hatched chicks that had been moved out of doors 1 week previously. Although all the chicks appeared to be eating well, this bird was found dead one morning.

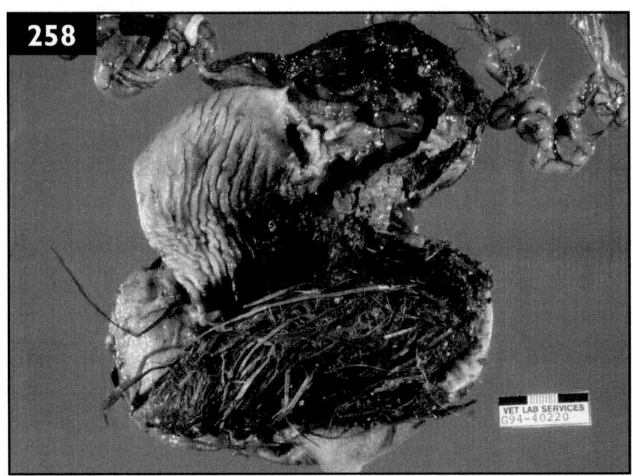

1 What abnormalities are present in this image?
2 How common is this problem in ratites?
3 What options are available for diagnosis and treatment of affected birds?

CASE 259 The head of a spermatozoon is shown (**259**).

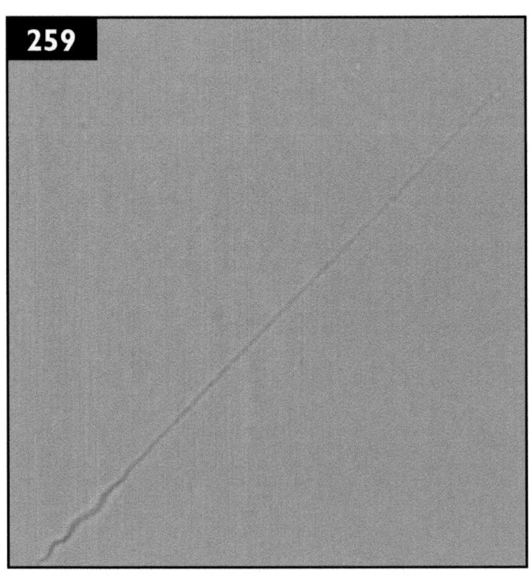

1 In which Order of birds is the head of the spermatozoa characteristically spiral in shape?
2 What are the main characteristics of the semen of birds of this Order?
3 The semen of members of this Order is stored at 4°C lower than the body temperature in what anatomic structures?
4 How do aviculturists use these structures to determine the sex of the birds?

CASE 260 This young psittacine chick is presented with a severely gas distended crop (**260**). It is obviously distressed and unable to eat.

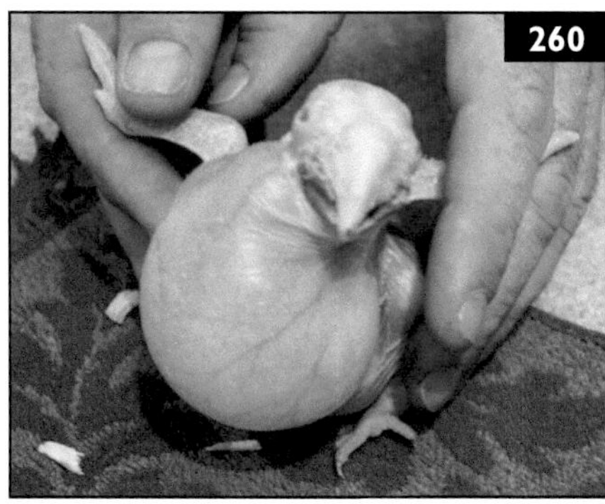

1 What is the cause of the problem?
2 What is the initial recommended treatment for this condition?
3 What further treatment may be necessary if the initial treatment fails?

CASE 261 An owner brings in their cockatiel (*Nymphicus hollandicus*) complaining of a nonhealing wound over the dorsal tail base. The gross appearance of the lesion after you remove overlying crusts is shown (**261**).

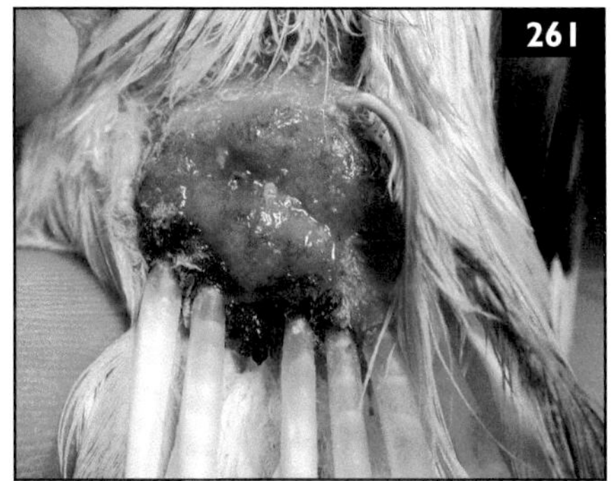

1 What is the main differential for this lesion?
2 What is a potential predisposing factor for this lesion?
3 What are treatment options for this lesion?

CASE 262 A juvenile call duck (*Anas platyrhynchus domesticus*) is presented for general examination showing blepharitis, epiphora, and upper respiratory signs (**262**). Infectious differential diagnoses for ocular and/or upper respiratory clinical signs in Anseriformes should include bacterial, viral, and fungal agents.

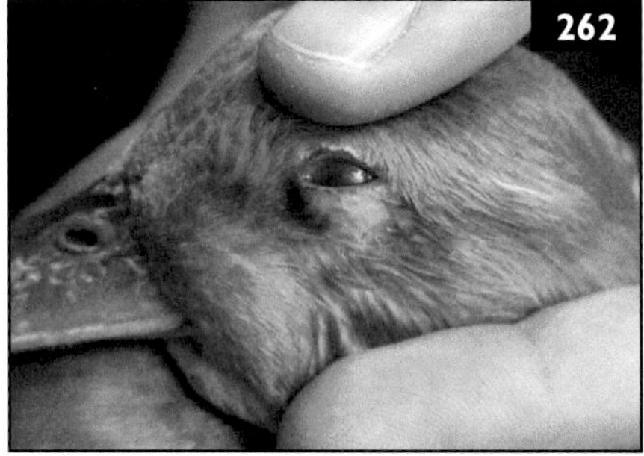

1 What bacterial etiologies are compatible with the observed clinical signs?
2 What viral etiologies are compatible with the observed clinical signs?
3 What fungal etiologies are compatible with the observed clinical signs?

CASE 263 A budgerigar (*Melopsittacus undulatus*) with a history of wasting, diarrhea and repeated vomiting is presented for postmortem examination. Caseous plaques are observed in the mucosa of the upper gastrointestinal tract (**263**).

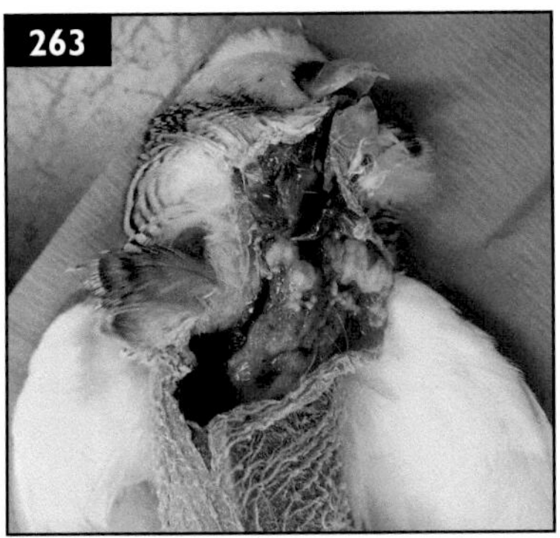

1 Which protozoal parasite would you consider as the most likely differential diagnosis?
2 How would you test the rest of the specimens housed in the same aviary?
3 What treatment and control measures would you use if other birds in the aviary are also affected?

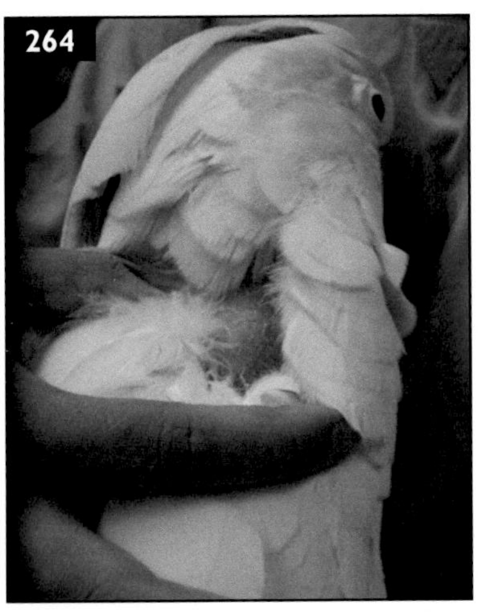

CASE 264 With regard to the bird shown (**264**).

1 Describe the different parts of the cervicocephalic air sac. What are their functions?
2 Why does hyperinflation of the cervicocephalic air sac occur in some birds?
3 How would you manage hyperinflation of the cervicocephalic air sac

CASE 265 Welfare for captive birds is always a compromise between several factors, and there is no single combination of variables that can claim to be the perfect model for the best avian welfare. A controversial topic with regard to avian welfare is the issue of flight restriction. One of the animal welfare tenants is 'the freedom to express normal behavior', and flying is a normal behavior for most birds. Many captive birds have restrictions on their ability to fly. There are several methods available for restricting flight or deflighting a bird, each with a varying degree of invasiveness. Some methods are permanent while others may be short term. Some techniques are illegal in some countries. Opinions as to the suitably of all methods will vary between individuals.

1 Provide a common form of flight restriction used with the following types of bird: caged psittacines and passerines; companion psittacines; cranes; falconry birds; flamingos in an outdoor exhibit.
2 List three positive welfare opportunities that trimming the remiges of a pet bird could provide.
3 List negative welfare aspects of preventing a bird from flying. Welfare may include physical, medical, as well as behavioral aspects.

CASE 266

1 What is the standard management of a broken blood feather with active hemorrhage (**266**)?
2 If bleeding has stopped or is minimal with a broken blood feather, how should the avian patient be managed?
3 Management of a bleeding broken blood feather on the wing should only involve pulling the feather as a last resort. Why should the feather be left in place, if possible?

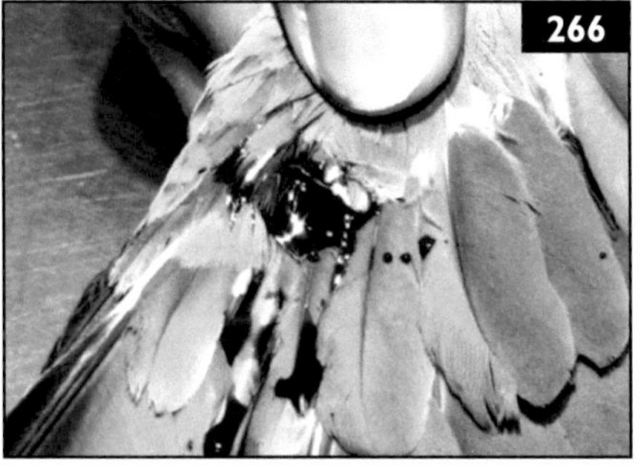
266

CASE 267 Most parrot species are highly social animals that establish strong pair bonds and often form gregarious flocks. A survey of parrot owners in the USA found that more than 50% of owners kept birds singly housed. Parrots housed alone may be more likely than those housed in pairs or groups to show feather damaging behavior, incompatibility with other parrots, screaming, and mating displays towards humans. Considering the welfare of a companion parrot, answer the following questions.

1 List three advantages for a bird's welfare to be housed with one or more of the same species.
2 Parrot owners may be concerned that socially housed parrots will bond to the other birds rather than to humans. Has this concern been validated or invalidated?
3 Species-specific characteristics must be taken into account when considering pair housing. What psittacine species is notorious for being prone to aggressive behavior toward conspecifics?

CASE 268 A juvenile Northern saw-whet owl (*Aegolius acadicus*) with a suspected history of head trauma is presented for ophthalmic examination as part of a complete physical examination. Intermittent anisocoria and lack of direct and indirect pupillary reflexes are observed (**268**).

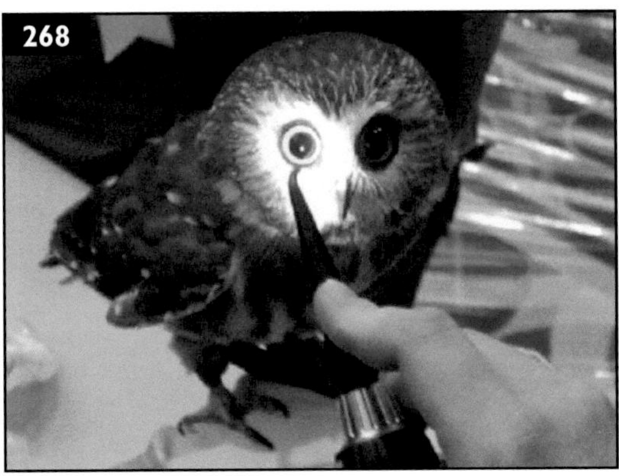
268

1 Why is intermittent anisocoria frequently observed in some birds?
2 How do you explain and interpret the diagnostic procedure shown in the image?
3 Why may directing the light source to one eye result in miosis in the contralateral eye?

CASE 269 A 7-year-old African grey parrot (*Psittacus erithacus*) escaped from his cage and was found by his owner in the kitchen, eating chocolate. The owner is very concerned about chocolate toxicity and rushes the bird to the nearest veterinary hospital for evaluation and treatment (**269a**).

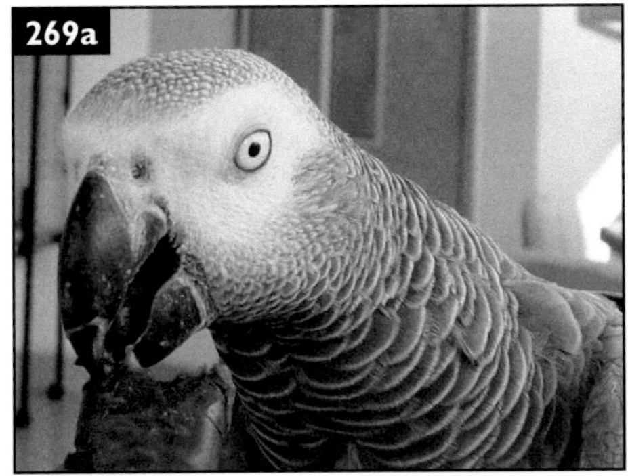
269a

1 What are the toxic agents in chocolate?
2 What are the expected clinical signs in cases of chocolate intoxication in birds?
3 How would you treat this bird in an emergency?

CASE 270 Feathers are the most distinctive feature of avian anatomy (270).

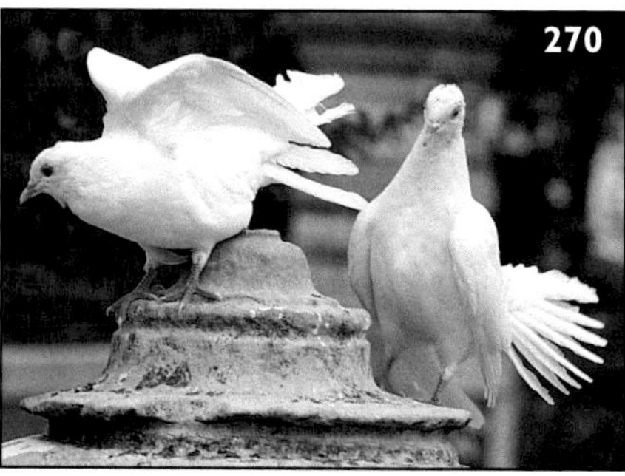
270

1 What are the three main functions of feathers?
2 Give a description of the function of the following feathers: flight feathers, down feathers, semiplumes, filoplumes, and bristles.

CASE 271 There is a growing interest in developing and implementing animal welfare assessment schemes for farms, zoos, aquaria, and laboratories. A welfare assessment is a tool for providing information, with the intention of improving the health and wellness of the birds, plus increasing the commitment of the caregiver and the veterinarian's relationship with clients and caregivers. The welfare assessment includes identification of both problems and attributes. It requires application of a system to evaluate the issues, followed by a re-evaluation of the welfare after changes have been implemented.

1 List key features to include in an avian welfare assessment.
2 Give examples of what resources can be objectively evaluated in an avian welfare assessment.
3 Give examples of what the veterinarian can do to determine the physical state of individual birds.
4 Evaluation of the mental state of a bird is the most abstract and subjective part of the overall welfare assessment. What kinds of questions are included in the assessment of a bird's mental state?

CASE 1

1 What are the main differential diagnoses? Differential diagnoses to be taken into consideration are: iron storage disease (ISD), bacterial hepatitis, diffuse fatty liver (hepatic lipidosis).

2 What complementary test would you request or perform? Liver biopsy would be the best way to confirm ISD. A complete blood panel would help to determine if the condition has an infectious origin. In this case, fine needle aspiration was performed and the presence of hemosiderin aspirate was suggestive of ISD.

3 How would you treat this condition? While this condition can be controlled by a low iron diet, the use of tannins and other oral compounds will not decrease the iron liver content once iron is already stored there; on the other hand, cycles of phlebotomies (2 mL of blood/kg once a week), coupled with the use of iron chelating agents, such as deferoxamine (100 mg/kg SC q24h) and deferiprone, has been described and looks a viable option. The latter act by binding free iron in the bloodstream and enhancing its elimination in the urine. Even if ISD can be treated, or at least controlled, both the cost of the treatment and the commitment asked of the owner are considerable.

Further reading

Cornelissen H, Ducatelle R, Roels S (1995) Successful treatment of a channel-billed toucan (*Ramphastos vitellinus*) with iron storage disease by chelation therapy: sequential monitoring of the iron content of the liver during the treatment period by quantitative chemical and image analyses. *J Avian Med Surg* 9(2):131–137.

CASE 2

1 What advice could you give to improve the reproductive success in this collection? Flamingos are colony breeders. A large group is needed to trigger breeding behavior. The zoo can try to acquire more individuals. Several artificial devices have been used successfully to mimic a larger flock: placing mirrors, loudspeakers with flock noise, placing artificial nests. Rainfall is also a powerful trigger. Nests are fashioned from mounds of soil. These should be removed after one breeding season and fresh mounds supplied at the start of the next, which also forms a trigger for nest building and breeding. Misting the area regularly may also be useful. Particular care must also be taken to select animals from the same species, since hybridization is common between flamingo species, the offspring being infertile.

2 List some possible causes of low egg fertility in flamingo flocks? What management techniques can be used to overcome this difficulty? Egg fertility in captive flamingo flocks is often low (30%). Several causes have been implicated. Flamingos in captive collections tend to be pinioned. Pinioning is believed to introduce additional physical difficulties for successful copulation in long legged and long winged species such as flamingos. While one option is to maintain fully flighted birds in large netted enclosures, such species are prone to flight injuries against the netting, so these enclosures are not ideal. Flamingos cannot be kept fully winged, unless enclosed. Viable chick numbers per breeding pair have been normalized by candling eggs at 10 days of incubation and removing all clear eggs. If an egg is removed at 10 days, the hen will recycle, giving the pair an additional chance to produce a viable fertile egg. The removal of clear eggs is carried out only on the first two cycles.

3 What management actions can be taken to reduce hand-reared chick mortality during the first days of life? Captive reared flamingo chicks are intensely aggressive towards each other immediately after hatching. Chicks should be kept individually in nest bowls until 5 days of age. At this time they may be mixed as a group of three (not two), in which situation aggression between chicks does not occur. Flamingo chicks are naturally long boned and fast growing. When hand-rearing chicks, a significant percentage seem to have a compulsive behavior to eat parts of the egg shell soon after hatching. When such ingestion occurs, a significant mortality level will occur, due to small intestine perforation caused by trauma from sharp edges of their own ingested egg shells.

Further reading

Batty M, Jarrett NS, Forbes N *et al.* (2006) Hand-rearing Greater Flamingos *Phoenicopterus ruber roseus* for translocation from WWT Slimbridge to Auckland Zoo. *Int Zoo Year Book* 40(1):261–270.

Wyss FS, Wenker C (2015) Phoenicopteriformes. In: *Fowler's Zoo and Wild Animal Medicine*, Vol. 8, 1st edn. (eds. RE Miller, ME Fowler) Elsevier, St. Louis, pp. 105–112.

CASE 3

1 What is your problem list, differential diagnosis, and most likely diagnosis? The problem list should include: malnutrition, intermittent vomiting, feather damaging behavior, obesity, possible ileus, coelomic pain, leukocytosis, hyperamylasemia, and hypercholesterolemia. The differential diagnoses could include the following: enteritis, hepatopathy, pancreatic disease, gastrointestinal foreign body, and neoplasia of coelomic organs. The most likely diagnosis, based on the hyperamylasemia, is pancreatic disease. This can be associated with toxins (zinc, mycotoxins), high fat diets and obesity, neoplasia, trauma, or infection (bacterial, viral, or chlamydial). Pancreatitis develops when there is activation of the digestive enzymes (trypsin, protease, and phospholipase amongst others) within the gland, with resultant pancreatic autodigestion.

2 What further diagnostics could be used to confirm your tentative diagnosis? Further diagnostic testing could include: (1) Radiographs. To assess for the presence of hepatomegaly, ileus, and, with contrast, gastrointestinal foreign bodies. Coelomic fat, effusions, or organomegaly can lead to reduced serosal detail, limiting the usefulness of this modality. (2) Ultrasound. To differentiate between fluid and soft tissue opacities and identify specific organs. (3) Endoscopy and biopsy. The pancreas is best evaluated via the right coelomic approach (e.g. caudal thoracic or abdominal air sac). (4) Coeliotomy and biopsy. The pancreas is readily accessible via a ventral midline approach.

3 **How would you treat this patient?** There is little evidence-based information on the treatment of pancreatitis in birds, and most treatment regimens are extrapolated from small animal medicine. They revolve around:

- Reducing the workload on the pancreas:
  - Conversion to a low-fat balanced diet (e.g. formulated diet and vegetables) reduces the amount of fat presented for digestion, and reduces the pancreatic workload.
  - Increasing the amount of exercise (e.g. through the introduction of foraging activities) will improve tissue perfusion, especially of the pancreas.
  - Supplementing the diet with pancreatic enzyme extracts is reported in people.
  - There is no indication for fasting a bird with pancreatitis; indeed, such an approach may well precipitate a hypoglycemic crisis, collapse, and even death.
- Analgesia. Pancreatic disease can be painful. NSAIDs (e.g. meloxicam) are usually avoided where there is potential gastrointestinal dysfunction, leaving opioids as the mainstay of therapy. As opioids may potentially exacerbate ileus, synthetic opioids such as tramadol may be a suitable choice.
- Anti-inflammatory therapy. In recent years omega 3 and 6 essential fatty acids have been used for their anti-inflammatory, lipid stabilizing, antineoplastic and other potential qualities.

Birds that survive a bout of acute pancreatitis should be regularly monitored for evidence of pancreatic insufficiency and diabetes mellitus, both well-recognized sequelae to acute pancreatitis in mammals. Regular weight checks and annual blood screening may detect complications before they become life threatening. Most pancreatic disease is diagnosed as end-stage pancreatic atrophy, usually found at necropsy. There is obviously scope for earlier intervention in these cases.

Further reading

Candeletta SC, Homer BL, Garner MM *et al.* (1993) Diabetes mellitus associated with chronic lymphocytic pancreatitis in an African grey parrot (*Psittacus erithacus erithacus*). *J Assoc Avian Vet* 7:39–43.

Doneley R (2001) Acute pancreatitis in parrots. *Aust Vet J* **79**:409–411.

Phalen DN, Falcon M, Tomaszewski EK (2007) Endocrine pancreatic insufficiency secondary to chronic herpesvirus pancreatitis in a cockatiel (*Nymphicus hollandicus*). *J Avian Med Surg* **21(2)**:140–145.

Schmidt RE, Reavill DR (2014) Lesions of the avian pancreas. *Vet Clin North Am Exot Anim Pract* **17**:1–11.

CASE 4

1 How should one interpret the complete blood cell count? The bird has a pancytopenia based on the low total leukocyte count and the severe anemia (in general the normal PCV of birds ranges between 35 and 55%). The refractometric total protein suggests a hyperproteinemia (in general the normal refractometric total protein of birds ranges between 35 and 55 g/L [3.5 and 5.5g/dL]); however, this was not indicated by the total protein value from the plasma biochemistry profile.
2 How should one interpret the image of the blood film (4)? The heterophil exhibits 3+ toxicity. The erythrocytes reveal hypochromasia.
3 What is the significance of the cells in the image of the blood film? The toxic (3+) heterophil is indicative of a severe inflammatory leukogram regardless of the actual total leukocyte count. The erythrocytes lack polychromasia, indicating a nonregenerative response to the anemia. The presence of hypochromatic erythrocytes is indicative of iron deficiency, which likely is associated with chronic inflammatory disease; however, nutritional deficiency leading to iron deficiency or chronic lead toxicosis should also be considered.

Further reading

Campbell TW (2015) Peripheral bood of birds. In: *Exotic Animal Hematology and Cytology*, 4th edn. Wiley Blackwell, Ames, pp. 37–66.

CASE 5

1 Describe suitable endoscopy instrumentation required for the following procedures:

- **Coelioscopy with kidney and liver biopsies in a 1 kg raptor.** The 2.7 mm, 30° telescope, housed within a 4.8 mm operating sheath to allow introduction of flexible instruments, is ideal and is the most popular system amongst avian and exotics veterinarians. 5-Fr biopsy forceps are used to obtain the kidney biopsy. Ideally, 5-Fr single-action scissors are required to first incise the air sac and hepatoperitoneal membrane prior to obtaining a liver biopsy using 5-Fr biopsy forceps.
- **Tracheoscopy in a 400 gram parrot.** Ideally, a 1.9 mm telescope with an integrated sheath would be used. In birds with smaller tracheas, a 1-mm semi-rigid endoscope is often required. However, in a medium sized parrot, it is often possible to use the 2.7 mm telescope without a protective sheath to reduce the diameter. The trachea acts as a biological sheath such that instruments can be passed down the trachea alongside the telescope.
- **Air sac tube placement in a 400 gram parrot.** Any endoscope 1–3 mm in diameter (including the 2.7 mm telescope without a protective sheath) can be used. The endotracheal tube is placed over the endoscope and once the endoscope is appropriately positioned within the caudal thoracic air sac, the endotracheal

tube can be pushed off the telescope and into the air sac. The size of the air sac tube should be comparable to the tracheal diameter, and for a 400 gram parrot, 4–5 mm would be appropriate.

- **Cloacoscopy in a 3 kg goose.** A 2.7 mm, 30° telescope, housed within a 4.8 mm operating sheath, is most popular, but other sizes may be suitable as long as ports are available for saline irrigation. Warm (39–41°C [103–105°F]) saline infusion is required for visualization, connected to the ingress port of the operating sheath.

2 Contrary to reptile and mammal coelioscopy/laparoscopy, why is CO_2 insufflation contraindicated and not required for avian coelioscopy? CO_2 insufflation is not required in avian coelioscopy as the endoscope is inserted into and operated within the air sac system, which provides a working space that is not present in other taxa. CO_2 insufflation is contraindicated as CO_2 inhalation results in immediate death, and is a recognized method of euthanasia in birds.

3 When performing endoscopy and endosurgery within the avian air sac system, why is it important to ensure that there is a snug skin–endoscope interface and that all sheath ports are closed? As the endoscope is operated within the air sac system, any air movement between the endoscope and the body wall, or through the operating sheath system, is tantamount to breathing around the endotracheal tube. Consequently, as gas exchange is uncontrolled, anesthetic depth can become unstable. In addition, if a pressure cycle ventilator is used for anesthesia, peak inspiratory pressure would never be achieved, as anesthetic gases continuously escape through the surgical site or the operating sheath ports, resulting in respiratory alkalosis.

Further reading

Divers SJ (2010) Avian diagnostic endoscopy. *Vet Clin North Am Exot Anim Pract* **13(2)**:187–202.

Divers SJ (2015) Endoscopy practice management, fee structures, and marketing. *Vet Clin North Am Exot Anim Pract* **18(3)**:579–586.

Touzot-Jourde G, Hernandez-Divers SJ, Trim CM (2005) Cardiopulmonary effects of controlled versus spontaneous ventilation in pigeons anesthetized for coelioscopy. *J Am Vet Med Assoc* **227(9)**:1424–1428.

CASE 6

1 What are your main concerns on initial evaluation? Assessing and stabilizing the patient's overall condition is the main priority. If the fracture is open, it is important to protect the exposed bone from devitalization by covering it with surgical lubricant and a dressing. If the fracture is closed, the clinician should be aware that any movement may result in the sharp bone ends lacerating the skin and creating an open wound.

2 Describe how you would initially stabilize this fracture? In humeral fractures, a body wrap may be used to temporarily stabilize the wing to the body. A figure-of-eight bandage is inappropriate for use in humeral fractures as it causes distractive forces at the fracture site and pushes the distal fragment towards the *propatagialis pars brevis* (minor patagial ligament). Alternatively, if the bird can be safely anesthetized, a temporary fixator can be placed and a body wrap applied.

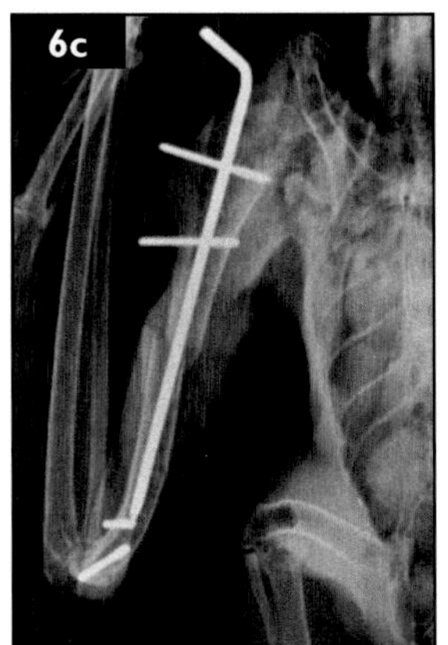
6c

3 What fixation method would you use for surgical repair? This fracture is well suited to the use of a hybrid fixator (ESF–intramedullary pin tie-in). Using a dorsal approach to the humerus, an intramedullary pin (IM pin) should be inserted retrograde (proximally). Two to four positive profile ESF pins are then inserted into the diaphysis from the lateral aspect. The IM pin is bent 90° and a connecting bar (e.g. Penrose filled with polymethylmethacrylate or other type) used to connect it to the ESF pins, creating an ESF–IM tie-in (**6c, d**).

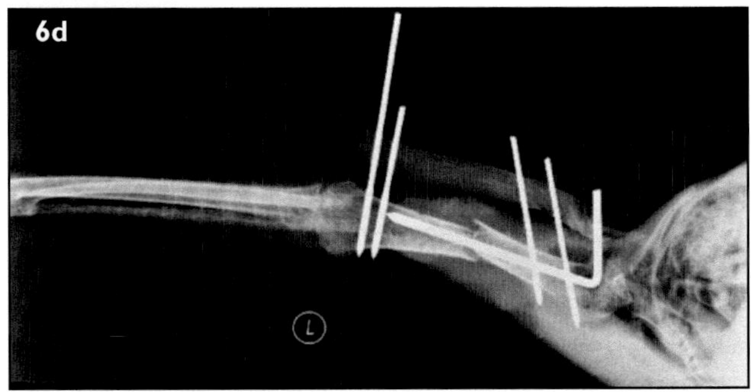

6d

Further reading

Bueno-Padilla I, Arent L, Ponder J (2011) Tips for raptor bandaging. *Exotic DVM* **12(3)**: 29–47.

CASE 7

1 Based on physical examination findings and the features of 7a, what is the cause of the coelomic distension in this hen? The ultrasound image illustrates the presence of a large volume of anechoic free fluid within the coelomic cavity, confirming that the distension is due to ascites.

2 Based on the clinical history, physical examination findings, ultrasound findings, and postmortem findings, what is the most likely diagnosis for this case? Due to the location and characteristics of the structure in **7b**, it is presumed to be a nodular mass originating from the ovary. The postmortem image illustrates a large nodular and firm ovary and smaller nodular lesions in the serosal surface of several coelomic organs. The most likely diagnosis for this case is ovarian neoplasia with secondary ascites and carcinomatosis.

3 What are the treatment options (medical and/or surgical) and prognosis for this case? The prognosis for advanced ovarian neoplasia with severe ascites and carcinomatosis is poor and euthanasia is recommended. The use of chemotherapy in cases of ovarian neoplasia is anecdotal. Early cases of reproductive neoplasia originating from the oviduct may have a fair prognosis with salpingohysterectomy. Ovariectomy is technically difficult and complete removal of ovarian neoplastic tissue even in early cases of neoplasia may be difficult. The ovary is tightly adhered to its dorsal attachments and poses significant risk of hemorrhage to the patient. The avian ovary is attached to the cranial renal artery by a short stalk and the attachment to the common iliac vein is intimate and extensive. There is a significant risk of damaging the left adrenal gland, significantly altering blood flow through the renal portal system and the cranial renal division, and damaging the overlying kidney and lumbar or sacral nerve plexus. Incomplete excision will result in recurrence of disease.

Further reading

Bowles H (2006) Evaluating and treating the reproductive system. In: *Clinical Avian Medicine*. (eds. GJ Harrison, TL Lightfoot) Spix Publishing, Palm Beach, pp. 519–539.

Mison M, Mehler S, Echols M *et al.* (2016) Selected coelomic surgical procedures. In: *Current Therapy in Avian Medicine and Surgery*. (ed. BL Speer) Elsevier, St. Louis, pp. 645–657.

CASE 8

1 How would you manage pain in this patient (1) during the preoperative period, (2) during the intraoperative period, and (3) during the postoperative period?

- **Preoperative period.** Combinations of an opioid and a NSAID are often administered to birds when initially presenting for orthopedic trauma. General anesthesia can cause hypotension and reduce renal perfusion, therefore it is still recommended to avoid NSAID administration in the immediate pre- and perioperative period. Opioids (e.g. butorphanol, 1–3 mg/kg) coupled with benzodiazepines (e.g. midazolam, 0.5–1 mg/kg) administered IM are frequently recommended for the immediate preanesthetic period and may assist in reducing the amount of volatile anesthetic needed for induction and maintenance of anesthesia.

- **Intraoperative period.** CRI using opioids (e.g. butorphanol, 1 mg/kg/hour IV) has been used as an adjunct to inhalation anesthesia for orthopedic pain. An effective local anesthetic block (e.g. lidocaine, 2 mg/kg) at the surgical site and splash blocks on nerves in the surgical area of the fracture can decrease sensitization and wind-up that might otherwise occur during tissue handling. Sciatic and femoral nerve block techniques with local anesthetics could be attempted with the aid of a nerve stimulator.
- **Postoperative period:**
  - Immediate postoperative period (24–48 hours). Assuming the patient is well hydrated, a combination of a NSAID (e.g. meloxicam, 1 mg/kg SC) and continued opioid CRI or parenteral opioid (e.g. butorphanol, 3 mg/kg q4h) administration with gradual reduction in doses during the 24–48-hour postoperative period are recommended. Adjunctive protocols including physical therapy and cold or warm thermal therapy may be included as needed. Cold therapy will help reduce swelling whereas warm therapy may stimulate blood flow to specific areas.
  - Later postoperative period. Opioid administration with titration to effect and gradual discontinuation. NSAIDS (e.g. meloxicam, 1.6 mg/kg PO q12h) or tramadol (30 mg/kg PO q8–12h) may be utilized when the patient returns to home care. Cold therapy of the affected regions should be continued for a minimum of 3 days if tolerated, at which point it can be alternated with heat therapy prior to stretching (with icing following these therapies).

Further reading

Hawkins H, Paul-Murphy J, Sanchez-Migallon Guzman D (2015) Recognition, assessment and management of pain in birds. In: *Current Therapy in Avian Medicine and Surgery*. (ed. BL Speer) Elsevier, St Louis, pp. 616–630.

CASE 9

1 Conduct a functional assessment of this African grey parrot's behavior. Include a description of the ABCs as well as a prediction of the parrot's behavior in your analysis. The following functional assessment can be made of this parrot's behavior:

- Antecedents (i.e. the events or conditions that immediately precede the behavior): the owner's hand approaches the parrot while it is sitting on top of its cage.
- Behavior: the parrot lunges towards the hand and bites.
- Consequences (i.e. the events or conditions that immediately follow the behavior): the owner retreats her hand and moves away from the cage.
- Prediction: the parrot will bite more often and/or more forcefully to prevent the owner from approaching the parrot with her hand.

2 Which of the following types has taken place in this situation? A behavior may increase or decrease in the future depending on the consequences that the behavior has produced in the past. Consequences that result in an increase of future behavior are referred to as reinforcers, whereas consequences that function to decrease future behavior are called punishers. Moreover, consequences can be termed positive (+) or negative (–) dependent on whether the behavior results in the addition or removal of a stimulus or condition (see below). In the situation as described, the parrot's behavior (i.e. lunging and biting) has increased, most likely due to the owner removing her hand following the biting, thus indicating negative reinforcement to have taken place.

		Function	
		Increase	Decrease
Operation	Addition	Positive reinforcement (rewards)	Positive punishment (discipline)
	Subtraction	Negative reinforcement (escape)	Negative punishment (fines)

3 Describe the different interventions that could be considered in this behavior modification plan to reduce the biting and/or prevent injury to the owner's hand. By careful observation and interpretation of the parrot's body language, the owner can learn to anticipate the bird's signals (e.g. backing away from the hand, raising a foot to fend off a hand) and avoid the bite with relative ease. Other methods that can help prevent biting include (a) giving the parrot something to place its beak on while stepping up onto the hand; (b) approaching the parrot with the hand from behind instead of the front or approaching with both hands simultaneously from both sides; (c) wearing a protective towel; (d) having the parrot step onto the perch or towel, avoiding the hand or arm altogether. In this particular situation, by changing the bird's position and increasing the bird's desire to climb onto a hand the bite can be avoided. To achieve this, place the parrot on the floor (using a stick or towel as a perch if necessary), then ask it to climb onto the hand. The owner should furthermore be made aware that birds use their beak as a hand, and may grab a hand more forcefully when it is pulled away, just to maintain its balance. Since biting imposing hands most commonly results from parrots being forced to do something that is not reinforcing to them in the past, behavior modification techniques (e.g. differential reinforcement of alternative, incompatible or other behavior) may be implemented to help shape the bird's behavior to a more desired behavior. Punishment of biting behavior (e.g. by 'laddering' or 'earthquakes') should be avoided as much as possible.

Further reading

Friedman SG, Edling TM, Cheney CD (2006) Concepts in behavior. Section I: the natural science of behavior. In: *Clinical Avian Medicine*, Vol. 2. (eds. GJ Harrison, TL Lightfoot) Spix Publishing, Palm Beach, pp. 46–59.

Welle KR, Luescher AU (2006) Aggressive behavior in pet birds. In: *Manual of Parrot Behavior*. (ed. A Luescher) Blackwell Publishing, Ames, pp. 211–217.

CASE 10

1 List the advantages and disadvantages of in-house laboratory testing. Advantages: (1) Rapid turnaround time. Many in-house machines, especially dry chemistry analyzers, have a turnaround time measured in minutes. (2) Accessibility at all times. These units are often left on or, if turned off, usually have a short warm-up period. The tests can be run at any time, morning or night, with minimal waiting. (3) Fresh sample. Blood can be collected from the patient and processed and placed into the analyzer within minutes of collection. This avoids many of the artifacts associated with transport delays and postage between collection and arrival at an external laboratory (hemolysis, prolonged contact time between erythrocytes and plasma). (4) Good correlation between in-house units and external laboratories. Several studies have validated the accuracy of some in-house units. (5) Instant results allow appropriate medication without delay, while any dubious results can still be forwarded to a quality controlled commercial laboratory. (6) Manual cell counts, differentials, and cytology can be performed by clinicians following appropriate training and experience, while referral to a clinical pathologist may still be sought on complex cases.

Disadvantages: (1) Limited range of tests. Many in-house units use either preprogramed profiles (e.g. rotors) or a profile has to be compiled using individual tests. Either system has an inherent inflexibility in the range of tests that can be run. Few have biochemistries such as cholesterol or triglycerides, which have recently been recognized as of value in avian medicine. (2) Labor costs. Each profile run on an in-house machine requires staff time to run the test and record the results. When multiple tests are being run each day this can represent a significant labor cost to the practice. (3) Lack of quality control. Many private practitioners do not invest in quality control, running their units continuously and never checking the accuracy and validity of the results they obtain. (4) Higher cost per profile. When the cost of the individual tests, purchase and depreciation of the equipment, loss of expired test rotors and reagents, and labor are taken into consideration, the cost per profile is significantly higher than similar profiles performed at an external laboratory. (5) Practitioner interpretation. The results from in-house units typically require the practitioner to make an interpretation. While many experienced avian practitioners can do this, new or inexperienced clinicians may misinterpret (or over interpret) the results they obtain. (6) Limited availability of species-specific normal ranges.

2 List the advantages and disadvantages of external laboratory testing. Advantages: (1) Wide range of tests. External laboratories have access to a wide range of biochemical tests and can often tailor a profile to the practitioner's requirements (or run extra tests as 'add-ons' on request). (2) Good quality control. As part of their accreditation, external laboratories run quality control tests at least once daily and often several times daily. This ensures that results given to practitioners are reliable and validated. (3) Lower cost per profile. The economy of scale means that external laboratories, running hundreds of profiles daily, can offer a lower cost per profile. (4) Clinical pathologist interpretation. Most laboratories include interpretation by a veterinary clinical pathologist in their fees.

Disadvantages: (1) Longer turnaround times. Delays in transporting the sample to the laboratory and then processing it can add hours – if not days – to the turnaround time. (2) Business hours availability. While some laboratories will offer an after hours service, most have business hours that do not fit in with the long hours of private practice. In some cases this adds to the long turnaround times experienced when sending samples out to an external laboratory. (3) Deterioration of sample in transport. Unless the sample is centrifuged and the plasma decanted and sent separately from the erythrocytes, prolonged contact time with erythrocytes will lead to artifacts in results for bile acids, bilirubin, LDH, CK, ALP, potassium, calcium, phosphorus, albumin, fibrin, and glucose.

Further reading

Ammersbach M, Beaufrère H, Gionet Rollick A *et al.* (2015) Laboratory blood analysis in Strigiformes - Part II: plasma biochemistry reference intervals and agreement between the Abaxis VetScan V2 and the Roche Cobas c501. *Vet Clin Pathol* **44**:128–140.

Doneley R (2015) Clinical technique: techniques in the practice diagnostic laboratory: a review. *Vet Clin North Am Exot Anim Pract* **18(1)**:137–146.

Greenacre CB, Flatland B, Souza MJ *et al.* (2008) Comparison of avian biochemical test results with Abaxis VetScan and Hitachi 911 analyzers. *J Avian Med Surg* **22(4)**:291–299.

CASE 11

1 What is the clinical significance of these radiographic findings? The bilateral bone structure in the propatagium is normal in this species. It appears in shearwaters and albatrosses, but not in fulmars.

2 What is the name for this structure? It is known as a sesamoid or sesamoides.

3 What is its function? The sesamoid comes off the *Processus ectepicondylaris* of the humerus and is imbedded in a fan of tendons in the propatagium. In the extended wing it is almost perpendicular to the long axis of the humerus and provides additional strength to the wing. The bone may be vestigial or a feature that other seabirds have lost through evolution.

Further reading

Seabird Osteology (2002–2013) Seabird wing anatomy figures and text. http://www.shearwater.nl/index.php?file=kop126.php

CASE 12

1 What is the most likely organ system involved and the cause of the presentation? The most likely cause is a reproductive disorder, which can include an infectious agent, metabolic disorder, dystocia, or neoplasia. In the current case, *Escherichia coli* was isolated from the oviduct and histopathology of the prolapsed tissue revealed salpingitis with intracellular bacteria consistent with *E. coli*.

2 What are the recommended diagnostic tests? Survey radiographs were performed to rule out the presence of an egg. Ultrasound did not reveal evidence of coelomic fluid or coelomitis. The cloaca was investigated and intestinal or renal involvement was ruled out. The prolapsed mass was gently removed and culture samples were collected.

3 What is the suggested treatment and underlying agent? Due to the initial clinical suspicion of reproductive disease, a deslorelin implant (Suprelorin, 4.7 mg implant) was placed subcutaneously in order to induce regression of the reproductive tract. Synthetic GnRH agonists, such as deslorelin implants, have a higher affinity to GnRH receptors (superagonists) and a longer half-life than endogenous GnRH. The effect of deslorelin implants in birds appears to be species specific. Suprelorin (4.7 mg implant) has been shown to suppress egg laying in chickens for approximately 6 months. In the reported case, this treatment was elected in order to suppress egg laying and reduce further damage to the oviduct. Based on the culture and sensitivity results, and histopathologic diagnosis of salpingitis with intracellular bacteria, oxytetracycline administration was initiated. *E. coli* salpingitis, also called coliform salpingitis/peritonitis/salpingoperitonitis or *E. coli* peritonitis syndrome, is a common condition reported in both backyard and commercial poultry. Salpingoperitonitis is the most common presentation, followed by salpingitis and peritonitis. Salpingitis can be the result of an ascending infection from the cloaca, and in layers salpingitis can cause egg peritonitis if yolk material has been deposited in the peritoneal cavity. *E. coli* is commonly involved in oviductal disease. Birds with salpingitis show an inflamed oviduct that is frequently distended, thin-walled, and filled with laminated, malodorous, caseous exudate consisting of fibrin, granulocytes, yolk, and shell material. This condition can lead to significant egg production decrease and potentially death if untreated.

Further reading

Bisgaard M, Dam A (1981) Salpingitis in poultry. II. Prevalence, bacteriology, and possible pathogenesis in egg-laying chickens. *Nord Vet Med* **33**:81–89.

de Matos R (2013) Investigation of the chemopreventive effects of deslorelin in domestic chickens with high prevalence of ovarian cancer. *Proc Int Conf Avian Herpetol Exot Mammal Med* **2013**:90.

Greenacre CB (2015) Reproductive diseases of the backyard hen. *J Exot Pet Med* **24**:164–171.

Heidemann Olsen R, Bisgaard M, Christensen JP *et al.* (2016) Pathology and molecular characterization of *Escherichia coli* associated to the avian salpingitis-peritonitis disease syndrome. *Avian Dis* **60(1)**:1–7.

Jordan FT, Williams NJ, Wattret A *et al.* (2005) Observations on salpingitis, peritonitis and salpingoperitonitis in a layer breeder flock. *Vet Rec* **157**:573–577.

Kabir S (2010) Avian colibacillosis and salmonellosis: a closer look at epidemiology, pathogenesis, diagnosis, control and public health concerns. *Int J Environ Res Publ Health* 7:89–114.

Landman WJ, Heuvelink A, van Eck JH (2013) Reproduction of the *Escherichia coli* peritonitis syndrome in laying hens. *Avian Pathol* **42**:157–162.

Mans C, Pilny A (2014) Use of GnRH-agonists for medical management of reproductive disorders in birds. *Vet Clin North Am Exot Anim Pract* 17:23–33.

Mete A, Giannitti F, Barr B *et al.* (2013) Causes of mortality in backyard chickens in Northern California: 2007–2011. *Avian Dis* **57**:311–315.

CASE 13

1 Would a red kite be able to carry away piglets? Red kites are predominantly carrion scavengers, but they also consume earthworms and insects. They have small and weak feet. They would not be capable of restraining and killing a live piglet and would be incapable of carrying away a normal sized piglet.

2 Would the red kite that had consumed a 6–7× LD50 of Mevinphos be able to fly 2 km following ingestion? If not, what other explanations are possible, and what further action would you take to investigate the case? Mevinphos is an organophosphate cholinesterase inhibitor and a fast acting and highly lethal toxin. There are no published data relating to this exact scenario; however, raptors consuming a lethal dose tend to show severe nervous signs and die rapidly, hence the numerous carcases very close to a source of toxin in many wildlife incidents. Poisoning can occur by ingestion, inhalation, or transdermally, the latter route taking longer to effect. It seems very unlikely that a bird ingesting a 6–7× LD50 dose would still be able to fly 2 km. Other explanations would be if the carcase was moved after death by a wild animal (e.g. a fox) or human, or if the poisoned bait was carried to the poisoned bird, who then ate it at a remote location. Further investigation of the circumstances, condition of the carcase, and location of the carcase is vital and potentially useful.

3 What relevance have the findings on the third bird? The feathers missing from the back of the neck and the presence of follicles developing on the ovary indicate breeding activity. On further assessment of the postmortem history, the carcase did not demonstrate any signs of bite wounds or other indication of being moved post mortem; however, on investigation it became apparent that the bird was found in a freshly built nest some 10 m off the ground. Putting these aspects together, it is apparent that the male bird could well have picked up poisoned bait on the farm and carried it in his talons (2 km) to the female on the nest, who then consumed it and died. It is possible that the male might have suffered transdermal poisoning some days later. Having unravelled the methodology of poisoning of this third kite, the court found the farmer guilty of poisoning all three birds.

Further reading

Mineau P (1991) (ed.) *Cholinesterase-inhibiting Insecticides: Their Impact on Wildlife and the Environment. Chemicals in Agriculture,* Vol. 2. Elsevier Science Publishing, Amsterdam.

CASE 14

1 Where are the blood sampling sites located in Spheniciformes? The jugular, the basilic, the medial metatarsal, and the interdigital veins can be used for blood sampling. A venous sinus is located on the dorsal aspect at the base of the tail and can also be used for sample collection (**14**).

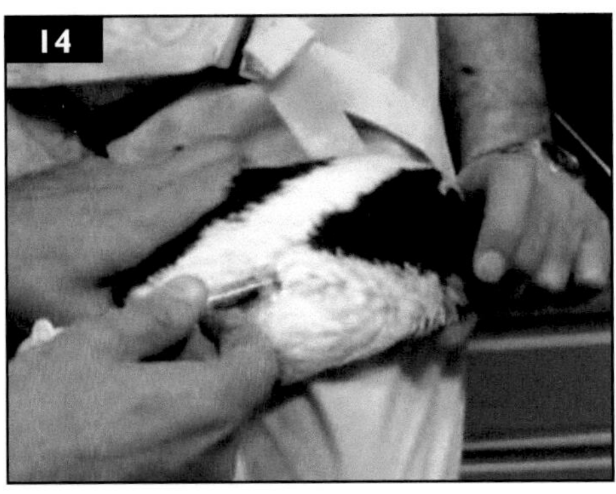

2 Which hemoparasites might be causing these clinical signs? *Plasmodium* spp. are pathogenic in penguins and can cause liver failure, biliverdinuria, and anorexia. This is usually caused by *P. relictum* or *P. elongatum.*

3 What diagnostic tests can be performed to screen for these hemoparasites? Traditionally, the examination of stained (Giemsa or Wright Rosenfeld) smears of peripheral blood samples has been used for the detection of *Plasmodium* spp. in penguins. However, it has been shown that this method is only 45% sensitive when compared with the examination of blood smears together with PCR testing in penguins.

Further reading

Kummrow M (2015) Ratites: Tinamiformes and Struthioniformes, Rheiiformes, Cassuariformes. In: *Fowler's Zoo and Wild Animal Medicine*, Vol. 8, 1st edn. (eds. RE Miller, ME Fowler) Elsevier/Saunders, St. Louis, pp. 75–82.

Vanstreels RET, da Silva-Filho RP, Kolesnikovas CKM *et al.* (2015) Epidemiology and pathology of avian malaria in penguins undergoing rehabilitation in Brazil. *Vet Res* **46**:30.

CASE 15

1 What route would you use to administer fluids in this patient? Ideally, oral or SC fluids should only be used in stable patients that require maintenance fluid therapy or patients with mild dehydration. IV or IO catheters are the routes of choice for the severely dehydrated or hypovolemic bird; however, the decision to place a catheter must be made on a case-by-case basis as the risk of the more intensive manual restraint or anesthesia can outweigh the benefits. In some patients, it may be beneficial to administer SC fluids along with other stabilization measures prior to subsequent handling, general anesthesia, or sedation for catheter placement. The choice between IV and IO catheters will depend on patient size and condition as well as personal preference and experience. IV catheters can be placed in birds the size of cockatiels and larger; however, bird veins can be difficult to access and the vessels are also prone to hematoma formation. Accessible veins for catheter placement include the basilic, medial metatarsal, and jugular veins. Keep in mind that no bird with an IV catheter should ever be left without continuous monitoring due to the risk of fatal hemorrhage if the bird should dislodge the catheter or chew the extension line connected to the catheter. IO catheters can be placed in birds as small as a finch or canary. The technique is generally faster and easier in the avian patient, and should be the technique of choice in an emergency situation, particularly when veins are collapsed or too small to allow IV catheterization.

2 What type of fluid, how much volume, and at what rate would be most appropriate? With hypotonic fluid loss as seen in this patient, an isotonic crystalloid solution with an osmolality close to 300–320 mOsm/L, such as Normosol-R, Plasmalyte-A, or NaCl 0.9%, is recommended.

Maintenance fluid requirements are generally estimated at between 50 and 100 mL/kg/day in medium size birds.

- Maintenance: 50 ml/kg/24 hours = 50 × 0.39 = 19.5 mL/kg/24 hours.
- Dehydration deficit: % dehydration × BW (kg) × 1,000 = 0.08 × 0.39 × 1,000 = 31.2 mL.
- Additional losses (e.g. blood loss, diarrhea): 0 mL.

Since fluid deficits were presumably incurred over days and not rapidly in this patient, fluid deficits can be replaced over 24–48 hours (e.g. half of the dehydration deficit over 24 hours).

$$\frac{(\text{Maintenance} + \tfrac{1}{2}\text{dehydration deficit})}{24 \text{ hours}} = \frac{(19.5+15.6)}{24 \text{ hours}} = 1.46 \text{ mL/hour}$$

A syringe pump is the safest method for delivery of IV or IO fluids. It is relatively easy to overhydrate the small avian patient if fluid administration is begun too aggressively. Also, urine output should be monitored to make sure the patient is not in anuric renal failure. The bird will need to be monitored closely for evidence of overhydration, such as serous nasal discharge, tachypnea, dyspnea, and excessive weight gain. Once or twice daily body weight measurement using a reliable gram scale is the most objective way to monitor hydration status, since daily changes in weight reflect fluid balance.

Further reading

Beaufrère H, Acierno M, Mitchell M *et al.* (2011) Plasma osmolality reference values in African grey parrots (*Psittacus erithacus erithacus*), Hispaniolan Amazon parrots (*Amazona ventralis*), and red-fronted macaws (*Ara rubrogenys*). *J Avian Med Surg* 25(2):91–96.

Carpenter JW, Marion CJ (2013) *Exotic Animal Formulary*. Elsevier Saunders, St. Louis, p. 332.

CASE 16

1 Based on the clinical history and gross postmortem findings, what are your differential diagnoses? Mycobacteriosis, amyloidosis, columbid herpesvirus 1, *Escherichia coli* septicemia.

2 What diagnostic test would you perform to confirm the diagnosis? Histopathology; bacteriology (culture and sensitivity testing); serology; PCR techniques; immunohistochemistry.

3 Is amyloidosis likely to be the cause of death? How can you treat amyloidosis? Can amyloidosis be prevented? Yes. There is currently no suitable therapeutic protocol for treating amyloidosis in falcons as it is technically impossible to remove the amyloid once it is deposited within the organs. Furthermore, very little is known of the causes and/or risk factors of amyloidosis in falcons. The cause(s) of primary amyloidosis in falcons remains unknown. However, secondary amyloidosis has been associated with chronic inflammation or infection (e.g. chronic bumblefoot).

Further reading

Hampel KR, Kinne J, Wernery U *et al.* (2009) Increasing fatal AA amyloidosis in hunting falcons and how to identify the risk: a report from the United Arab Emirates. *Amyloid* 16(3):122–132.

CASE 17

1 What abnormality is visible on this feather, and what is its cause? There are small white structures on the feather barbs near the rachis. These are the eggs (nits) of *Struthiolipeurus struthionis*, the ostrich feather louse. Infestation tends to be heaviest on the wings and neck. *S. struthionis* is present on captive ostriches worldwide.

2 What is the significance to the individual ostrich and to the flock? Infestation with *S. struthionis* has been reported to cause feather loss and a decrease in feather quality as a result of feather picking due to irritation. A controlled study on the effect of lice infestation in ostriches in South Africa showed no effect on production parameters or skin/leather quality.

3 What management actions are required to deal with the problem illustrated? *S. struthionis* is spread by direct contact between birds. Insecticidal treatment, in particular topical treatment with synthetic pyrethroids, can be used to reduce or eliminate infestation.

Further reading

Engelbrecht A, Cloete SWP (2012) Preliminary investigations into the effect of ostrich feather lice (*Struthiolipeurus struthionis*) on production and leather quality. *Anim Prod Sci* 52(5):347–353.

CASE 18

1 What is the most likely cause of this bird's seizure? Hypocalcemia is frequently seen in African grey parrots and can cause neurologic clinical signs ranging from weakness and ataxia to seizures. These birds have evidence of parathyroid gland hyperplasia on necropsy and have elevated serum concentrations of parathyroid hormone (PTH). Therefore, nutritional secondary hyperparathyoidism due to inadequate dietary calcium and vitamin D_3 has been suspected as well as increased dietary fat, which decreases the bioavailability of calcium from the intestines, and inadequate exposure to ultraviolet B light. More recently, hypomagnesemia has also been postulated as a cause of secondary hyperparathyroidism in these patients.

2 If hypocalcemia is suspected based on clinical signs and history, but total calcium levels are within normal limits, what additional test should be considered? Ionized calcium. Total serum calcium measures ionized, protein bound, and anion bound calcium, but ionized calcium alone is physiologically active, hence only measuring ionized calcium is useful in this situation. African grey parrots with clinical signs of hypocalcemia could have normal total serum calcium levels but low ionized calcium levels necessitating calcium therapy. In this patient, both the total calcium and ionized calcium levels were below normal. The ionized calcium was 0.9 mmol/L (3.61 mg/dL), (normal 0.96–1.22 mmol/L [3.84–4.88 mg/dL]).

3 What other analyte should be evaluated in this patient if initial treatment to increase the calcium levels is not effective? Magnesium. Magnesium is an essential dietary element that is needed for appropriate calcium homeostasis. Magnesium activates enzymes responsible for formation of the active form of vitamin D (calcitriol) and is needed for proper PTH receptor function. Therefore, hypomagnesemia must be corrected with parenteral supplementation before a normal calcium status can be reached. In this patient, the magnesium was decreased at 0.7 mmol/L (1.8 mg/dL) (normal 0.8–1.1 mmol/L [2.0–2.6 mg/dL]). In cases of refractory hypocalcemia, kidney function should also be checked since renal secondary hyperparathyroidism could also cause hypocalcemia.

4 What treatment should be given immediately to prevent another seizure? If the patient is actively having a seizure, initial stabilization should include midazolam (0.5–2 mg/kg IV or IM) or isoflurane to control the seizures. Once a diagnosis of hypocalcemia is confirmed, parenteral calcium gluconate can be administered slowly and to effect to stop the seizures. Constant monitoring of the heart rate and rhythm is recommended with an ECG if IV or IO administration is performed. As this patient has hypomagnesemia as well as hypocalcemia, she needs parenteral magnesium sulfate administered IM. As African grey parrots with this syndrome typically have low serum vitamin D_3 levels, parenteral vitamin D should be administered IM. Once the patient is more stable and can swallow, oral calcium glubionate supplementation can be administered. Close monitoring of calcium and magnesium levels is necessary to determine if additional supplementation is needed.

Further reading

de Carvalho FM, Gaunt SD, Kearney MT *et al.* (2009) Reference intervals of plasma calcium, phosphorus, and magnesium for African grey parrots (*Psittacus erithacus*) and Hispaniolan parrots (*Amazona ventralis*). *J Zoo Wildl Med* **40(4)**:675–679.

Fudge AM (2000) Laboratory reference ranges for selected avian, mammalian, and reptilian species. In: *Laboratory Medicine Avian and Exotic Pets.* (ed. AM Fudge) WB Saunders, Philadelphia, pp. 375–400.

Kirchgessner MS, Tully Jr TN, Nevarez J *et al.* (2012) Magnesium therapy in a hypocalcemic African grey parrot (*Psittacus erithacus*). *J Avian Med Surg* **26(1)**:17–21.

Stanford M (2007) Clinical pathology of hypocalcaemia in adult grey parrots (*Psittacus e erithacus*). *Vet Rec* **161(13)**:456.

CASE 19

1 What is the name of this claw? In which digit is it found? Toilet claw. Digit 3.

2 How many phalanges integrate this digit? Four.

3 What are the two main anatomic structures in the claws of birds of prey? The claws of birds of prey are integrated by a hard dorsal casing and a soft ventral casing.

Further reading

King AS, McLelland J (1984) Integument. In: *Birds: Their Structure and Function.* (eds. AS King, J McLelland) Baillière Tindall, Eastbourne, pp. 23–42.

CASE 20

1 What would be the differential diagnoses based on the clinical presentation? Mycotic keratitis, microsporidian keratitis, traumatic keratitis, toxic keratitis (soot), bacterial keratitis (e.g. *Pseudomonas* spp. and *Mycobacteria* spp.), poxvirus keratitis.
2 What is your diagnosis based on the corneal cytology? Fungal keratitis, a yeast etiology based on the pseudohyphae (red arrows). Fungal keratitis is an uncommon disease in avian patients, but different organisms have been reported to be involved including *Aspergillus* spp. and *Candida* spp. Most cases of fungal keratitis are thought to be related to damage to the cornea, typically resulting from a traumatic event. Traumatizing agents may be of plant or animal matter, and may either directly implant fungal organisms in the corneal stroma or abrade the epithelium. After a traumatic incident, the fungal organisms are able to adhere to the exposed corneal stroma and penetrate more deeply, which can lead to corneal perforation. These lesions may then extend into the anterior segment but rarely progress into the posterior part of the eye.
3 What additional diagnostics and treatment would you pursue in this case? Obtain a fungal culture and susceptibility as described for the cytology. Medical and surgical management can be used in the treatment of fungal keratitis, with medical management preferred. Topical ophthalmic treatment is preferred because of its benefits, including higher drug concentrations at the site of infection, no hepatic metabolism, and fewer adverse systemic side-effects. The most commonly prescribed antifungal medications used for topical treatment are amphotericin B, miconazole, and voriconazole. Treatment with topical voriconazole (1 drop OD q4–6h; 200 mg/vial suspended in preservative-free saline for a final concentration of 10 mg/mL) could be initiated while awaiting for the results of the culture and susceptibility, and switch to oral voriconazole (12–18 mg/kg PO q12h) later on when the lesions are resolving. Therapy should be maintained for at least 6 weeks as resolution can be slow. Meloxicam (1 mg/kg PO q12h) should be administered initially to treat the inflammation and associated pain. One of the editors (NF) has treated two avian fungal keratitis cases using F10 antiseptic solution at 1:1,000 dilution, achieving complete resolution in 5 days without any apparent adverse effects.

Further reading

Canny CJ, Ward DA, Patton A *et al.* (1999) Microsporidian keratoconjunctivitis in a double yellow-headed Amazon parrot (*Amazona ochrocephala oratrix*). *J Avian Med Surg* 13(4):279–286.

Hoppes S, Gurfield N, Hammer K *et al.* (2000) Mycotic keratitis in a blue-fronted Amazon parrot (*Amazona aestiva*). *J Avian Med Surg* **14(3)**:185–189.

Sadar MJ, Sanchez-Migallon Guzman D, Burton AG *et al.* (2014) Diagnosis and treatment of mycotic keratitis in a khaki Campbell duck (*Anas platyrhynchos domesticus*). *J Avian Med Surg* **28(4)**:322–329.

CASE 21

1 What additional examination could you perform to assess the thickness of the overgrown keratin layer? Radiographic evaluation of the beak will allow differentiation between the length and thickness of the bone as well as the overlying keratin. The length of the normal beak can be measured as well as the thickness of the beak.

2 How would you treat this condition? The beak needs to be trimmed in length with a burring device such as Dremel tool. The keratin (tip and outer edge) is trimmed from the tip to the commissure. Next the ventral (internal) part of the rhinotheca is burred, paying attention to correcting the tomium and checking that the occlusal plane is level and sufficiently deep to accommodate the tip of the gnathotheca. The gnathotheca is trimmed in a similar fashion, checking that the tip is not overlong for its insertion in the rhinotheca. Care must be taken in reducing the length of both the rhinotheca and gnathotheca, as each possesses a rich supply of sensory nerve endings. Sedation or general anesthesia might be advisable to correct severe overgrowth, and in some instances treatment might need to be staged in multiple procedures or corrected over time. Analgesia should be provided with butorphanol and meloxicam as appropriate.

3 What pathologies may result in excessive beak growth in psittacine birds? Liver pathology has been associated with beak overgrowth, so blood tests for AST, LDH, CK, and bile acid may be indicated. Psittacine beak and feather disease may be evident by a loss of powder down on the beak (it appears shiny rather than dusty in a cockatoo). Neoplasia of the beak will cause abnormal beak growth; however, such growth will not be symmetrical. Increased and abnormal beak growth are also commonly seen in budgerigars with long-standing *Cnemidocoptes* spp. mite infestation.

Further reading

King AS, McLelland J (1984) Integument. In: *Birds: Their Structure and Function*, 2nd edn. Baillière Tindall, London, pp. 23–26.

CASE 22

1 What is the most likely diagnosis? A cerebrovascular accident, such as a hemorrhagic or ischemic stroke, likely secondary to atherosclerosis. With cerebrovascular accidents, neurologic deficits develop abruptly and depend on the location of the vascular insult. For instance, motor deficit, cognition impairment, and monocular vision loss might be present.

2 What additional test would you perform to confirm your diagnosis? MRI is indicated to evaluate soft tissue and has been found very useful for visualizing and evaluating various parts of the central nervous system, including the cerebral hemispheres, cerebellum, optic chiasm, brainstem, and spinal cord. Cerebrovascular accidents, such as hemorrhagic or ischemic strokes, require differentiation through MRI for specific medical treatment.

3 How would you treat this bird? Treatment of ischemic stroke includes thrombolytic agents, which are contraindicated in cases of hemorrhagic lesions. Surgical treatment for hemorrhagic stroke or vascular aneurysm might not be currently feasible in birds because of size limitations. Supportive treatment after a cerebral infarct or hemorrhage is aimed at maintaining adequate tissue perfusion and oxygenation and managing neurologic and non-neurologic complications. The seizures are managed long term with antiepileptic drugs, which should be introduced at the second convulsive epileptic seizure. Phenobarbital, based on pharmacokinetic studies in African grey parrots, requires dosages higher than 20 mg/kg PO q12h. Peak and trough serum levels should be checked 2–3 weeks after initiating therapy or changing the dose until significant therapeutic levels are reached (10–45 mg/mL) or seizures are controlled. Potassium bromide can be used alone or in conjunction with phenobarbital when phenobarbital alone does not work to control the seizures adequately. Based on clinical reports in psittacines, 80 mg/kg PO q24h is recommended but pharmacokinetic studies are lacking. It might take 2–3 months to reach a steady state, and peak and trough serum levels should be checked (1–3 mg/mL). Levetiracetam is a newer antiepileptic drug and based on pharmacokinetic studies in Hispaniolan Amazon parrots, 50–100 mg/kg PO q8–12h is recommended. Long-term monitoring requires a detailed log of the number of seizures and duration, adjusting therapy with antiepileptic drugs as needed to control seizures. An attempt at tapering off the antiepileptic drug can be done when the bird has been seizure-free for more than 2 years. The tapering of medication should be done slowly over several months before discontinuation of the treatment. If the epilepsy is structural, with an obvious demonstrated lesion, the epileptic focus rarely disappears spontaneously and the antiepileptic drugs are continued indefinitely.

Further reading

Beaufrère H, Nevarez J, Gaschen L *et al.* (2011) Diagnosis of presumed acute ischemic stroke and associated seizure management in a Congo African grey parrot. *J Am Vet Med Assoc* **239(1)**:122–128.

CASE 23

1 What is your assessment of this diet? The diet is likely unbalanced and does not provide all the required nutrients for the bird's needs. Nutritional studies that analyzed the dietary composition of psittacine diets found that diets comprised of less than 75% as commercial pellets are nutritionally inadequate and may lead to nutritional deficiencies.

2 What are the potential nutritional deficiencies that psittacines fed such a diet may be presented with? How would they manifest clinically? Common potential nutritional deficiencies in psittacine diets include calcium, phosphorus, sodium, iron, zinc, lysine, and vitamin A. Calcium and phosphorus deficiencies may manifest clinically as poor bone quality, brittle bones, or skeletal deformities. Calcium deficiency may also have a neurologic manifestation or may reduce egg shell quality or cause dystocia in females. Zinc deficiency may cause a decrease in skin and feather quality as well as retarded growth in growing chicks. Iron deficiency may typically cause anemia, although this is less commonly seen in birds compared with other species. Changes in plumage pigmentation may also result from iron deficiency. Sodium deficiency can lead to severe systemic effects in very severe cases, but more commonly, signs are subtle and nonspecific. Lysine deficiency signs may also be nonspecific, such as decreased growth and reproductive success, although changes in feather coloration have also been described. Clinical vitamin A deficiency is relatively common in companion psittacines. It can cause squamous metaplasia and result in blunting of the choanal papillae, oral plaques, a decrease in skin and feather quality, upper respiratory signs, and renal tubular disease.

3 What would be your recommendation in terms of this bird's diet? Commercial formulated pellets should comprise at least 75% of the diet. The remainder may be composed of produce, nuts, and other treats. High fat and energy food items should be provided sparingly as these may easily unbalance the diet. Fruit and vegetables make great treats as they are usually not calorically dense and thus may be provided in higher quantities. The commercial pellets should be fed by their due date and be kept in a sealed container until feeding to prevent nutrient deterioration and lipid oxidation, which may decrease both palatability and nutritional value.

Further reading

Brightsmith DJ (2012) Nutritional levels of diets fed to captive Amazon parrots: does mixing seed, produce, and pellets provide a healthy diet? *J Avian Med Surg* **26**(**3**):149–160.

CASE 24

1 Describe the normal anatomic structures that can be found in the area of the soft tissue structure, taking into consideration both radiographic views. List five differential diagnoses for the soft tissue structure seen in the radiographs.

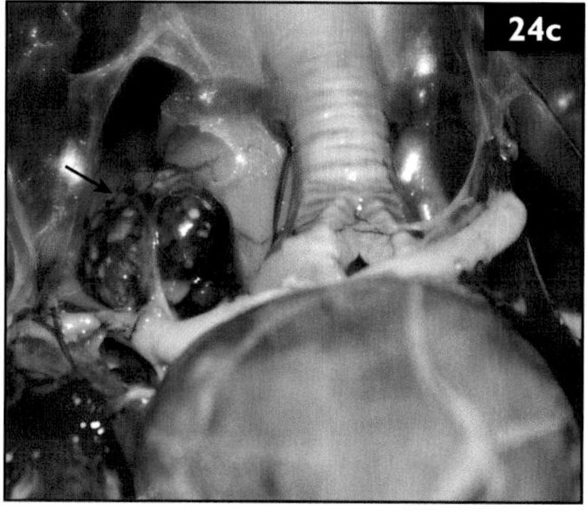

Anatomic structures in this area include the thyroid, parathyroid, and ultimobranchial glands, great vessels, nerves, and thoracic inlet skeletal muscles; the structure could also be associated with the trachea or esophagus (extraluminal) or the thoracic girdle bones. Differential diagnoses for the soft tissue structure seen include granuloma (fungal, bacterial), abscess, gland hyperplasia, cyst, and neoplasia.

2 What other diagnostic tests should be considered to further evaluate the nature and identity of the soft tissue structure seen on the image? Other diagnostic tests to be considered include CT scan with contrast, MRI, endoscopy via the clavicular air sac approach and possible biopsy, or postmortem examination if euthanasia is elected or death occurs. Measurement of T_4 pre- and post-thyroid-stimulating hormone administration and possibly measurement of total T_4 and free T_4 can be considered if the presence of a functional thyroid mass is suspected. In this case, the mass was a productive follicular carcinoma.

3 If the mass affects the thyroid gland, what is the most likely diagnosis? Neoplasia because of the unilateral presentation; hyperplasia (goiter) or thyroiditis secondary to disseminated mycobacteriosis can also cause enlargement of the thyroid gland, but this is typically bilateral.

Further reading

Brandão J, Manickam B, Blas-Machado U *et al.* (2012) Productive thyroid follicular carcinoma in a wild barred owl (*Strix varia*). *J Vet Diagn Invest* **24(6)**:1145–1150.

Helmer P (2006) Advances in diagnostic imaging. In: *Clinical Avian Medicine.* (eds. GJ Harrison, TL Lightfoot) Spix Publishing, Palm Beach, pp. 653–659.

King AS, McLelland J (1984) Endocrine system. In: *Birds, Their Structure and Function*, 2nd edn. Baillière Tindall, Eastbourne, pp. 200–213.

Lierz M (2006) Diagnostic value of endoscopy and biopsy. In: *Clinical Avian Medicine.* (eds. GJ Harrison, TL Lightfoot) Spix Publishing, Palm Beach, pp. 631–652.

Orosz S, de Matos R, Monks D (2016) Clinical endocrinology of the protein hormones. In: *Current Therapy in Avian Medicine and Surgery.* (ed. BL Speer) Elsevier, St. Louis, pp. 378–399.

CASE 25

1 What disease is demonstrated in each image? The saker falcon is suffering from a 'wet form' of pox, while the raven is suffering from a 'dry form' of pox.

Avian poxviruses (*Avipoxvirus* spp.) are large DNA viruses that cause disease in over 200 species of domestic and wild birds. There are currently 10 different species of poxvirus, for each of whom different bird species are the natural hosts.

2 What is the etiology? Avian pox occurs worldwide and is typically an endemic, mild, and self-limiting disease. Outbreaks may occur in captive situations, such as zoos and game farms, where bird densities are high. Epizootics among endemic birds on remote islands (e.g. Hawaiian Islands, Galapagos Archipelago, Canary Islands, and Falkland Islands) are characterized by high morbidity and mortality and indicate the invasive nature of avian pox. Pox is transmitted by ingestion of contaminated food, water, and aerosols, biting insects (mosquitoes are the commonest vector), arthropods, or by any means that brings viruses into direct contact with living epithelial cells. There are two alternative common forms of clinical signs. Cutaneous pox signs are most common. They appear as wart-like growths around the eyes and other apterylae (feather-free) areas, sometimes in large clusters. Diphtheritic, or wet, pox is characterized as raised yellow blemishes on the mucous membranes of the mouth, esophagus, trachea, and lungs, or areas of transparency on the skin, which change to brown scabs as they mature.

3 What treatment and preventive actions should be taken? The recommended method of preventing transmission of poxvirus is to prevent standing water in the environment (i.e. to prevent mosquitoes) and decontaminate feeders, perches, cages etc. (i.e. to reduce or prevent direct contact between individual birds). Vaccines have been developed from strains of the virus for fowlpox, canarypox, pigeonpox, and quailpox to help prevent infection in captive and domestic bird populations. Poxviruses tend to be taxon specific, so vaccines derived from one poxvirus species tend to be ineffective or only render partial resistance to alternative strains. Avipoxvirus acts as an immune suppressant, leading to secondary bacterial infections, for which antibiotic therapy is recommended. Iodine–glycerine applications may assist lesions to heal, as may vitamin A supplementation.

Further reading

Gerlach H (1994) Viruses. In: *Avian Medicine: Principles and Applications*. (eds. BW Ritchie, GJ Harrison, LJ Harrison) Winger's Publications, Lake Worth, pp. 862–948.

CASE 26

1 What are the abnormal radiographic findings? The radiographs show marked air sac lines, abnormal air filling lines on the lateral view, and general increased opacity of the air sacs on the ventrodorsal view. The heart measurements are comparable to other birds of the same species, but the long axis is slightly increased compared with what has been published as reference values in mid-size psittacine birds (African greys, Pionus and Amazon parrots), as heart width as a proportion of thoracic width should be 51–61% and heart length as a proportion of sternal length should be 35–41%. These findings are consistent with an airsacculitis, most commonly caused by aspergillosis.

2 **How do these findings explain the clinical pathology finding?** The persistent elevated hematocrit is consistent with polycythemia. In this case secondary polycythemia is suspected as a response to hypoxia, resulting in an increased production of erythropoietin. Disease conditions that lead to secondary polycythemia include chronic respiratory disease, cardiac disease, or renal neoplasia. As the bird had been treated with antibiotics and antifungal therapy prior to blood testing, it is not surprising that the white blood cell count was normal. The elevated AST and GLDH, with normal CK result, may well correlate with *Aspergillus* spp. aflatoxin production affecting the liver parenchyma.

3 **What further diagnostic tests might be beneficial?** Echocardiography and ECG are required to rule out cardiac disease. Endoscopy or CT would be useful to further quantify pulmonary disease. Sagittal and coronal CT cross-sections are shown (**26c–e**), which are consistent with marked pulmonary fibrosis (arrows) and scarring secondary to fungal infection (arrowheads).

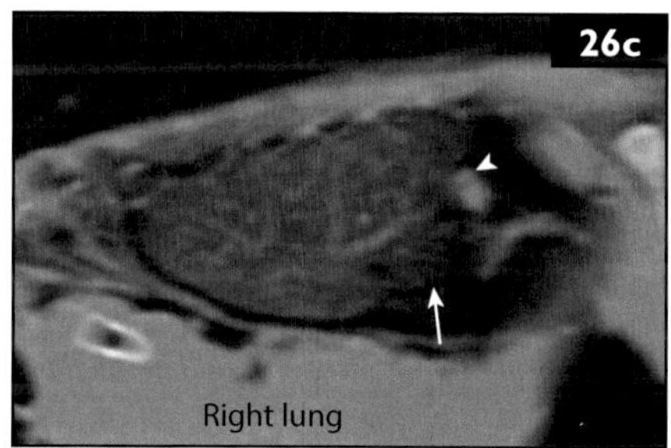

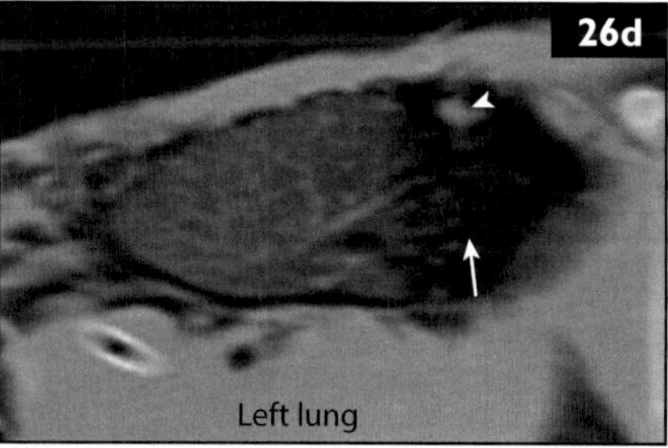

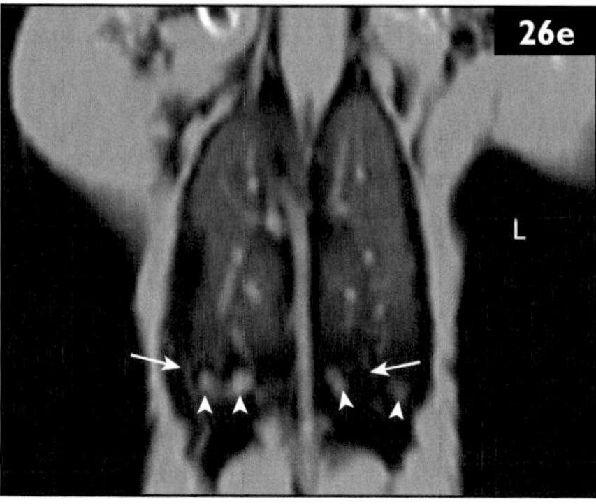

Further reading

Jones M (2015) Avian hematology. *Vet Clin North Am Exot Anim Pract* **18(1)**:51–61.
Straub J1, Pees M, Krautwald-Junghanns ME (2002) Measurement of the cardiac silhouette in psittacines. *J Am Vet Med Assoc* **221(1)**:76–79.

CASE 27

1 What diseases could cause these clinical signs? Which one is most likely? Infectious bronchitis virus (IBV) caused by a coronavirus, avian influenza (AI) caused by an orthomyxovirus, infectious laryngotracheitis (ILT) caused by a herpesvirus, infectious coryza (IC) caused by the gram-negative bacterial rod *Haemophilus paragallinarium*, or mycoplasmosis (MG) caused by the bacterium *Mycoplasma gallisepticum*. IBV is most likely since there is respiratory disease with concurrent egg shell abnormalities. The signs are consistent with IBV in that there are rales but also mild coughing. Anytime there are deaths in a flock, especially a flock showing signs of respiratory disease, AI should be on the differential list and the appropriate authorities contacted. ILT is usually associated with more coughing. MG is more chronic. IC is generally associated with swollen infraorbital sinuses and less mortality. IBV affects only chickens and has a worldwide distribution. The younger and more immunosuppressed a chicken is the worse the clinical signs. Typically, all birds within a flock will develop clinical signs within 36–48 hours and the signs last approximately 4 days, or longer if secondary infections develop. Hens show a 5–10% drop in egg production for about 10–14 days, with irregular and roughened eggshells. Tests include virus neutralization, hemagglutination inhibition, or ELISA. The best method to control this highly contagious disease is to cull the flock, then disinfect (most disinfectants and heat and sunlight) and repopulate. Vaccination, although available, is not recommended since it can revert to a virulent form and cause disease, or it may not protect due to multiple serotypes.

2 How would you euthanize these birds? Backyard poultry are generally euthanized instead of slaughtered. These chickens were rendered unconscious with isoflurane gas anesthesia while being held in a towel, and then administered an overdose of sodium pentobarbital in the right jugular vein. It is very important to collect a blood sample and a choanal swab for subsequent testing, prior to euthanasia. The carcase should ideally also be submitted for a complete necropsy.

3 What diagnostic test would you perform? Serum samples were submitted to a poultry laboratory for serologic testing and were found to be negative for AI, ILT, IC, and MG, but positive for IBV. Histopathology and necropsy confirmed this finding.

Further reading

Gallardo RA, Hoerr FJ, Berry WD *et al.* (2011) Infectious bronchitis virus in testicles and venereal transmission. *Avian Dis* **55(2)**:255–8.

CASE 28

1 List the five principal factors that control the amount of lateral heat damage occurring in a radiosurgical incision. (1) Frequency. It has been shown that 3.8–4.0 MHz is the optimum frequency for tissue incision. This frequency, with its short waveform, provides a precision focus of the energy in a minimal area. (2) Power setting. If the power setting is too high, there is excessive sparking and lateral heat damage. If it is too low, the 'electrode' drags and actually tears tissue, causing excessive lateral heat and damage. (3) Waveform. If the waveform is fully filtered, it is less pulsatile in nature and there is minimal lateral heat. (4) Electrode size. The greater the noninsulated surface area of the electrode, the more energy is radiated from it and therefore more lateral heat is generated. A very small diameter fine-wire electrode provides an incision with the least lateral heat damage to adjacent tissue. (5) Time. The longer the tissue is exposed to the energy, the more lateral heat is created in the tissue. A smooth rapid stroke is necessary to minimize tissue damage. The operator should not return to cut the same tissue within 7 seconds if using a fine, straight wire electrode or within 15 seconds if using a loop electrode.

2 What are the advantages of bipolar over monopolar radiosurgery? The radiofrequency is focused between the tips of the forceps, which allows a higher concentration of the energy in a smaller area. As a result, it is possible to apply more energy to a desired area with little collateral heat damage to adjacent tissue. This is useful when coagulating small vessels. Monopolar coagulation is ineffective in a fluid (wet) field, while bipolar is effective even in a wet field. One technique described utilizing bipolar forceps for cutting, with a modified bipolar forceps with a fine and angled tip; however, this is generally contraindicated if the tissue is required to heal (as opposed to being removed), as the use of bipolar forceps causes additional lateral heart and tissue damage. Bipolar probes do not require a ground plate.

3 What special considerations occur during the preparation of a potential surgical field if radiosurgery is to be used? All combustible solutions can ignite on initiating the current (a particular risk when using a volatile agent in oxygen via face mask). If alcohol is used in skin preparation, it is essential to permit it to evaporate totally prior to radiosurgery. Failure to do this can lead to combustion of the patient.

Further reading

Forbes NA, Altman RB (1998) *Self-Assessment Colour Review of Avian Medicine*, 1st edn. Manson Publishing, London, pp. 103–104.

CASE 29

1 What is the most likely diagnosis? The signalment, clinical signs, leukopenia, and suspected hepatic disease are consistent with African grey parrots naturally infected with psittacine beak and feather disease virus (PBFD virus, psittacine circovirus) suffering the peracute form. Birds with peracute PBFD infection commonly are presented to the veterinarian before they are 6 months of age with the following signs: anorexia, weight loss, vomiting, and weakness. Feather abnormalities are seldom observed. Anemia and leukopenia are presumed to be circoviral induced.

2 What additional test would you perform to confirm your diagnosis? Whole blood and oropharyngeal and cloacal swabs submitted for psittacine circovirus PCR testing. Leukopenia also has been reported to be responsible for false-negative PCR test results in some cases.

3 How would you treat this disease? What is the prognosis? Young African grey parrots with peracute PBFD infection may die within 2 weeks of clinical presentation despite treatment. Postmortem examination and histologic evaluation usually reveal lymphocellular depletion and atrophy of the bursa of Fabricius, extensive hepatocellular necrosis, and secondary bacterial and fungal infections. Supportive care with fluid therapy, nutritional support, antibiotics, and antifungals for secondary infections is needed. The use of filgrastim (Neupogen®) (10 IU/kg IM q24h for 3 days), a man-made form of granulocyte colony-stimulating factor, has been used anecdotally in some cases with some degree of success. The administration of interferon of avian origin derived from poultry cell cultures (10^6 IU IM for 90 days), together with nebulization for 15 minutes once daily of F10SC (Health and Hygiene) (1:125), in African greys with PBFD (unknown age of the birds and form of the disease) is reported to have resulted in clearance of the infection in seven out of 10 birds.

Further reading

Schoemaker NJ, Dorrestein GM, Latimer KS *et al.* (2000) Severe leukopenia and liver necrosis in young African grey parrots (*Psittacus erithacus erithacus*) infected with psittacine circovirus. *Avian Dis* **44(2)**:470–478.

Stanford M (2004) Interferon treatment of circovirus infection in grey parrots (*Psittacus erithacus*). *Vet Rec* **154**:435–436.

CASE 30

1 What is *Hexamita meleagridis* (*Spironucleus meleagridis*)? *Hexamita meleagridis* is a single celled protozoan; it has a single flagellum, which helps to make it motile. It inhabits the gastrointestinal tract of both pheasants and partridges and is often found in healthy birds in very low numbers, but its population will dramatically increase in sick animals. These protozoa can only be seen via a microscope.

2 What are the clinical signs observed in partridges and pheasants, and why do these signs occur? Pheasants and partridges would both show similar signs including weak staggering birds, a 'tucked up' appearance, diarrhea, severe weight loss, and increased mortality. Although there has been very little work undertaken on the life cycle and pathogenicity of this protozoan, it is understood from serology taken during a study from the Game & Wildlife Conservation Trust (GWCT) that birds suffering with this disease enter a period of starvation when they do not eat or drink and eventually die. On postmortem examination, the birds are emaciated and severely dehydrated and their ceca are often enlarged and gaseous (30).

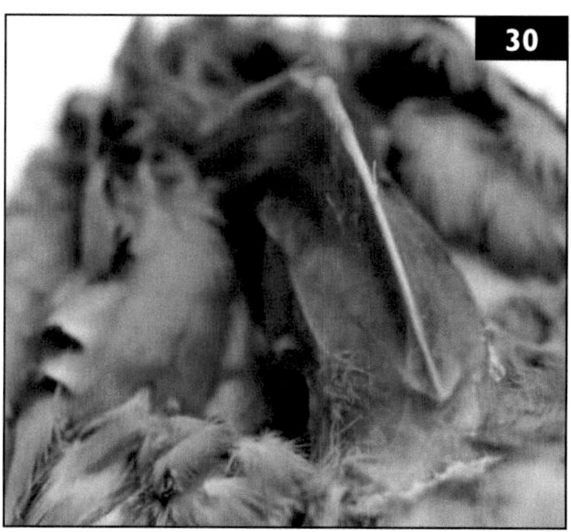

3 How is this disease diagnosed and controlled? Clinical signs are often highly suggestive; however, the only diagnostic method currently available is to necropsy the bird and perform an intestinal scrape at four points along the digestive tract: duodenum, jejunum, ileum, and ceca. Examination of the scrapes under the microscope usually reveals a high concentration of motile protozoa in the shape of a tear drop; usually the single flagellum can also be seen. Control can often be challenging as there is no licenced product in the UK to treat the disease. For this reason, emphasis should be placed on preventing the disease. This disease is often secondary to stress, so understanding the management of game birds and how to reduce stress is key to controlling this disease. The only treatment that shows efficacy in the majority of cases is tiamulin in food or water, often combined with a tetracycline based antibiotic for 5–7 days.

Further reading

Wood M, Smith HV (2005) *Spironucleosis* (Hexamitiasis, Hexamitosis) in the ring-necked pheasant (*Phasianus colchicus*): detection of cysts and description of *Spironucleus meleagridis* in stained smears. *Avian Dis* **49(1)**:138–143.

CASE 31

1 Based on the physical examination findings and the features of the ultrasound images, what is the cause of the coelomic distension in this hen? **31a** illustrates the presence of a large elliptical mixed echogenicity mass with a layering appearance. **31b** illustrates the same structure seen in **31a** just caudal to a normal ovarian follicle, supporting normal ovarian activity. The presumptive diagnosis in this case is oviduct impaction.

2 What is the proposed pathophysiology of this condition in laying hens? Oviduct impaction can occur secondary to salpingitis, metritis, dystocia, cystic hyperplasia of the oviduct (with secondary excessive production of mucin or albumin), or accumulation of inspissated egg material. In chickens, the condition is most commonly seen in older laying hens and presumed to be secondary to weakening of the oviduct muscle due to repeated laying, resulting in increased probability of bacterial migration from the cloaca during egg development and/or oviposition. Several bacteria have been implicated including *E. coli*, *S. aureus*, *Klebsiella pneumoniae* and *Salmonella* spp.

3 **Describe the treatment options (medical and/or surgical) for this case.** Supportive treatment should be initiated with parenteral fluid therapy, nutritional support, and broad-spectrum antibiotic therapy (pending results of culture and sensitivity of the inspissated yolk material). Due to the caseous nature of the material impacting the oviduct (**31c**), medical management alone is not likely to be successful. Surgical removal of the yolk material via salpingotomy and possible salpingohysterectomy is recommended and is often successful for treatment in cases without yolk peritonitis and adhesions.

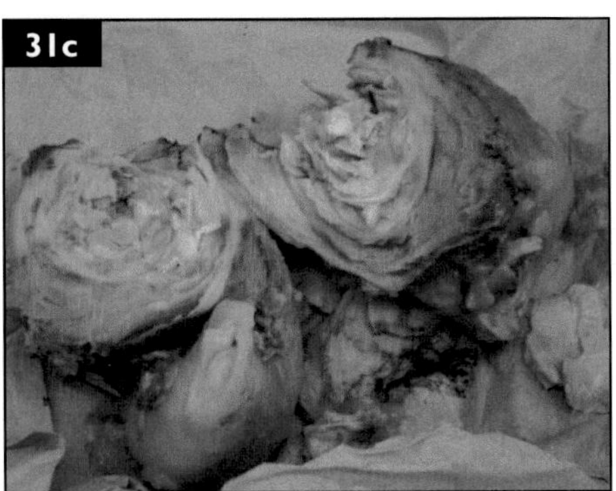
31c

Further reading

Bowles H (2006) Evaluating and treating the reproductive system. In: *Clinical Avian Medicine*. (eds. GJ Harrison, TL Lightfoot) Spix Publishing, Palm Beach, pp. 519–539.

Gingerich E, Shaw D (2015) Reproductive diseases. In: *Backyard Poultry Medicine and Surgery*. (eds. C Greenacre, T Morishita) Wiley, Ames, pp. 169–180.

Mison M, Mehler S, Echols M *et al.* (2016) Selected coelomic surgical procedures. In: *Current Therapy in Avian Medicine and Surgery*. (ed. BL Speer) Elsevier, St. Louis, pp. 645–657.

CASE 32

1 **What are your main differential diagnoses?** The findings are suggestive of bacterial pneumonia and septicemia. Other possible causes of acute pneumonia that should be ruled out are toxicity (e.g. Teflon), and viruses (e.g. paramyxovirus, orthomyxovirus).

2 **How would you confirm them?** A sterile swab was taken from the lung and pericardium and cultured by standard technique. There was a pure growth of

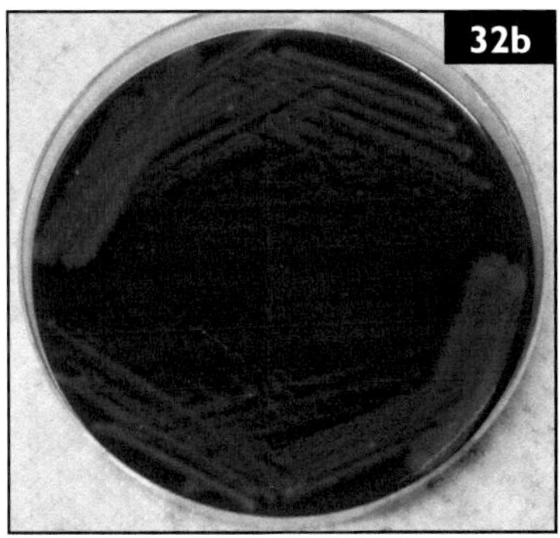
32b

large, irregular, greenish colored colonies (shown is blood agar plate after 24 hours of incubation [**32b**]). The bacterium was strongly oxidase positive and had a marked grape smell. Biochemical testing confirmed the presumptive diagnosis of *Pseudomonas aeruginosa*. Furthermore, histopathology

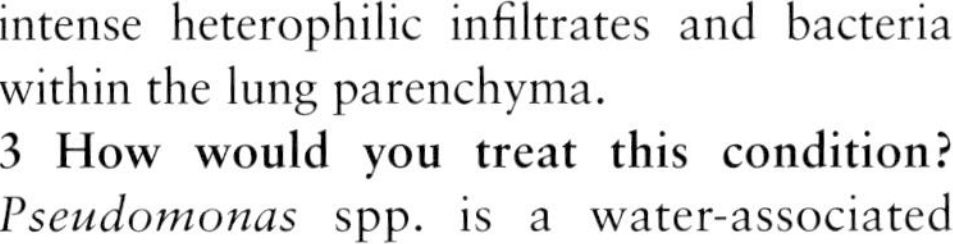

showed a severely congested lung, with intense heterophilic infiltrates and bacteria within the lung parenchyma.

3 How would you treat this condition? *Pseudomonas* spp. is a water-associated bacterium. Although it is an opportunistic pathogen, it can cause severe disease and even peracute death. Even with aggressive supportive therapy and appropriate antibiotic treatment, the prognosis is always guarded. The use of piperacillin, alone or in combination with tazobactam and/or with aminoglycosides (e.g. amikacin), is recommended; however, amikacin is associated with renal damage and must be used with care. Investigations in respect of water source, storage, and delivery (e.g. hosepipes, natural water supplies, untreated water, and uncovered storage tanks) and hygiene (especially during warmer months) are required.

Further reading

Garner M (2003) Aeromoniasis and pseudomoniasis. In: *Zoo and Wild Animal Medicine*, 5th edn. (eds. RE Miller, MR Fowler) Elsevier, St Louis, pp. 702–705.

Ritchie BW (1995) Paramyxoviridae and Orthomyxoviridae. In: *Avian Viruses: Function and Control*. (ed. BW Ritchie) Wingers Publishing, Inc., Lake Worth, pp. 253–283, 351–364.

CASE 33

1 How long should avian patients be fasted prior to anesthesia? Fasting duration is related to species, food consumption, and clinical status of the bird. Small birds (canaries, budgerigars, lovebirds) may be fasted for 3–6 hours. Large birds (>500 g) may be fasted for 12 hours or longer in some cases. Water is offered up to 2–3 hours before induction. The aim is to avoid anesthetizing any bird that does not have an empty crop, except in emergency situations. Birds with significant crop content may require their crop to be emptied using a gavage tube. Otherwise, the head should be kept elevated above the crop during induction and intubation, and packing of the pharynx should be performed.

2 What preanesthetic evaluation should be considered? Prior to anesthesia, a comprehensive history and a complete physical examination should be conducted. Initial assessment should focus on evaluating the cardiopulmonary function (mucous membranes, vein refill time, auscultation, respiratory rate), body condition, and hydration status. As a generalization, the minimal clinicopathologic database includes PCV, total protein, and blood glucose. CBC, chemistry panel, and other tests are performed according to the bird's condition. Each patient should be considered individually and the clinical approach should be adjusted accordingly.

3 What premedication may be considered? Depending on the procedure anticipated, prior to gas induction, analgesia may be provided with butorphanol. Butorphanol has been shown to lower the minimum anesthetic concentration (MAC) in some parrot species. Benzodiazepines produce dose-dependent sedative-hypnosis and muscle relaxation. They are used as anxiolytics to facilitate induction and for minor nonpainful procedures. Midazolam may be administered (0.1–1 mg/kg SC or IM) for sedative purposes. Midazolam given IN (0.5–2 mg/kg) provides fast and reliable sedation in budgerigars. In Hispaniolan Amazon parrots, administration of midazolam IN yields sedative effects within 3 minutes of administration, with vocalization, flight, and defense responses significantly reduced during capture. If surgery or procedures involving the head, eyes, or neck of the patient are anticipated, glycopyrrolate (0.01 mg/kg SC, IM, or IV) or atropine (0.02–0.08 mg/kg SC, IM or IV) is advised in order to prevent vagal induced bradycardia.

Further reading

Heard DJ (2000) Avian anesthesia. In: *Manual of Avian Medicine*. (eds. GH Olsen, SE Orsoz) Mosby, St. Louis, pp. 464–492.

Mans C, Guzman DS, Lahner LL *et al.* (2012) Sedation and physiologic response to manual restraint after intranasal administration of midazolam in Hispaniolan Amazon parrots (*Amazona ventralis*). *J Avian Med Surg* **26**(3):130–139.

Sadeg AB (2013) Comparison of intranasal administration of xylazine, diazepam, and midazolam in budgerigars (*Melopsittacus undulatus*): clinical evaluation. *J Zoo Wildlife Med* **44**(2):241–244.

CASE 34

1 Based on the history and clinical findings described, list three significant differential diagnoses. (1) Pseudomoniasis, caused by *Pseudomonas aeruginosa*; (2) trichomoniasis, caused by *Trichomonas gallinae*; (3) candidiasis, most likely caused by *Candida albicans*.

2 What diagnostic tests would you perform to confirm the diagnosis? (1) Stain wet smears obtained from the oropharynx using a rapid stain (e.g. Diff-Quik™), methylene blue stain, or Giemsa stain. (2) Bacterial and fungal culture.
3 Microbiological cultures yielded pure growths of *Pseudomonas aeruginosa*, which were suspected to have occurred subsequent to a prior *Trichomonas* infection. What therapeutic management would you establish for the *Pseudomonas* spp. infection? Provide nutritional support by gavage feeding two or three times a day as necessary in order to maintain or gain weight. Based on the sensitivity test, the antibiotics recommended included piperacillin (100 mg/kg q12h) on its own or in combination with tobramycin (10 mg/kg IM q12h for 7–10 days). Débride the caseous masses and spray the oropharynx with a 1% povidone–iodine mouthwash preparation. In birds with unilateral or bilateral sinusitis, use a solution of chlorhexidine (0.2 ml of a 5% preparation diluted to 20 ml with sterile saline) or F10 (Health and Hygiene) (1:250) to flush the affected sinus q12h for 3–5 days.

Further reading

Samour J (2000) *Pseudomonas aeruginosa* stomatitis as a sequel to trichomoniasis in captive saker falcons (*Falco cherrug*). *J Avian Med Surg* **14(2)**:113–117.

CASE 35

1 What common diseases could produce anorexia and the passing of green urates in falcons? Columbid herpesvirus 1, lead toxicosis, amyloidosis, *Escherichia coli* septicemia, aspergillosis.
2 What laboratory diagnostic tests you would require to establish a definitive diagnosis? Essential testing includes hematology, blood chemistry, and survey radiographs. Additional testing includes endoscopy and liver biopsy together with histopathology, microbiology, PCR testing, and serology testing.
3 How would you proceed in the light of these findings? Avian influenza is an infectious disease transmitted by a virus of the family Orthomyxoviridae and is a notifiable disease. Avian influenza virus phenotypes H5, H7, and H9 represent a high pandemic potential. The relevant authorities should be notified of the findings. The virus is commonly transmitted through direct contact with feces and aerosols from infected birds and through contaminated water in overcrowded ponds and lakes. Adequate disinfection of the premises where the falcon was examined and housed overnight should be undertaken.

Further reading

Samour J, Naldo JL, Wernery U *et al.* (2007) Avian influenza infection in saker falcons (*Falco cherrug*). *Proc Europ Assoc Avian Vet Conf*, Zurich, pp. 155–162.

CASE 36

1 What is the most likely cause for the elevated AST in this patient? AST is found in both the liver and muscle, as well as in red blood cells. Therefore, elevations in this parameter could correlate with disease in either system. With the severe elevation in CK, which is only found in muscle, the AST elevation is most consistent with recent muscle damage due to trauma from the dog bite. In birds, the half-life of AST is twice as long as the half-life of CK, which is also longer than in LDH. Therefore, depending on the time interval between muscle injury and blood collection, the CK may have returned to normal while the AST is still elevated.

2 Can liver disease be ruled out as a cause for the elevated AST? What other values could be tested to rule in or out liver disease? Liver disease cannot be ruled out as the bird could have concurrent muscle and liver damage. Blood should also be collected to look at other liver parameters such as bile acids, which will give additional information on liver function. However, it is common to have active liver cellular damage prior to any effect on liver function (bile acid). Other liver values such as GGT could be measured, although GGT is not a very sensitive indicator of liver disease. A very sensitive indicator of liver injury, LDH would not be helpful to differentiate between liver and muscle damage, as LDH is found in liver and muscle and also the half-life is too short to be of significant value.

3 Apart from muscle trauma such as a dog bite, in what other situations is it common to see elevated CK levels in avian patients? CK concentrations will also be elevated following IM injections and in situations where a patient is losing body mass (e.g. weight reduction due to muscle breakdown).

Further reading

Fudge AM (2000) Laboratory reference ranges for selected avian, mammalian, and reptilian species. In: *Laboratory Medicine Avian and Exotic Pets*. (ed. AM Fudge) WB Saunders, Philadelphia, pp. 375–400.

Lumeij JT, De Bruijne JJ, Slob A *et al.* (1988) Enzyme activities in tissues and elimination half-lives of homologous muscle and liver enzymes in the racing pigeon (*Columba livia domestica*). *Avian Pathol* **17(4)**:851–864.

Lumeij JT, Meidam M, Wolfswinkel J *et al.* (1998) Changes in plasma chemistry after drug-induced liver disease or muscle necrosis in racing pigeons (*Columba livia domestica*). *Avian Pathol* **17(4)**:865–874.

CASE 37

1 Which species of *Aspergillus* are causative agents of respiratory aspergillosis in psittacine birds? What is the commonest source of infection? *Aspergillus fumigatus, A. flavus, A. niger, A. terreus*. The commonest source of infection in parrots is contaminated seed-based diets that have been harvested or stored with a moisture content of >17%. Seed batches with weevil contamination are at particular risk.

The weevil lays eggs in the sunflower seed. When the egg hatches, the weevil beetle bores its way out of the seed, leaving a hole for moisture to enter and create a suitable environment for *Aspergillus* spp. spores to develop.

2 How you would treat a psittacine bird with respiratory aspergillosis? What should be considered regarding the different drugs? Combination therapy using systemic and topical or nebulized agents is beneficial for the treatment of aspergillosis. Administration of amphotericin B is advised initially as an IV bolus, due to its rapid fungicidal effect, but care should be taken in dehydrated patients or those with pre-existing renal disease as amphotericin B is potentially nephrotoxic. Further systemic therapy options include agents of the azole family (e.g. voriconazole, itraconazole). The modern avian licensed itraconazole formulation (Fungitraxx®, Petlife International) has a far superior respiratory tissue level compared with the human version previously used in birds. Systemic drugs may be used in conjunction with topical nebulizable agents such as F10 (Health and Hygiene) or enilconazole (Imaverol: Elanco) delivered 3–4 times daily for periods of 15–20 minutes. Direct application of antifungal drugs such as clotrimazole, enilconazole, or F10 to endoscopically visualized fungal plaques is also beneficial in controlling lesions. As aspergillosis often occurs in birds with immunosuppression, environmental conditions should always be improved as well (housing, nutrition, treatment of concurrent diseases, air hygiene).

3 Which antifungal drug has been shown to cause adverse reactions in African grey parrots suffering from aspergillosis? Which alternate systemic antifungal drugs may be used for aspergillosis in these birds? The first-generation triazole itraconazole has been shown to be poorly tolerated in some psittacine birds and may be toxic in affected species. The second-generation triazole voriconazole (VFend®, Pfizer) and the allylamine drug terbinafine hydrochloride may be used in sensitive patients (e.g. African grey parrots) and seem to be well tolerated.

Further reading

Girling SJ (2005) Respiratory disease. In: *BSAVA Manual of Psittacine Birds*, 2nd edn. (eds. N Harcourt-Brown, J Chitty) British Small Animal Veterinary Association, Gloucester, pp. 170–179.

CASE 38

1 What would be included in your differential diagnoses for this case? Differential diagnoses for chronic regurgitation and crop enlargement include infectious diseases affecting the upper gastrointestinal system, gastrointestinal foreign bodies, traumatic injuries or burns, heavy metal toxicity, neoplasia, or crop stasis as a result of metabolic and systemic conditions such as dehydration or renal disease. Increased respiratory effort that is mostly expressed in inspiration indicates upper respiratory tract disorders. Differentials for this include infectious diseases of the trachea or the nasal cavity, mechanical obstruction by foreign material, exposure to irritating substances (such as smoke or aerosols), trauma, stricture of the trachea or nares, granuloma, and neoplasia. Mechanical tracheal compression may result from enlargement of the thyroid gland. Thyroid goiter of a nutritional etiology is the most common thyroid pathology in birds, and has been described primarily in budgerigars. Budgerigars with goiter usually do not present with clinical signs of hypothyroidism; presentation is rather a progressive dyspnea, commencing with a clicking noise as the bird breathes.

2 What diagnostic tests could be of aid in diagnosis? Radiographs may demonstrate compression and even displacement of the trachea by a soft tissue mass. Due to lack of specific diagnostic tests, diagnosis of goiter relies on clinical signs, diet history, and presentation. Budgerigars suffering from goiter do not have clinical signs or changes in thyroid levels characteristic of hypothyroidism, therefore there would be little use for a thyroid hormone panel.

3 What would be included in your treatment plan? This bird presented with increased respiratory effort and might benefit from oxygen until stabilized. Long-term supplementation of iodine solution, such as Lugol's iodine (1 drop of 0.3% Lugol solution per 20 mL of water daily for the first week, three times a week for the second week, then weekly), may be used to restore iodine status, which will lead to a decrease in the thyroid size and resolution of clinical signs. A conversion to a diet based on at least 75% commercial formulated pellets is recommended to decrease the risk of concurrent nutritional deficiencies.

Further reading

Merryman JI, Buckles EL (1998) The avian thyroid gland. Part two: a review of function and pathophysiology. *J Avian Med Surg* **12**:238–242.

CASE 39

1 Describe the radiographic findings. What should the radiographic size for the heart be in medium to large-size parrots? What is the radiographic appearance of the heart in cockatoos? There is a severe enlargement of the cardiac silhouette visible on both the ventrodorsal and lateral views. There is no evidence of ascites and the pulmonary field appears clear or with a slight parabronchial pattern (honeycomb appearance more marked). In medium to large-size Psittaciformes, the radiographic cardiac size on a ventrodorsal radiographic view should comprise 51–61% of the thoracic width at its widest point. This may be slightly affected by respiratory stage at the time of obtaining the radiographs. In large cockatoos, an air sac diverticulum from the interclavicular air sac is seen between the heart and the sternum, which is visible on a lateral radiographic view. In this cockatoo, the air space between the heart and the sternum is diminished and the heart is in contact with the sternum, which is abnormal for the species.

2 Describe the echocardiographic findings. What do you know about the reliability of echocardiographic measurements in birds? What is the differential diagnosis for these findings? What is the likely cause for the respiratory signs? There is a severely enlarged left atrium and mild pericardial effusion. The ventricles are considered to be of normal size. On the color Doppler images (not shown), there was a large amount of turbulence at the left atrioventricular valve. Together, these changes may be caused by left atrioventricular insufficiency or stenosis. The most likely cause for the dyspnea noted at presentation would be pulmonary edema or decreased cardiac output. The bird was eventually euthanized and necropsy confirmed the presence of left atrioventricular stenosis and pulmonary edema. Echocardiographic measurements in birds have been shown to be of low reliability overall with low interobserver agreement. This is due to the small structures imaged and the fast heart rate. Consequently, published reference values should be used with caution.

3 What other clinical signs are common in companion psittacine birds with this condition? In pet birds, right heart or bilateral heart failure is typically common and classically manifests with exercise intolerance, ascites, hepatic congestion, pericardial effusion, dyspnea from air sac compression, and valvular insufficiency.

Further reading

Beaufrere H, Pariaut R, Rodriguez D *et al.* (2012) Comparison of transcoelomic, contrast transcoelomic, and transesophageal echocardiography in anesthetized red-tailed hawk (*Buteo jamaicensis*). *Am J Vet Res* **73**(**10**):1560–1568.

Krautwald-Junghanns M-E, Pees M, Schroff S (2011) Cardiovascular system. In: *Diagnostic Imaging of Exotic Pets*. (eds. M-E Krautwald-Junghanns, M. Pees, S. Reese, T. Tully) Schlutersche Verlagsgesellschaft mbH & Co., Hanover, pp. 84–91.

Pees M, Krautwald-Junghanns M-E (2009) Cardiovascular physiology and diseases of pet birds. *Vet Clin North Am Exot Anim Pract* **12**(**1**):81–97.

CASE 40

1 What is your presumptive diagnosis? Protozoal enteritis, possibly due to *Giardia* spp. Several typical flagellate trophozoites and cysts can be observed in the fecal cytology. Budding yeasts are also apparent.

2 What additional examination would you request? PCR testing of the stools confirmed the diagnosis of giardiasis. A complete blood panel would help to assess the overall clinical condition of the bird and, more importantly, the severity of the anemia due to the blood loss.

3 How would you treat this condition? This condition should be treated with metronidazole (50 mg/kg PO q12h for 5 days) and supportive therapy. In severe cases of anemia (PCV <15% [0.15 L/L]), blood transfusions may be necessary. The yeast infection also requires treatment with nystatin (300,000 IU/kg PO q12h for 7–14 days). Fecal cytology should be used to monitor the response to the treatment.

Further reading

Dislich M (2014) Piciformes. In: *Tratado de Animais Selvagens*, 2nd edn. (eds. ZS Cubas, JCR Silva, JL Catão-Dias) Roca, São Paulo, pp. 598–625.

CASE 41

1 What initial data, information, and material do you request? All breeding records should be requested. This should include the numbers and identification of all male and female breeding birds, the dates and numbers of eggs laid by each female and the outcome of each egg (fertile, not fertile, hatch, or dead in shell), the dates of all artificial inseminations (in this case all nonhatched eggs had been stored and were made available for postmortem examination), and all closed-circuit television footage from the whole breeding season. For each falcon, calculate the numbers of eggs laid and the fertility and hatchability levels. Then calculate the fertility and hatchability levels for both naturally breeding falcons and imprint (artificially inseminated) falcons during all three periods of time (prior to over fly, during incubation at time of overfly, laid and incubated after over fly). In this case, there was no change in fertility between the three time periods, but a dramatic increase in dead in shells, which only affected eggs under parents, but not those in incubators, at the time of the over fly. Examination of closed-circuit television footage from the date showed eggs being deserted for an average of 6.5 hours, an excessive period for gyr eggs during the first third of incubation. It is well reported that birds react more to helicopters than other aircraft. The disturbance is greater when they are not habituated to overflights, and the lower the aircraft the greater the effect. A repeated fly over in close succession will have a greater effect than the sum of two individual events.

2 At what stage of incubation are eggs most likely to suffer? Helicopter over flights have been shown to cause egg losses due to vibration and chilling subsequent to parental desertion. Both forms of loss are commonest during the first third of incubation, as eggs are most sensitive to these effects at this stage.

3 You realize that you cannot accurately calculate the losses. Why? Acceptance of liability (and number of chicks lost) and agreement on quantum are two entirely different stages of the process. The value of juvenile gyrfalcons is very much dependent on the exact parentage (i.e. species of hybrid, if not pure gyr), the sex, and the color. As in all diurnal raptors, the female is 30% larger and hence more desirable and valuable for hunting. Moreover, in respect of the color of pure gyr, gray is ordinary, white is special, and black extremely special. So performing egg autopsies and calculating the number of eggs lost is just part of the story and egg autopsy material must not be discarded. DNA analysis should be used to verify parentage and sex, as this is highly relevant in respect of the quantum of financial losses. A pure bred black gyrfalcon (i.e. female) is likely to be worth up to 15 times more than a gray gyrkin (male).

Further reading

Manci KM, Gladwin DN, Villella R *et al.* (1988) *Effects of Aircraft Noise and Sonic Booms on Domestic Animals and Wildlife: A Literature Synthesis.* U.S. Fish and Wildlife Service National Ecology Research Center, Fort Collins, NERC-88/29.

Ruddock M, Whitfield DP (2007) *A Review of Disturbance Distances in Selected Bird Species.* A Report from Natural Research (Projects) Ltd to Scottish Natural Heritage.

CASE 42

1 What is the most likely differential diagnosis in this case? Lead toxicity is the main differential as metallic opacities are visualized in the coelom in association with compatible clinical signs such as hemoglobinuria and digestive and neurologic signs. The metallic opacities are most likely ingested heavy metal-containing particles.

2 What complementary test do you perform to confirm this suspicion? Blood lead concentration should be measured: in Psittaciformes, a concentration higher than 0.2 ppm (0.97 µmol/L or 20 µg/dL) is suggestive of toxicity and concentrations higher than 0.4 ppm (1.93 µmol/L or 40 µg/dL) with compatible clinical signs are considered diagnostic. If the bird is seen as an emergency and this test is not readily available, the level of suspicion can be raised by a complete blood cell count showing anemia, variable level of polychromasia, and displaced erythrocyte nuclei. A mild leukocytosis is a common feature in lead toxicity cases. Basophilic stippling is rare in lead-intoxicated birds compared with mammals.

3 What treatment would you recommend? (1) Preventing further absorption. If particles are in the crop or proventriculus, then with the bird anesthetized and intubated, a red-rubber tube is passed PO into the proventriculus. With the tail elevated in relation to the head, the gastrointestinal tract is flushed with warm saline. This procedure is straightforward and relatively safe. An alternative is endoscopic removal through the oropharyngeal cavity, but this would be limited to the upper gastrointestinal tract since the intestines could not be reached. Any particles remaining after the above procedures could potentially be managed medically with gavage feeding with almond butter, peanut butter, magnesium sulfate, and psyllium. Fine grit has been shown to facilitate lead fragmentation of small particles in the ventriculus. Surgery of the gastrointestinal tract would be a last resort.

(2) Providing antidote. Chelation of the lead salts with calcium disodium EDTA (35–50 mg/kg SC daily maintained until 5 days after the last particles are eliminated from the gastrointestinal tract) is the preferred treatment. If not available, D-penicillamine (30 mg/kg PO q12h PO) or dimercaptosuccinic acid (25–35 mg/kg PO q12h) may be administered until the lead concentration is within normal limits.

(3) Providing supportive care. Seizure control, fluid therapy, and nutritional support as needed.

Further reading

Campbell TW (2015) Peripheral blood of birds. In: *Exotic Animal Hematology and Cytology*, 4th edn. (ed. TW Campbell) Wiley-Blackwell, Ames, pp. 40–44.

Denver MC, Tell LA, Galey FD *et al.* (2000) Comparison of two heavy metal chelators for treatment of lead toxicosis in cockatiels. *Am J Vet Res* **61(8)**:935–940.

Dumonceaux G, Harrison GJ (1994) Toxins. In: *Avian Medicine: Principles and Application*. (eds. BW Ritchie, GJ Harrison, LR Harrison) Wingers Publishing, Lake Worth, pp. 1030–1052.

Lupu C (2009) Comparison of treatment protocols for removing metallic foreign objects from the ventriculus of budgerigars (*Melopsittacus undulatus*). *J Avian Med Surg* **23(3)**:186–193.

CASE 43

1 Name the primary bony abnormality present. There is a sequestrum, or necrotic bone fragment, present (**43c, d,** arrows)

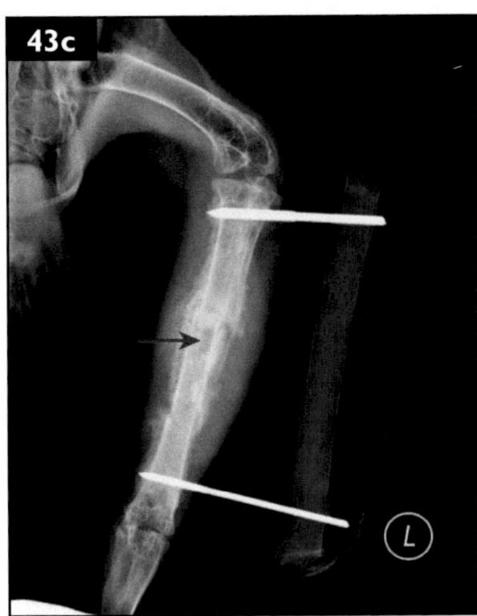

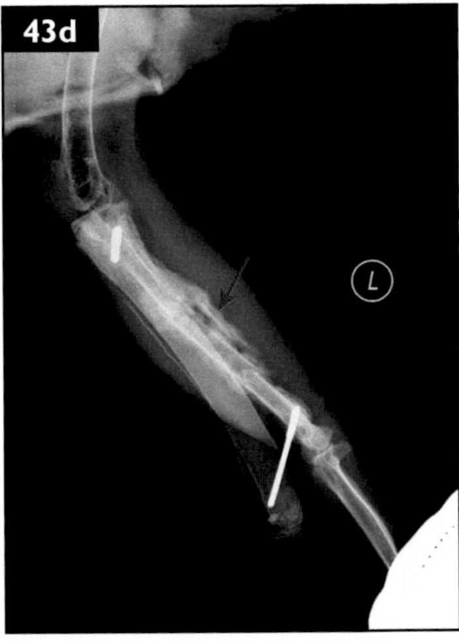

2 How would you treat this problem? A sequestrum forms when a lack of soft tissue attachments and adequate blood supply leads to bone fragment death. This necrotic fragment causes delayed bone healing and may lead to a nonunion. For small sequestra, treatment options include maintaining the fixator for a longer period of time, allowing for a delayed healing process, or surgical intervention to remove the necrotic bone fragment. Larger sequestra are more likely to require surgical removal. Infection may be associated with sequestra, and any bone fragments removed during surgery should be cultured.
3 How would you minimize the risk of developing this problem? Maintaining a sterile field during surgery, if a compound fracture, leaving no implants at the fracture site (e.g. use a traditional hybrid fixator pattern, but with two pins in each extremity). Once IM and ESF placement is complete, and alignment is assured, the IM element is removed so there is no foreign material close to where infection is likely to be present. Treating all soft tissue carefully, considering the risks associated with excessive tissue handling (loss of blood supply and introduction of infection), achieving longitudinal, lateral and rotational stability while minimizing all iatrogenic tissue damage. Removal of nonviable bone fragments during fracture fixation. Minimizing surgical time, so that the risk of tissue desiccation is reduced. The use of appropriate systemic or local antibiotics (e.g. antibiotic impregnated calcium sulfate beads) to treat potential osteomyelitis.

Further reading

Redig PT, Ponder J (2016) Management of orthopedic issues in birds. In: *Avian Medicine*, 3rd edn. (ed. J Samour). Mosby, St. Louis, pp. 312–350.

CASE 44

1 Which protozoal organism would you consider as a differential diagnosis? Extraintestinal *Isospora* spp., previously described as *Atoxoplasma* spp., a coccidian parasite with a complex life cycle that includes invasion of both the reticuloendothelial system and the intestinal epithelium. Birds become infected after ingesting sporulated oocysts. Merogony (asexual reproduction) occurs in both intestinal and lymphoid–macrophage cells, resulting in the presence of merozoites in the mononuclear leukocytes of the peripheral blood and dissemination to other viscera. Gametogenesis occurs in the intestinal cells of the same host. *Atoxoplasma* infections have been observed in a wide variety of passerine birds including canaries, sparrows, finches, mynahs, starlings, and thrushes.
2 How would you evaluate whether the rest of the flock is affected by the same parasite? Standard fecal flotation using centrifugation with Sheathers's sugar solution will allow visualization of coccidial oocysts in the feces, but due to the lack of correlation between the presence of oocysts in feces and the infected lymphocytes

by merozoites, it is advisable to examine a blood smear or a buffy coat smear to allow detection of the parasites infecting lymphocytes. At necropsy, impression smears of the liver, spleen, and lungs should be made. The parasite merozoites can then be identified, appearing crescent shaped in the nucleus of the host cell. PCR techniques from blood, feces, or tissue may be more sensitive.

3 What treatment would you consider, and what is the main limitation of this treatment? Toltrazuril (12.5 mg/kg PO or 2 mg/L drinking water for 2 consecutive days each week) or sulfachloropyrazine or sulfachlorpyridazine (150–300 mg/L for 5 consecutive days per week) for prolonged periods (1 month or more) have been proven to reduce the number of oocysts in the feces, but will not affect the intracellular parasites. There is still no effective treatment that completely clears isosporid coccidians from extraintestinal stages within a host species. Quarantine, population control, improved hygiene, and suspended flights are recommended. Hand-rearing may under certain circumstances be a viable control method.

Further reading

Greiner EC (2014) *Isospora, Atoxoplasma*, and *Sarcocystis*. In: *Parasitic Diseases of Wild Birds*. (eds. CT Atkinson, NJ Thomas, DB Hunter) Wiley-Blackwell, Ames, pp. 108–119.

CASE 45

1 What would be your nutritional assessment of this diet? The current diet is most likely unbalanced and does not provide the necessary nutrients for adequate growth of a young chick. Appropriate diet formulation requires knowledge and expertise to avoid deficiencies, therefore most home-prepared diets are usually inadequate unless formulated by a professional to ensure adequacy. While the current diet may be tolerated by the bird and provides energy and fat, which are necessary for survival, other nutrients that are necessary for growth are likely deficient.

2 What would be your dietary recommendation in light of the presentation? Commercial bird hand-rearing products are formulated according to known avian requirements for growth. One study found that commercial diets may be lower in several minerals and amino acids than samples of wild macaw crop content. Even so, the likelihood of nutritional deficiencies is much higher in home-prepared diets compared with formulated commercial products. The presented bird may benefit from transition to a commercial diet, especially in light of the delay in development.

3 List the important considerations in the diet preparation and feeding regimen of a young macaw chick? Water content, temperature, and consistency are important factors in preparation of hand-rearing formulas. It is also important that the diet is well mixed and prepared just prior to feeding to avoid separation of the solids, as this may lead to delayed crop emptying and impaction. Temperature is critical for acceptance and to prevent thermal damage with 100–105°F (37.8–40.6°C) the recommended temperature range. Method of feeding may be by spoon, syringe, or by a tube inserted into the crop. Tube insertion should be performed by experienced breeders or handlers to avoid risk of placing the tube in the trachea. Younger birds should be fed more often than older birds. Birds 1–5 days old should be fed 5–6 times daily. One- to two-week-old birds may be fed 4–5 times a day and birds older than 3 weeks may be fed three times a day. This regimen may be altered according to development and weight gain, and more frequent feedings may be needed to meet energy requirements. Regular assessment of body weight and body condition and regular physical examinations are necessary to establish if the energy and nutritional requirements are being met.

Further reading

Cornejo J, Dierenfeld ES, Bailey CA *et al.* (2013) Nutritional and physical characteristics of commercial hand-feeding formulas for parrots. *Zoo Biol* **32**:469–475.

CASE 46

1 What disease process is suspected in this patient? Is there an additional biochemical analyte that should be checked? Based on the elevated AST and LDH values with a normal CK, liver disease is suspected. The additional finding of an elevated cholesterol with the clinical signs, history of an all seed diet, presence of obesity, and lipomas makes hepatic lipidosis likely. Bile acids should be submitted to further support the suspicion of liver disease because they are a specific and sensitive indicator of hepatic function. Elevations in bile acids have been shown to have the highest correlation with confirmed compromise of liver function when compared with AST and LDH. This patient's bile acid concentration was significantly elevated at 161.9 mmol/L (63.56 mg/mL) (reference interval in *Amazona* spp. 33–154 mmol/L [12.96–60.5 mg/mL]), further supporting the suspicion of hepatic disease.

2 How do the yellow urates correlate with the blood work findings? Hepatic dysfunction can lead to biliverdinemia, which can cause biliverdinuria, or a yellow–green discoloration to the urates and/or urine. Because birds lack biliverdin reductase, they do not produce bilirubinemia or bilirubinuria as seen in mammals with hepatic dysfunction.

3 What additional diagnostic tests could be performed to confirm the suspected disease in this patient? For a definitive diagnosis of hepatic lipidosis, fine needle aspiration or biopsy (either surgically, endoscopically, or ultrasound guided) is required. Caution must be taken with liver sample collection as animals with hepatic dysfunction may also have impaired clotting ability, leading to excessive bleeding.

Further reading

Beaufrère H, Cray C, Ammersbach M *et al.* (2014) Association of plasma lipid levels with atherosclerosis prevalence in psittaciformes. *J Avian Med Surg* **28(3)**:225–231.

Cray C, Gautier D, Harris DJ *et al.* (2008) Changes in clinical enzyme activity and bile acid levels in psittacine birds with altered liver function and disease. *J Avian Med Surg* **22(1)**:17–24.

Fudge AM (2000) Laboratory reference ranges for selected avian, mammalian, and reptilian species. In: *Laboratory Medicine Avian and Exotic Pets.* (ed. AM Fudge) WB Saunders, Philadelphia, pp. 375–400.

Grunkemeyer, Vanessa L (2010) Advanced diagnostic approaches and current management of avian hepatic disorders. *Vet Clin North Am Exot Anim Pract* **13(3)**:413–427.

CASE 47

1 What is the most likely diagnosis? The radiographs were consistent with diskospondylitis. The extent of the condition was confirmed by CT. The lower spinal structures are affected. The common site for this presentation in birds is at the level of the one mobile vertebra in a bird's back, typically L3, a natural hinge point between the notarium and the synsacrum (**47c**).

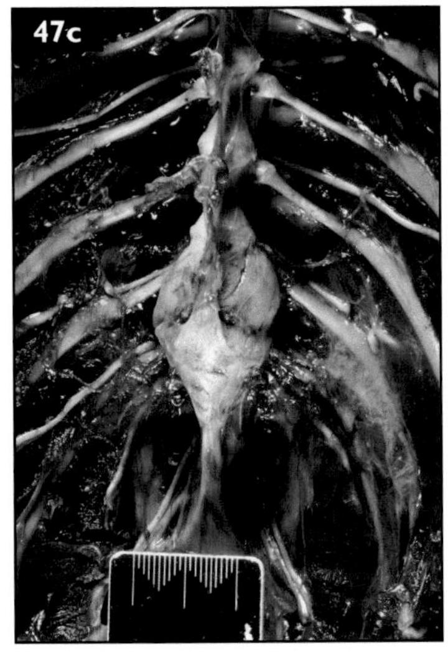
47c

2 What is the prognosis for this condition? Poor, once severe neurologic deficits (e.g. loss of deep pain perception) develop.

3 What is the most likely etiology? The diskospondylitis in this penguin was located at the mobile vertebra of the vertebral column between the notarium and the synsacrum. This single mobile vertebra in the bird's mid-spine (from notarium cranially to synsacrum caudally) region is a naturally weak point of the vertebral column; the vast majority of trauma and infection arises at this location. The reasons for this predisposition are unknown but higher vascularization, microtrauma, or a hinge effect between the notarium and the synsacrum can be speculated.

Further reading

Bergen DJ, Gartrell BD (2010) Discospondylitis in a yellow-eyed penguin (*Megadyptes antipodes*). *J Avian Med Surg* **24(1)**:58–63.

CASE 48

1 List some disadvantages and advantages associated with endosurgery compared with the more traditional open coeliotomy. Disadvantages: (1) The surgeon's hands are more distant from the bird to facilitate triangulation, resulting in reduced tactile feedback. (2) The surgeon has to use a 2-D monitor, making depth perception more difficult. (3) There are extra costs required in terms of equipment, additional training requirements, and the need for a mechanical arm or assistant to support the telescope.

Advantages: (1) There is reduced surgical access to the coelom resulting in less trauma to the coelomic body wall and air sac system. (2) The air sac system is not open and therefore improved intraoperative respiratory function is maintained. (3) The surgeon is able to perform the procedure using magnification and a focused light source for improved visualization. (4) Postoperative recoveries tend to be faster following endosurgical procedures.

Further reading

Divers SJ (2010) Avian endosurgery. *Vet Clin North Am Exot Anim Pract* **13(2)**:203–216.

CASE 49

1 How you would treat the grade 1/5 lesion? In a grade 1 lesion, there is no infection, simply a localized inflammatory response. In such cases, so long as the underlying cause is found and addressed, and the lesion treated topically (e.g. application of Preparation H or F10 Barrier Cream, daily for 7–10 days), it will resolve.

2 How would you treat the grade 3/5 lesion? In grade 3 lesions, infection is present, which is no longer just localized to the initial lesion. In this case there is significant firm caseous exudate between digits two and three that appears to have occurred following a penetrating wound to the plantar aspect. Where possible, bacterial culture and sensitivity testing should be conducted prior to surgery; this may not be possible in this case. The bird's general health should be assessed, in particular checking for any pathology on the contralateral leg, which might account for excessive weight bearing on this foot. The lesion is assessed and if deemed possible that there is any bone involvement, a radiograph of each foot should be taken and compared. The bird is anesthetized and the foot prepared for aseptic surgery. A tourniquet (e.g. finger of a surgical glove, clamped with hemostat forceps and twisted tight around the distal tarsometatarsus) may be required. An elliptical incision is made around the lesion on the plantar aspect, taking care not to alter the physiologic digital architecture. An attempt should be made to remove the lesion *in toto* by surgical and blunt dissection, without rupturing the capsule and thereby contaminating the surrounding tissue. If contamination does occur, the tissues should be irrigated and cleansed (e.g. saline, followed by F10 disinfectant [1:250, Health and Hygiene]). The wound edges are closed. A dressing is applied, akin to a large corn plaster, to relieve pressure from the area of the surgical site, instead taking weight on the bases of each digit. Systemic antibiotics are recommended. After removal of the exudate and infected tissue, part of the pyogenic membrane is submitted for culture and sensitivity testing. Once correct antibiotic therapy is assured, it is maintained for 3 weeks. Dressings are changed weekly, being kept dry in the interim.

3 How would you treat the grade 4–5/5 lesion? In grade 4–5/5 lesions, there is widespread infection and disruption of the bone and tendinous architecture of the foot. Radiographs should be taken to check for evidence of osteomyelitis. Culture and sensitivity testing is required prior to surgery. Surgery is then performed, the aim being to change an infected site into a clean site, which will heal by primary or secondary intention. If deeper structures are affected, the prognosis is at best poor. Success rates are optimized by the use of antibiotic impregnated bone cement or calcium sulfate beads (using an antibiotic in line with culture and sensitivity results). Pressure relieving dressings are mandatory following surgery (**49d**). Antibiosis should be maintained for at least 2 weeks after apparent healing and normality. The underlying cause of the problem needs to be considered and addressed.

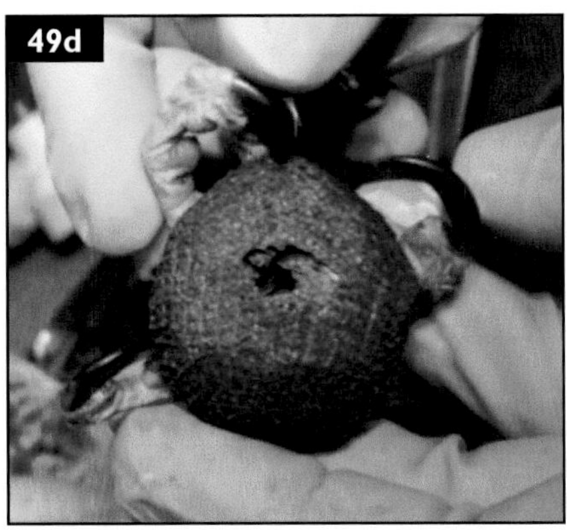
49d

Further reading

Bailey T, Lloyd C (2008) Raptors: disorders of the feet. In: *BSAVA Manual of Raptors, Pigeons and Passerine Birds*. (eds. J Chitty, M Lierz) British Small Animal Veterinary Association, Gloucester, pp. 176–189.

Remple JD, Forbes NA (2000) Antibiotic impregnated polymethyl methacrylate beads in the treatment of bumblefoot in raptors. In: *Raptor Biomedicine III*. (eds. JT Lumeij, JD Remple, PT Redig *et al*. Zoological Education Network, Palm Beach, pp. 255–266.

CASE 50

1 What physical examination findings can you use to estimate the hydration status? Decreased skin turgor is seen with dehydration; however, normal bird skin is relatively inelastic and will also be more difficult to assess in cachectic or obese patients. The skin turgor in birds can be evaluated in the upper eyelid. Dry or tacky oropharyngeal mucosa will also be seen with severe dehydration. Thick, stringy mucus may also be visualized within the oropharynx. Since birds have the ability to absorb significant amounts of ureteral water in the colon and ceca, dehydration can also lead to changes in the appearance of the droppings. Sunken eyes can be observed with profound (10%) dehydration. Therefore, in this patient, estimated to be 8–10% dehydrated, there is tackiness of the oropharyngeal mucosa with thick, stringy mucus visible, and the eyes are mildly sunken with a reduction in skin turgor appreciable.

2 What laboratory findings can help you confirm your findings from the physical examination? Hemoconcentration or an increase in PCV and total protein levels is consistent with dehydration. Elevations in BUN levels are a sensitive indicator of dehydration. Although BUN has little value in diagnosing renal disease in most birds, up to 99% of BUN undergoes tubular reabsorption in the dehydrated bird. Therefore, levels typically rise from negligible to 1.07–2.14 mmol/L (3–6 mg/dL). In contrast, uric acid excretion is largely independent of urine flow and therefore is unaffected by mild to moderate decreases in glomerular filtration; however, moderate to severe elevations in uric acid can be seen with severe dehydration and are also seen in carnivorous birds within 24 hours of consuming a meal. Hypernatremia is also consistent with fluid losses, as many clinical conditions associated with hypernatremia reflect hyperosmolality and hypertonicity of the extracellular fluid. Plasma osmolality can also help to confirm dehydration. Comparison of osmolality values in mammals and values reported in birds suggest that plasma osmolality is slightly higher in parrots than in mammals. Urine specific gravity (USG) is not very useful in birds, because the bird's ability to concentrate urine is limited and postrenal modification occurs with fluid absorption in the colon. USG collected directly from the ureters can range from 1.005 to 1.020 but is highly variable among species.

Further reading

Beaufrère H, Acierno M, Mitchell M *et al.* (2011) Plasma osmolality reference values in African grey parrots (*Psittacus erithacus erithacus*), Hispaniolan Amazon parrots (*Amazona ventralis*), and red-fronted macaws (*Ara rubrogenys*). *J Avian Med Surg* 25(2):91–96.

Carpenter JW, Marion CJ (2013) *Exotic Animal Formulary*. Elsevier Saunders, St. Louis, p. 332.

CASE 51

1 Provide at least three characteristic historical findings that are noted in many of the cockatoos presented with cloacal prolapse. In cockatoos with cloacal prolapse, characteristic historical findings may include: hand-rearing; delayed weaning; bonding to a specific person; and display of behaviors such as continued begging for food, sexual arousal and/or a tendency to hold feces for a prolonged period of time (which may have been stimulated further by potty training by the owner).

2 Describe the various treatment options that may be considered for these patients. Initial treatment should be aimed at maintaining tissue viability and restoring normal anatomy. Careful cleaning, irrigation, and lubrication (e.g. using a water-based lubricant) are deemed essential. Topical administration of dextrose 50% or dimethyl sulfoxide (DMSO) may be considered to reduce tissue swelling. Following reduction of the prolapse, placement of temporary or permanent stay sutures in the cloacal sphincter may be considered to prevent recurrence. It is important to ensure that the placed sutures allow the bird to defecate normally. Persistent or recurrent prolapses may require more extensive surgical intervention such as cloacopexy or cloacoplasty. In addition, the underlying cause should be addressed to prevent recurrence. In cases of cloacal prolapse that are suspected to have a behavioral origin, treatment requires modifications to the bird's living environment to derail the reproductive drive (e.g. adjusting photoperiod, diet, curtailing cavity seeking and courtship behaviors, and providing opportunities for physical exercise) as well as changes to the owner–bird relationship, whereby the owners should prevent their bird from excessively bonding to one person. Physical contact needs to be kept to a minimum, while reinforcing the bird for appropriate social interactive and food acquisition behaviors. In particular, stroking of the back and/or tail, cuddling and/or hand feeding need to be avoided. To ameliorate hormone-related behavior, hormone therapy using GnRH agonists (e.g. leuprolide acetate, deslorelin) may also be considered.

3 Which complication may commonly be seen in cockatoos with chronic cloacal prolapse, and how would this condition best be treated? The continued straining and cloacal prolapse may often result in distension and flaccidity of the cloacal sphincter. To correct this condition, a cloacoplasty (ventplasty) may be performed. Other complications that may occur include secondary (bacterial) infections, necrosis, and/or difficulties with urination and defecation.

Further reading

Bowles HL (2006) Evaluating and treating the reproductive system. In: *Clinical Avian Medicine*, Vol. 2. (eds. GJ Harrison, TL Lightfoot) Spix Publishing, Palm Beach, pp. 519–539.

van Zeeland YRA, Friedman SG, Bergman L (2016) Behavior. In: *Current Therapy in Avian Medicine and Surgery*. (ed. BL Speer) Elsevier, St. Louis, pp. 177–251.

Wilson L, Lightfoot T (2006) Concepts in behavior. Section III: Pubescent and adult psittacine behavior. In: *Clinical Avian Medicine*, Vol. 2. (eds. GJ Harrison, TL Lightfoot) Spix Publishing, Palm Beach, pp. 73–83.

CASE 52

1 What anatomic structure of the beak is present in *Falco* spp., but is absent in *Accipiter* spp. and *Buteo* spp.? Tomial tooth.

2 This structure allows members of the Falconiformes to perform what task when hunting? Dislocate the neck of the prey.

3 What is the ancient falconry term used for trimming the beak of falconry birds? Coping.

Further reading

Samour J (2006) Management of raptors. In: *Clinical Avian Medicine*, Vol. 2. (eds. GJ Harrison, TL Lightfoot) Spix Publishing, Palm Beach, pp. 915–956.

CASE 53

1 What is the possible cause for the bone marrow suppression? The benzimidazoles bind to the parasitic tubulin, thus inhibiting microtubule polymerization in the parasite cytoskeleton. The affinity of benzimidazole anthelmintics to parasitic tubulin is higher than to that of mammals, although it has been demonstrated to have effects in mammals, birds, and reptiles. Bone marrow suppression is attributed to the inhibition of mitosis in rapidly dividing cells.

2 What other system may be affected? The rapidly dividing mucosal cells of the gastrointestinal tract.

3 What other condition could enhance the toxicity of fenbendazole? A coccidial infestation may be responsible for mucosal epithelial necrosis, as coccidia complete part of their lifecycle within the intestinal mucosal epithelium. Damage to the intestinal mucosa may facilitate a greater drug absorption, resulting in toxic levels of fenbendazole even for doses within anecdotal reference ranges for domestic pigeons.

Further reading

Gozalo AS, Schwiebert RS, Lawson GW (2006) Mortality associated with fenbendazole administration in pigeons (*Columba livia*). *J Am Assoc Lab Anim Sci* **45**(6):63–66.

Rivera S, McClearen J, Reavill D (2000) Suspected fenbendazole toxicity in pigeons (*Columba livia*). *Proc Assoc Avian Vet Conf*, Portland, pp. 207–209.

CASE 54

1 What type of plant is shown? *Philodendron* spp.

2 What is the mechanism of toxicity for this plant? What are the expected clinical signs? *Philodendron* as well as *Dieffenbachia* species contain insoluble crystals of calcium oxalate called raphites, which are needle-like crystals and cause irritation

of the mucosa of the gastrointestinal tract. Chewing or ingestion of the plant releases the crystals, which penetrate tissue resulting in injury. Irritation of the oropharyngeal cavity and crop result in hypersalivation, difficulty swallowing, and regurgitation. Ingestion of large quantities can result in severe gastrointestinal upset, convulsions, and death.
3 **What is the recommended treatment?** Hospitalization and SC (or IO or IV) fluid therapy until dehydration has been corrected. Consider oral antibiosis to reduce secondary bacterial overgrowth (e.g. amoxicillin) if increased numbers of bacteria are present on crop cytology.

Further reading

Dumonceaux G, Harrison GJ (1994) Toxins. In: *Avian Medicine: Principles and Application.* (eds. BW Ritchie, GJ Harrison, LR Harrison) Wingers Publishing, Lake Worth, p. 1041.

CASE 55

1 **How would you confirm your diagnosis?** Myelography, while described in birds, is rarely used in clinical avian practice. Its limited use in birds is likely because of the rare clinical indications, lack of familiarity with the technique, fear of iatrogenic injury to the spinal cord, and concern about potentially fatal complications of the procedure. The cerebellomedullary cistern is very small in many avian species and directly overlies a large venous plexus. It is considered by some authors that injection of contrast medium into the subarachnoid space in the cerebellomedullary cistern cannot be consistently repeated and trauma to the spinal cord near the brainstem can result in death. This technique has been described in pigeons and postmyelographic complications were not observed and the quality of the myelogram was considered acceptable. However, the cistern is relatively larger in pigeons than in some other avian species and accommodates a needle for injection of contrast medium. The fused vertebrae of the synsacrum, the glycogen body, and the absence of a cauda equina interfere with the typical mammalian technique of lumbosacral puncture for subarachnoid access, necessitating a thoracolumbar approach. This technique has been evaluated in chickens, resulting in complications leading to death in several birds. CT, MRI, or nuclear scintigraphy would be able to provide more information, but these diagnostic modalities are rarely performed in wildlife rehabilitation because of the cost.
2 **How would you treat this bird?** Medical treatment is aimed at preventing further primary injury by careful handling and strict restriction of activity, and to prevent secondary injury to the spinal cord. If needed, sedation or general anesthesia is recommended to facilitate handling and restrict activity. Intravenous fluid therapy is recommended to improve tissue perfusion and oxygenation. Opioid drugs are recommended to treat pain secondary to the trauma. NSAIDs, gastrointestinal

protectants, and nutritional support should be considered. Corticosteroids such as methylprednisolone sodium succinate have been used historically in the treatment of spinal cord injuries for their anti-inflammatory and free radical scavenging properties. However, corticosteroids can cause severe side-effects in birds, including hemorrhage, gastrointestinal ulceration, and immunosuppression, and are not currently recommended in most cases. Surgical stabilization is indicated for an unstable spinal fracture or subluxation with decompensating neurologic signs, but has not been reported successfully in birds. Once the fracture has stabilized, physical therapy with passive range of motion is recommended to regain normal function.

3 What is the prognosis? Birds with mild to moderate neurologic deficits like the ones described in this case may regain neurologic function with time and appropriate treatment, and would have to be evaluated daily for progression of the neurologic deficits. Two weeks is recommended to provide a definitive prognosis in these cases. More severe cases, with loss of deep pain perception for 24 hours, have a poor prognosis.

Further reading

Sanchez-Migallon Guzman D (2016) Systemic diseases: disorders of the neurological system. In: *Avian Medicine*, 3rd edn. (ed. J Samour) Elsevier, St Louis, pp. 421–433.

CASE 56

1 What anatomic structure is depicted by the arrows in this parrot's heart (56)**?** This is the right atrioventricular valve. This valve is very different from its mammalian counterpart as it is muscular, not held by chordae tendinae. It is an extension of the right ventricular myocardium and possesses its own innervation. Its function is not completely understood but it is speculated that it participates in actively closing the right atrioventricular aperture.

2 What other anatomic differences are there between the avian and mammalian heart? Other cardiovascular anatomic and physiologic peculiarities of birds include the following: poorly defined left atrioventricular valve, muscular ring around the aortic valve, negative cardiac mean electrical axis (except broiler chickens and Pekin ducks), ring of Purkinje fibers around the aorta and right atrioventricular valve, depolarization of epicardium precedes endocardium; higher heart rate, arterial blood pressure, cardiac output; larger heart, smaller cardiac muscle fibers, absence of T-tubules in cardiac myocytes, absence of M-bands connecting myosin filaments, ascending aorta on the right, brachiocephalic arteries larger than the aorta, cartilage at base of aorta, the majority of myocardium vascularization derived from deep coronary arteries.

3 What are the clinical implications of these differences for diagnostic tests?

- Cardiac auscultation. The heart is located in the concave side of the sternum, therefore the stethoscope bell may be positioned right on top of the keel for auscultation. Due to the presence of large air sac diverticulae, cardiac sounds may appear muffled in some species, in particular Pelecaniformes.
- Electrocardiography. The fast heart rate of birds requires the use of a paper speed of 100 mm/sec for optimal assessment. The fact that ventricular depolarization travels from the epicardium to the endocardium results in an overall negative mean electrical axis in most species in the form of a QRS of the type (Q)rS rather than the type qRs.
- Echocardiography. The location of the heart in an indentation of the keel and surrounded by the air sac system 'shields' it from echocardiographic assessment. As a consequence, in most birds, only a median sonographic window through the liver allows echocardiographic planes. In addition, B-mode echocardiography is not possible through the transcoelomic approach in the majority of birds. In response to these challenges, a transesophageal approach has been developed in birds using a transesophageal ultrasound probe and has been shown to be superior to the standard transcoelomic approach but limited in smaller birds. The small size of many birds and the extremely fast heart rate render transcoelomic echocardiographic measurements grossly inaccurate.
- Angiography. The relatively fast heart rate and high cardiac output in birds lead to an extremely fast distribution of intravenous radiographic contrast agents through the arterial system. Consequently, angiographic imaging (CT angiography, radiographic angiography) must be performed within seconds or almost immediately after contrast administration. In addition, it may be difficult to differentiate the arterial phase from the venous phase.

Further reading

Baumel JJ (1993) Systema cardiovasculare. In: *Handbook of Avian Anatomy: Nomina Anatomica Avium*, 2nd edn. (eds. JJ Baumel, AS King, JE Breazile, HE Evans, JC Vanden Berge) Nuttall Ornithological Club, Cambridge, MA, pp. 407–476.

Beaufrère H, Nevarez JG, Holder K *et al.* (2011) Characterization and classification of psittacine atherosclerotic lesions by histopathology, digital image analysis, transmission and scanning electron microscopy. *Avian Pathol* **40**(**5**)**:**531–544.

Beaufrère H, Pariaut R, Nevarez JG *et al.* (2010) Feasibility of transesophageal echocardiography in birds without cardiac disease. *J Am Vet Med Assoc* **236**(**5**)**:**540–547.

Beaufrèere H, Pariaut R, Rodriguez D *et al.* (2012) Comparison of transcoelomic, contrast transcoelomic, and transesophageal echocardiography in anesthetized red-tailed hawk (*Buteo jamaicensis*). *Am J Vet Res* **73**(**10**)**:**1560–1568.

Krautwald-Junghanns M-E, Pees M, Schroff S (2011) Cardiovascular system. In: *Diagnostic Imaging of Exotic Pets*. (eds. M-E Krautwald-Junghanns, M Pees, S Reese, T Tully) Schlutersche Verlagsgesellschaft mbH & Co., Hanover, pp. 84–91.

Lumeij, JT, Ritchie BW (1994) Cardiology. In *Avian Medicine: Principles and Applications.* (eds. BW Ritchie, GJ Harrison, LR Harrison) Wingers Publishing, Lake Worth, pp. 695–722.
Smith FM, West NH, Jones DR (2000) The cardiovascular system. In: *Sturkie's Avian Physiology*. (ed. GC Whittow) Academic Press, London, pp. 141–232.
West NH, Langille BL, Jones DR (1981) Cardiovascular system. In: *Form and Function in Birds*, Vol. 2. (eds. AS King, J McLelland) Academic Press, London, pp. 235–339.

CASE 57

1 What could cause the clinical signs seen in these chicks? Selenium toxicosis. Lethargy, stunting, and death can be caused by a variety of diseases including malnutrition. A common cause of diarrhea in birds this age is coccidial infection, but a fecal float was negative. Coelomic effusion can have multiple causes but in chicks this young, heart disease, salt toxicity, or selenium toxicosis are the top differentials. On further questioning, it was found that the facility had been making its own feed for years, but had just recently purchased a different brand of mineral mix that on closer inspection had a higher level of selenium in it than the previously used mix. The maximum tolerable concentrations for selenium in most livestock feed is considered to be 2–5 ppm, and these chicks were receiving approximately 14 ppm. Selenium causes an oxidation of lipid layers of cell membranes lining the capillary walls, resulting in increased permeability, and then fluid exudes into the subcutaneous tissues.

2 How would you confirm the diagnosis? Confirmation of selenium toxicosis requires measuring elevated serum and/or liver selenium levels. The liver levels in the two necropsied chicks were elevated. No further problems were identified after changing to a diet with normal selenium levels. If the fecal float had been positive for coccidia, then any one or more of more than nine species of *Eimeria* spp. could have been detected. The most severe clinical signs are seen with *Eimeria tenella*, commonly associated with hematochezia. Cecal coccidiosis is more pathogenic as it typically causes bloody droppings and is associated with higher mortality, while intestinal coccidiosis is typically more chronic in nature but is associated with lower mortality. The clinical signs of coccidiosis are severe in young (4–16 weeks of age) chickens, commonly presenting with bloody diarrhea, pale combs, lethargy, tendency to huddle, partial anorexia, weight loss, dehydration, and variable levels of mortality. As chickens get older they become more resistant and show few or no clinical signs, but can act as carriers to later exposed young chicks. Poultry coccidiosis is commonly prevented and treated with medicated starter feeds that contain amprolium or individually treated with direct oral administration of sulfa medications such as sulfadimethoxine. Other antiparasiticides are not labeled for use in chickens, which are considered a food animal, therefore proper use of any extra-label medication used in chickens should be investigated through the Food Animal Residue Avoidance Databank (FARAD) at farad.org. Some antiparasiticides such as metronidazole are prohibited for use in chickens.

Further reading

Hall J. Selenium toxicosis. In: *Merck Manual On Line* at http://www.merckvetmanual.com/mvm/toxicology/selenium_toxicosis/overview_of_selenium_toxicosis.html
http://www.farad.org

CASE 58

1 What are the preanesthetic considerations for a tracheoscopy? Patients that are in respiratory distress or have a change in or loss of voice due to a tracheal disease/obstruction require stabilization prior to anesthesia. This requires oxygen therapy and often an air sac tube needs to be placed to improve respiratory function. The air sac tube also facilitates anesthesia and tracheoscopy.

2 A tracheoscopy is being performed in this cockatoo. An abnormal finding is encountered (58a). What are the differential diagnoses for this finding? An obstruction is visualized in the tracheal lumen. Differential diagnoses for this structure include a fungal granuloma, bacterial exudate, a foreign body, neoplasia, or, very rarely, a parasitic (*Cyathostoma* spp., *Serratospiculum* spp., *Syngamus trachea*) granuloma.

3 What are the immediate diagnostic and therapeutic steps that should be undertaken? Foreign bodies should be retrieved; endoscopic retrieval is ideal if feasible. Granulomas should be biopsied for histopathology and bacterial and fungal cultures; however, intraoperative impression smears often permit differentiation between fungal and bacterial disease. Impression smears/cytologic samples should be evaluated promptly, particularly for infectious agents, to allow targeted topical treatment at the time of tracheoscopy. Débridement of granulomas to restore lumen patency should be performed using biopsy forceps, keeping in mind that mucosal damage due to débridement or the disease process itself can predispose to stricture formation and stenosis. Although controversial, topical corticosteroids can be considered if inflammation is severe.

4 An intraoperative impression smear was evaluated in this case (58b). Describe the cytologic finding. What is the most likely diagnosis? In this case, fungal elements were seen on Romanowsky stain (Diff-Quik™) cytology, allowing topical amphotericin B, enilconazole, or F10®SC 1:250 (quaternary ammonium and biguanide antiseptic solution: Health and Hygiene) therapy at the time of tracheoscopy, followed by nebulization (enilconazole or F10®SC 1:250 for 30 minutes q8h together with systemic antifungal therapy [itraconazole 10 mg/kg PO q12h or voriconazole 10 mg/kg PO q12h for a 2-month period in most species) pending culture results. Because of the variety of *Aspergillus* strains and the variability of response of avian species to antifungal agents, choice of therapy, dosage, and duration of treatment should be based on sensitivity data, minimum inhibitory concentration, clinical response, and species of bird and should ideally follow the guidelines of peer-reviewed studies if available. Culture results confirmed aspergillosis.

Further reading

Divers SJ (2010) Avian diagnostic endoscopy. *Vet Clin North Am Exot Anim Pract* 13(2):187–202.

CASE 59

1 What is the likely origin of the *Pseudomonas* spp. infections, and how could this be best prevented? *Pseudomonas* is a serious pathogen that is almost always found growing in a contaminated water source such as an uncovered header or storage tank, water standing in hose pipes in sunlight, or use of untreated water. In the Middle East, while some falconers will have access to chlorinated water, even so, water will tend to be stored in large metal drums, kept in direct sunlight (i.e. warm), refilled from time to time but not cleaned out or disinfected prior to refilling. *Pseudomonas* is a common contaminant, and yet by correct water hygiene management, using disinfection of the containers prior to refilling or even while in use (e.g. F10 SC disinfectant [Health and Hygiene]), this incidence could be greatly reduced or eliminated.

2 What is the likely origin of the *E. coli* infections, and how could this be best prevented? *E. coli* is most likely derived from food that has not been prepared, defrosted, or delivered to birds in a hygienic manner, or due to handlers' contaminated hands (i.e. poor personal hygiene). It is vital that food fed to falcons is killed and fed fresh, stored for short periods in a refrigerator, or rapidly frozen after killing, then defrosted in a refrigerator prior to feeding. Food should not be provided to excess, so that it is eaten quickly when offered. Good hygiene practices, in particular in relation to food, should reduce or avoid such infections.

3 What is the likely origin of the *Staphylococcus* spp. infections, and how could this be best prevented? *Staphylococcus* is not a natural contaminant of free living falcons. It is common in captive falcons, being the most common pathogen in bumblefoot cases. This infection is derived from the hands of falconers (i.e. those who handle and care for the birds, *Staphylococcus* spp. being natural commensals on human hands). Good personal hygiene will help to reduce incidence; however, contamination seems inevitable, therefore 1–2 times weekly application of a suitable disinfectant cream to the feet to control this undesirable contamination is advised (e.g. F10 Barrier Cream [Health and Hygiene]).

Further reading

Ali M, Al-Karkhi IM, Pakola B (2014) Trend of bacterial and fungal diseases in falcons in Qatar. In: *Proceedings Veterinary Medicines for Falconry into the 21st Century Conference*, Doha, p. 47.

CASE 60

1 What radiographic abnormalities are shown? The radiographs show moderate dilation of the proventriculus and ventriculus. On the ventrodorsal view, the 'hourglass' is asymmetrical and dilated on the left side. The proventriculus extends laterally beyond the liver margin (the perpendicular line dropped from the scapula to the acetabulum) at the expense of air sac space on the left side. Also, on the lateral view, the proventriculus and ventriculus are severely gas distended.

2 How can proventricular size be evaluated radiographically in psittacines? The proventricular size can be evaluated radiographically in birds using the proventriculus:keel height ratio. The proventricular diameter (PV) is measured at the level of the junction between the last thoracic vertebra and the synsacrum and perpendicular to the long axis of the proventriculus, while the keel height (K) is measured as the maximum dorsoventral height of the keel of the sternum (**60c**). In this case the proventriculus:keel height ratio is 1.4. A ratio value <0.48 indicates that the proventricular diameter is normal, whereas ratios >0.52 are consistent with proventricular disease. The sensitivity and specificity of the ratio for detection of proventricular enlargement were both 100% in one study, and a follow-up study evaluating the prognostic value of the proventriculus:keel ratio found that 39% of

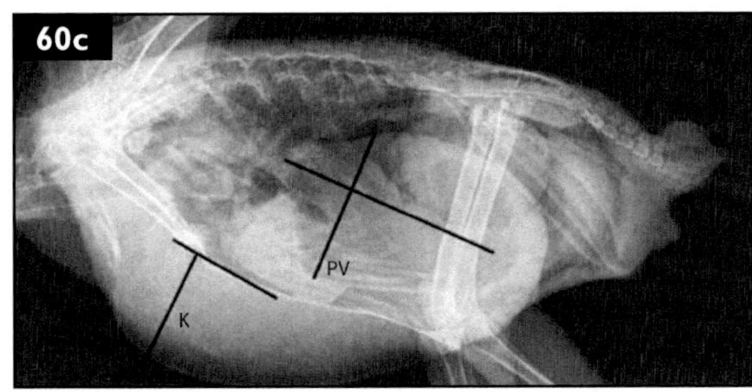

parrots with enlarged proventriculus succumbed to the disease within 1 month of diagnosis. The effects of anesthesia, positioning, time, feeding, and interobserver variation on the proventriculus:keel height ratio of clinically healthy parrots have been evaluated, resulting in no significant effect due to anesthesia, feeding, fasting, or repeated imaging through an 8-hour period. Interobserver agreement for measurability and correlation for the proventriculus:keel height ratio values was considered high.

3 What diseases could result in similar abnormal radiographic findings? Proventricular enlargement in radiographs can be seen with proventricular dilatation disease, nonspecific proventriculitis, heavy metal toxicosis, foreign body, koilin dysplasia, proventricular neoplasia, *Macrorhabdus ornithogaster* infection, and helminth infection.

Further reading

Dennison SE, Adams WM, Johnson PJ *et al.* (2009) Prognostic accuracy of the proventriculus: keel ratio for short-term survival in psittacines with proventricular disease. *Vet Radiol Ultrasound* 50(5):483–486.

Dennison SE, Paul-Murphy JR, Adams WM (2008) Radiographic determination of proventricular diameter in psittacine birds. *J Am Vet Med Assoc* **232**(5):709–714.

Dennison SE, Paul-Murphy JR, Yandell BS (2010) Effect of anesthesia, positioning, time, and feeding on the proventriculus:keel ratio of clinically healthy parrots. *Vet Radiol Ultrasound* **51**(2):141–144.

CASE 61

1 **What is the most likely diagnosis?** Chronic lymphocytic leukemia (CLL), which originates from bone marrow and affects the blood before disseminating later on to multiple organs including coelomic viscera. CLL is a neoplastic clonal proliferation of small and mature appearing lymphocytes that manifests as a persistent, often marked, peripheral lymphocytosis. Lymphoma, a lymphoid neoplasia of solid organs, can become leukemic and may appear similar to CLL that has begun to infiltrate solid organs. In contrast to lymphoma, lymphocytic leukemia appears to be rare in birds. CLL can be further classified as having a T-cell or B-cell origin by immunophenotyping. Most immunophenotyping is performed with monoclonal antibodies. CD3 is highly conserved across many species and anti-CD3 antibodies have been shown to accurately stain T cells in chickens. In contrast, the anti-B-cell antibodies tested (CD79a and BLA.36) are not able to accurately identify B cells in birds.

2 **What additional test would you perform to confirm your diagnosis?** Coelomic ultrasound, coelomic endoscopy, and bone marrow aspirate to stage the disease. The abnormal hematologic results with progressively increasing lymphocytic leukocytosis and anemia and the presence of a monomorphic population of well-differentiated lymphocytes in the bone marrow aspirate confirmed the diagnosis in this bird.

3 **How would you treat this disease?** Although treatment for CLL is not always indicated in birds without clinical signs, individual factors such as the lymphocyte count, organ involvement, cytopenia, and secondary infections influence the decision whether to begin therapy. Treatment choice depends on the staging of the disease, the molecular profile of the individual tumor, patient age, and the performance status of the patient. Chlorambucil and prednisone, cyclophosphamide and prednisone, lomustine, L-asparaginase, and whole body radiation have been use to treat birds with CLL. Bone marrow suppression, thrombocytopenia, and hepatotoxicity are common adverse effect of chlorambucil, and thrombocyte counts should be monitored. Gastrointestinal toxicity is a known adverse effect of cyclophosphamide. Antibiotics and antifungals should be administered as needed, especially if there is evidence of immunosuppression. Reported survival times for CLL in avian species are usually short, up to approximately 2 months after starting treatment. However, those birds that showed lasting response to treatment had survival times of at least 6 months (including this swan) up to more than a year.

Further reading

Sinclair KM, Hawkins MG, Wright L *et al.* (2015) Chronic T-cell lymphocytic leukemia in a black swan (*Cygnus atratus*): diagnosis, treatment, and pathology. *Avian Med Surg* **29(4)**:326–335.

CASE 62

1 Vaccines exist for protection against four different infectious agents in pigeons. What is known about the preventive efficacy of each of these vaccines? The four different infectious agents for which vaccination exists in pigeons are: avian paramyxovirus serotype 1 (APMV-1), pigeon pox, pigeon herpesvirus, and *Salmonella typhimurium* var. Copenhagen. Vaccination against APMV-1 (killed vaccine) and pigeon poxvirus (modified live vaccine) is considered to be fully protective. Vaccination against *Salmonella typhimurium* var. Copenhagen (killed vaccine) is partially protective, while there are no scientific reports available on the efficacy of the vaccine against pigeon herpesvirus (killed vaccine).

2 Which routes are used for administration of the aforementioned vaccines in pigeons? Vaccination against APMV-1, avian poxvirus, and *Salmonella typhimurium* var. Copenhagen can all be performed subcutaneously in the neck. There are also vaccines against avian poxvirus available that need to be applied topically into the feather follicles of plucked feathers.

3 What are 'the recommended vaccination protocols' for each vaccine? Vaccination of squabs is possible from 3 weeks onwards to prevent APMV-1. Vaccination to prevent avian pox, *Salmonella*, and herpesvirus is possible from 5 weeks onwards. A booster vaccination 2–4 weeks later is needed for the *Salmonella* and herpesvirus vaccination. A booster vaccination is not necessary for the APMV-1 vaccination. Yearly revaccinations are recommended for all these pathogens at least 3 weeks prior to their first flight during the racing season.

Further reading

Hooimeijer J (2006) Management of racing pigeons. In: *Clinical Avian Medicine*, Vol. 2. (eds. GJ Harrison, TL Lightfoot) Spix Publishing, Palm Beach, p. 853.
http://www.pharmagalbio.sk/en/products/pigeons/pharmavac-columbi-2/

CASE 63

1 What is the most likely cause of the hypercalcemia and hyperproteinemia seen in this cockatiel? This cockatiel is laying eggs as evidenced by the medullary hyperostosis of the femurs and the egg in her coelom. Increased estrogen levels during egg laying lead to osteoblast activation to form nonstructural medullary bone, which starts 2 weeks before egg laying. When actively laying, calcium is readily absorbed from the intestinal tract and mobilized from the medullary bone to go to the shell gland for eggshell formation, leading to increased serum levels. In addition to its effect on calcium, estrogen also induces the production of proteins needed for yolk formation such as albumin and precursors of vitellogenin and lipoproteins. Therefore, the increased formation of proteins for egg production also leads to an increased serum calcium concentration due to an increase in protein-bound calcium.

2 What other parameter could be measured to evaluate this bird's calcium status? Ionized calcium should be measured because this is not affected by increased or decreased concentrations of calcium binding proteins, which is seen during egg laying. Additionally, ionized calcium is the only physiologically active form of calcium and up to 40% of calcium can be bound to albumin and vitellogenic protein in birds.

3 Does this cockatiel still require calcium supplementation even though her serum calcium levels are so high? Yes, oral calcium supplementation should still be given to this bird. During egg formation, calcium sources include the diet and medullary bone. Medullary bone is able to supply enough calcium for only one egg. When egg laying, calcium is readily absorbed from the intestinal tract (up to 70% absorption), so oral supplementation is adequate if the bird is healthy enough to take oral supplementation. Egg laying cockatiels require a diet that is 0.35% calcium.

Further reading

de Matos R (2008) Calcium metabolism in birds. *Vet Clin North Am Exot Anim Pract* **11**(1):59–82.

Fudge AM (2000) Laboratory reference ranges for selected avian, mammalian, and reptilian species. In: *Laboratory Medicine Avian and Exotic Pets.* (ed. AM Fudge) WB Saunders, Philadelphia, pp. 375–400.

Scholtz N, Halle I, Flachowsky G *et al.* (2009) Serum chemistry reference values in adult Japanese quail (*Coturnix coturnix japonica*) including sex-related differences. *Poultry Sci* **88**(6):1186–1190.

CASE 64

1 Is there any advantage of urine mixing with feces in the lower intestine? Avian kidneys differ in structure and function from those of reptiles or mammals. Urine produced by the kidneys mixes with fecal components in the lower intestine where additional water can be reabsorbed as needed.

2 What is the advantage of excretion of nitrogen wastes in the form of uric acid in birds, as opposed to the excretion of nitrogen as urea in mammals? The most conspicuous physiologic adaptation for promoting water economy in birds is the excretion of nitrogenous wastes in the form of uric acid. The white crystals are synthesized in the liver and give bird droppings their characteristic color; 90% of its secretion is via tubular secretion from reptilian-type nephrons and therefore largely independent of urine flow. Excretion of nitrogen as urea, in mammals, in aqueous solution requires flushing by large quantities of water but uric acid can be excreted as a semi-solid suspension – a colloidal solution – in which each molecule of uric acid contains twice as much nitrogen as a molecule of urea. Therefore, birds require only 0.5–1.0 ml of water to excrete 370 mg of nitrogen as uric acid, whereas mammals require 20 ml of water to excrete the same amount of nitrogen as urea. Birds concentrate uric acid to amazing levels in the cloaca, just prior to defecation. It can be up to 3,000 times the uric acid level in their blood. Uric acid is 'insoluble' and so can be safely stored in an egg during incubation without resulting in toxicity. In mammals, 'soluble' nitrogenous waste is excreted across the placenta.

CASE 65

1 What is your anesthetic plan for premedication, induction, and maintenance of this patient? The patient may be premedicated using midazolam and butorphanol (1–3 mg/kg IM). Anesthesia is induced using either isoflurane or sevoflurane in oxygen (200 mL/kg/min) using a face mask followed by intubation with an uncuffed endotracheal tube. Intraoperative administration of fluid may be achieved through a venous (ulnar or medial metatarsal vein) or intraosseous (distal ulna, proximal tibiotarsus) catheter at a rate of 5–10 ml/kg/hour. An arterial catheter may be placed in the ulnar artery for direct blood pressure monitoring and blood gas analysis. Monitoring may be completed using end-tidal CO_2, oximetry, temperature probe, and electrocardiogram. Mechanical ventilation or manual intermittent positive pressure ventilation must be initiated with peak inspiratory pressure not exceeding 15 cm of H_2O prior to paralysis.

2 How would you paralyze and monitor systemically the bird intraoperatively? The ischiatic nerve is stimulated with a train-of-four (TOF) pattern. A TOF pattern stimulates the nerve with four equal electrical stimulations. This leads to four muscle twitch responses of equal strength of the adjacent fibularis longus muscle. Cis-atracurium (0.1–0.25 mg/kg IV) may then be administered and twitch responses are monitored until a loss of all four twitches in response to a TOF stimulation indicates effective neuromuscular blockade. Blood gas analysis may be used to monitor ventilation throughout the anesthetic episode. The duration of action of cis-atracurium in mammals is usually less than 1 hour. If required, edrophonium (0.5 mg/kg) may be administered following administration of atropine (0.04 mg/kg) to counter any undesirable parasympathetic effects. Once TOF stimulation is restored, mechanical ventilation may be discontinued and the patient recovered from anesthesia as usual.

3 What are the potential anesthetic complications associated with ocular surgery? Sensory stimulation of the eye and orbital areas results in stimulation of the vagal nucleus in the brainstem, thus causing a reflexive slowing of the heart. The afferent arc of the reflex involves the sensory branches of the ophthalmic division of the trigeminal nerve (CN V) to its sensory nucleus. The efferent arc is via the vagus nerve (CN X) to the heart. The most common effect of the reflex is bradycardia, but other clinically significant effects are cardiac arrest and ventricular fibrillation. This is the reason that prior to commencing with ocular surgery in avian species, it is important to have prepared parasympatholytic drugs (atropine) and other emergency drugs in the event that such a vagal response is observed.

Further reading

Barsotti G, Briganti A, Spratte JR *et al.* (2010) Mydriatic effect of topically applied rocuronium bromide in tawny owls (*Strix aluco*): comparison between two protocols. *Vet Ophthalmol* **13:**9–13.

Barsotti G, Briganti A, Spratte JR *et al.* (2010) Bilateral mydriasis in common buzzards (*Buteo buteo*) and little owls (*Athene noctua*) induced by concurrent topical administration of rocuronium bromide. *Vet Ophthalmol* **13:**35–40.

Loerzel SM, Smith PJ, Howe A *et al.* (2002) Vecuronium bromide, phenylephrine and atropine combinations as mydriatics in juvenile double-crested cormorants (*Phalacrocorax auritus*). *Vet Ophthalmol* **5:**149–154.

Petritz OA, Guzman DS, Gustavsen K *et al.* (2016) Evaluation of the mydriatic effects of topical administration of rocuronium bromide in Hispaniolan Amazon parrots (*Amazona ventralis*). *J Am Vet Med Assoc* **248(1):**67–71.

Ramer JC, Paul-Murphy J, Brunson D *et al.* (1996) Effects of mydriatic agents in cockatoos, African gray parrots, and blue-fronted Amazon parrots. *J Am Vet Med Assoc* **208:** 227–230.

Verschueren CP, Lumeij JT (1991) Mydriasis in pigeons (*Columbia livia domestica*) with D-tubocurarine: topical instillation versus intracameral injection. *J Vet Pharmacol Ther* **14:**206–208.

CASE 66

1 What is the preferred surgical treatment for this condition? Ocular evisceration of the affected eye is the recommended treatment modality, given the loss of the eye's integrity and internal structural collapse. After standard sterile preparation, including careful plucking of the feathers along and adjacent to the eyelid margins, a limbal stab incision was made with a beaver #65 blade or a #15 scalpel blade. The cornea is excised using Wescott tenotomy scissors. The iris, lens, vitreous body, retina, and uvea are removed using gentle blunt dissection with a lens loupe, exposing the white-colored scleral shell. The upper and lower eyelid edges are excised.

2 Why is this technique recommended? Owls use hearing in hunting, which may account for increased survival of one-eyed owls post release compared with diurnal raptors (hawks and falcons). A technique that decreases the chance of rostral deformity, with fewer changes to the facial disk and hearing, is preferable. Enucleation, with complete removal of the globe, is deforming to the rostrum and facial disk, and may affect the animal's ability to hunt by sound. Post-release follow-up indicates better survival of owls subjected to ocular evisceration than to enucleation.

3 What are the release criteria once the procedure is completed? Criteria for release vary according to each country's laws and wildlife regulations. It is generally accepted that birds with poor sight or blindness in one eye should not be released. Nocturnal and crepuscular owl species may be released after careful evaluation for hunting ability under nighttime conditions.

Further reading

Murray M, Pizzirani S, Tseng F (2013) A technique for evisceration as an alternative to enucleation in birds of prey: 19 cases. *J Avian Med Surg* **27(2)**:120–127.

CASE 67

1 What is the clinical diagnosis based on the available information? Acute anemia due to gastrointestinal bleeding and hepatopathy. The animal's low hematocrit and total plasma protein in conjunction with a normal body condition are highly suggestive of hemorrhagic or acute hemolytic anemia. The black discoloration of the feces is also suggestive of melena. The green discoloration of the urates is consistent with biliverdinuria, secondary to impaired liver function (or excessive blood breakdown products), of unknown etiology.

2 You perform an occult fecal blood test. How do you interpret the result (67b), and what is the mechanism of action of this test? How sensitive and specific are commercially available occult fecal blood tests in birds? The occult blood test is strongly positive, based on the dark blue discoloration of the filter paper. This test is able to detect hemoglobin in fecal samples. Hemoglobin has peroxidase activity, which catalyzes the oxidation of guaiac, which is impregnated in the filter paper. Blue chromogen is formed after the developer solution (hydrogen peroxide) is applied, and the intensity of blue coloration is proportional to the amount of hemoglobin present in the fecal sample. Chromogen tests have been shown to have a high sensitivity and an acceptable specificity *in vivo* in psittacines and are recommended over the cytologic evaluation of fecal samples in order to detect gastrointestinal bleeding in birds. Several fecal samples should be tested in order to decrease the risk of a false-positive or false-negative diagnosis, and therefore increase specificity and sensitivity.

3 What factors can interfere with fecal occult blood test results? False-positive results can occur following ingestion of hemoglobin-containing animal products (including in processed form) as well as following ingestion of peroxidase-rich plants (e.g. broccoli, cauliflower, turnips, melons). Since droppings in birds exit through the cloaca, which is also the terminus of the urinary and reproductive tracts, bleeding from any of these organs could lead to positive test results despite the source of bleeding not being gastrointestinal. False-negative results can occur consequent to the ingestion of large amounts of ascorbic acid rich fruits (e.g. citrus) or juices.

Further reading

Gibbons PM, Tell LA, Kass PH *et al.* (2006) Evaluation of the sensitivity and specificity of four laboratory tests for detection of occult blood in cockatiel (*Nymphicus hollandicus*) excrement. *Am J Vet Res* **67**:1326–1332.

CASE 68

1 Based on the history provided, what is the most likely diagnosis? What are the predisposing factors for this condition in this flock? Nutritional secondary hyperparathyroidism, hypocalcemia, osteoporosis, and 'caged layer fatigue'. Inadequate calcium intake (high ratio of forage and fresh greens, low ratio of pelleted diet, and the use of a maintenance chicken diet instead of a layer diet), in association with high egg production, typical of the breed, results in inadequate calcium levels in the blood, with secondary excessive secretion of parathyroid hormone and clinical disease associated with calcium deficiency.

2 What other clinical signs may be seen with this condition? What gross lesions would you expect to see on postmortem examination in an affected bird? Other clinical signs include paralysis due to spinal fractures; neurologic signs, ranging from weakness and ataxia to seizures can be seen in the more advanced stages of the disease when calcium blood levels are low.

Postmortem lesions may be limited to soft bones, deformed keels, and pathologic fractures of the long bones, ribs, or spine.

3 What recommendations would you provide to the owner of this flock? Adjusting the diet by offering a chicken layer diet and not adding chopped greens to avoid diluting the calcium content of the diet is recommended. Oral calcium supplementation can be provided initially to clinically affected birds to address calcium deficiencies immediately. Supplementation of the food with oyster shell is commonly used as a long-term calcium supplement. Birds should be allowed outside for exposure to UV-B light for activation of vitamin D. In the initial stages of the treatment, the perches in the coop should be lowered and birds handled with care to prevent development of pathologic fractures.

Further reading

de Matos R (2008) Calcium metabolism in birds. *Vet Clin North Am Exot Anim Pract* **11**:59–82.

CASE 69

1 What investigations should be carried out to determine if the spots are blood? Initial testing with phenolphthalein (turns purple in presence of blood) will validate if these are blood spots. Further blood spatter analysis is a specialist field, but can be very useful in determining the activity and nature of blood loss.

2 How can you differentiate between canine and avian blood? Individual discrete blood drops should be cut away from the surface and submitted for cytology and PCR testing by an independent certified forensic laboratory. Avian erythrocytes will be nucleated and nonavian erythrocytes will not be nucleated.

3 How can you determine if the blood is associated with cock fighting? Full analysis of the blood spatter will assist greatly. The whole 'pit wall' should be submitted for analysis. Careful collection and analysis of multiple individual blood spots will determine if all the blood spots are avian, whether they were poultry, their sex, and whether the blood samples are from numerous different birds rather than from one or a small number. In a cock fighting pit, one would expect all blood spots to be from cockerels, and these to represent samples from numerous different individuals.

Further reading

Merck MD (2012) (ed.) *Veterinary Forensics: Animal Cruelty Investigations*, 2nd edn. Wiley-Blackwell, Ames.

CASE 70

1 Describe your gross findings. This bird appears to be severely overweight. Gross examination suggests increased fat stores subcutaneously over the sternum and in the intracoelomic space. The liver is enlarged and pale.

2 What are the main differential diagnoses? Fatty tumors (lipoma or, less likely, liposarcoma) and hepatic lipidosis.

3 Describe a common cause for these lesions. High-fat diet. Generally, budgerigars with this condition have been fed an all seed diet. If detected antemortem, dietary change, liver support, additional vitamins, and the addition of L-carnitine to the diet will effect an improvement over time.

Further reading

De Voe RS, Trogdon M, Flammer K (2004). Preliminary assessment of the effect of diet and L-carnitine supplementation on lipoma size and bodyweight in budgerigars (*Melopsittacus undulatus*). *J Avian Med Surg* **18(1)**:12–18.

Hochleithner M, Hochleithner C, Harrison LD (2006) Evaluating and treating the liver. In: *Clinical Avian Medicine*, Vol. 1. (eds. GJ Harrison, TL Lightfoot) Spix Publishing, Palm Beach, pp. 441–449.

CASE 71

1 What is this condition called in birds? Valgus rotation of the distal wing resulting in dorsolateral rotation of the primary flight feathers is known by numerous colloquial terms: angel wing, slipped wing, healed-over wing, crooked wing, sword or spear wing, rotating wing, airplane wing, straw wing, flip wing, or dropped wing.

2 What is the cause of this condition? The etiology involves a valgus deformity of the growing metacarpal bones or a rotation in the carpal joints resulting in dorsolateral rotation of the primary flight feathers, which protrude when the wing is folded to the body during rest. The condition can occur either unilaterally or bilaterally. Angel wing is most frequently described in larger waterfowl, such as geese and swans, both captive and wild. It is believed to be caused by consumption of a diet containing excessive levels of protein, which lead to increased growth rates. Compromised calcium and phosphorus intake is also likely to be involved in the pathophysiology. Consequently, the body size increases at a faster rate than bone ossification. The weight of the growing flight feathers places excessive force on the muscles and ligaments of the carpal joint and the inadequately mineralized metacarpal bones, thus exacerbating the condition. Affected waterfowl are usually those species that should naturally be eating grass containing a crude protein content of only 17%–18%. The condition increases in prevalence when these birds are fed grower pellets or cereals (or bread) with a relatively higher protein content.

3 How can this condition be treated/managed? This musculoskeletal problem can be very easily corrected if it is recognized in the early stages by gently wrapping the wing with an elastic bandage around the humerus and distal wing for 3–7 days to provide external support, while reducing the rate of growth and dietary protein level. However, once the wing is fully developed, as in the juvenile swan in this case, the problem is not easily corrected. In some cases an osteotomy of the common or major metacarpus, placement of an intramedullary pin, and de-rotation of the distal wing may effect a correction, although in many cases secondary malalignments of primary feather insertions still prevent normal flight. In uncorrected cases, annual trimming of primary flight feathers may be necessary to prevent feather trauma when the wings are flapped, especially against the enclosure wire.

Further reading

Kreeger TJ, Walser MM (1984) Carpometacarpal deformity in giant Canada geese (*Branta canadensis maxima delacour*). *J Wildlife Dis* **20**:243–245.

CASE 72

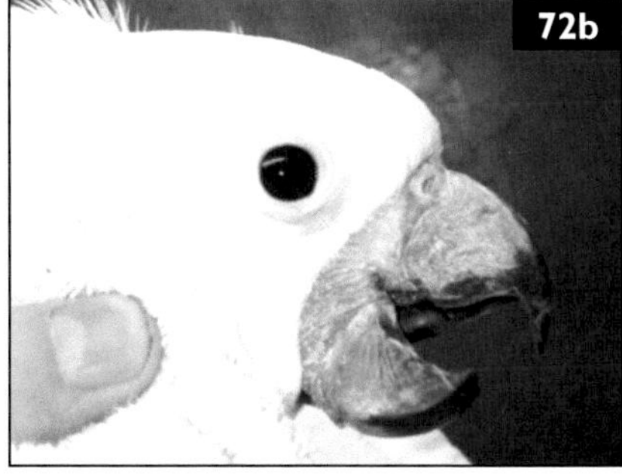
72b

1 What is your immediate concern regarding this bird? What disease is likely to be resulting in this abnormality? The bird has an abnormally shiny black beak compared with a normal cockatoo (**72b**). This finding is typically associated with psittacine beak and feather disease (PBFD), due to loss of powder down feathers (the first feathers to be affected in the feather dystrophy form of the disease). The disease is caused by psittacine circovirus. These feathers are ordinarily ground up by the bird to form a dry powder spread during preening.

2 How would you confirm your diagnosis, and what action can you take to clear infection from a collection? Most commonly, diagnosis is made by real-time PCR testing of feather pulp or blood samples. Feather plumes themselves should not be used, as false positives can occur due to contamination from an infected environment. Histopathologic examination of the bursa of Fabricius shows extensive necrosis of lymphoid follicles with lymphocytolysis, medullary cysts, and hemorrhage. This disease can be diagnosed on electron microscopic examination of feather pulp tissue, electron dense viral particles forming nonmembrane-bound paracrystalline arrays, whorls, semicircles, or concentric circles. Inclusion-bearing lesions are widely disseminated but often closely associated with the alimentary tract. There is no effective treatment for birds with consistent clinical signs that test positive. Birds testing positive but with no clinical signs should be retested 30 days later. Some individuals will clear the infection and test negative at 30 days. If still positive at 30 days, they will go on to develop clinical disease at some point in the future. All other in-contact birds should be tested. A test and removal policy is advised in a breeding collection.

3 What action must be taken to eliminate the pathogen from the environment and prevent the disease spreading? As a positive bird has been in your facility, all areas, clothes, and other fomites must be identified and effectively disinfected. Clinical areas cannot be used until effectively disinfected. The infection is spread in feather dust (i.e. is air borne), therefore disinfection should be carried out by fogging with a disinfectant of proven efficacy against this virus and deliverable via this route (e.g. F10 [Health and Hygiene]). If uncontrolled, viral material remains infectious in the environment for up to 2 years. It is not uncommon for subclinically infected birds to visit your premises and potentially contaminate your facility, creating a 2-year long risk of infection to other patients. Regular weekly fogging with a suitable disinfectant and record keeping of all clinical areas is recommended.

Further reading

Shearera PL, Sharpa M, Bonnea N *et al.* (2009) A quantitative, real-time polymerase chain reaction assay for beak and feather disease virus. *J Virol Methods* **159(1)**:98–104.

Stanford M (2004) Interferon treatment of circovirus infection in grey parrots (*Psittacus e erithacus*). *Vet Rec* **154**:435–436.

www.meadowsah.com/home/assets/.../f10.../The%20Facts-Issue%202.pdf

CASE 73

1 How would you initially stabilize this bird? Treatment of cardiac disease first requires stabilization of the patient. Coelomocentesis and O_2 supplementation should be considered if severe ascites is present and the bird shows increased respiratory effort. Administration of furosemide would be controversial, since it is contraindicated in cardiac tamponade because it decreases cardiac preload, which is necessary in this disease to support ventricular filling and maintain cardiac output. Finally, furosemide should be used with caution in patients with renal diseases.
2 How would you perform pericardiocentesis in a bird? Endoscopically guided pericardiocentesis under general anesthesia should be considered when severe pericardial effusion results in diastolic heart failure. The midline approach is recommended so no fluid leaks into the air sacs. An endoscopic needle is used with its sheath and should only protrude by 1–2 mm to prevent puncturing the heart during the procedure. A permanent surgical window or partial pericardectomy can be performed if necessary.
3 How would you treat this bird long term? Diuretics are indicated to reduce fluid overload, edema, and effusion. Furosemide (0.1–2 mg/kg PO, IM q12–24h) is the most commonly used diuretic. It should not be used alone long term because it further activates the renin–angiotensin–aldosterone system. Electrolytes and renal parameters (e.g. uric acid) should be monitored when using furosemide chronically and hypokalemia is a frequently reported side-effect. Angiotensin-converting enzyme (ACE) inhibitors block the formation of angiotensin II. They promote venous and arterial vasodilation and limit aldosterone production. As a result, they decrease preload and afterload, with a risk of hypotension and hyperkalemia. Enalapril (1.25–5 mg/kg PO q12h) is the most commonly used ACE inhibitor in birds and has been reported to be safe and effective in companion psittacine birds. Positive inotropes are used to enhance cardiac contractility. They are contraindicated in hypertrophic cardiomyopathy and aortic and pulmonic stenosis. Pimobendan is a positive inotrope and arterial vasodilator (inodilator), with its action from calcium sensitization of myofibrils and phosphodiesterase III inhibition. Pimobendan (10 mg/kg PO q12h) has been evaluated in psittacine birds, and it is recommended that the tablet is compounded so that a larger amount of the drug is absorbed. Pimobendan pharmacokinetics is likely very different in other avian groups (e.g. raptors, 0.25 mg/kg PO q12h) and dosages might not be able to be extrapolated.

Further reading

Beaufrère H, Sanchez-Migallon Guzman D (2016) Systemic diseases (Disorders of the cardiovascular system). In: *Avian Medicine*, 3rd edn. (ed. J Samour) Elsevier, St. Louis, pp. 395–407.

CASE 74

1 How would you surgically manage this fracture? A type-II ESF using centrally threaded half-pins (**74c**) would be appropriate for managing a simple fracture of the tarsometatarsus in a raptor or other large bird. Pin placement must be accurate and careful to avoid entrapment of the extensor tendons cranially or flexor tendons caudally. Use of a traditional ESF-intramedullary (ESF-IM) tie-in fixator is not possible in tarsometatarsal fractures due to the lack of a medullary canal in this bone, decreased circulation to the extremities, and the strong forces exerted by the digital flexors. Type-I ESFs with unilateral support are also ineffective as they do not provide enough support in weight-bearing bones.

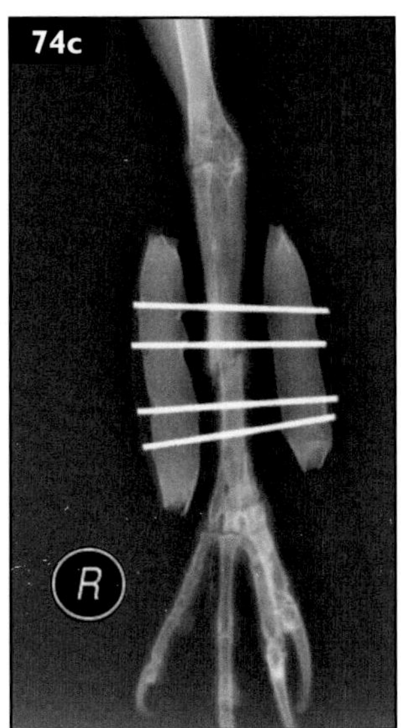

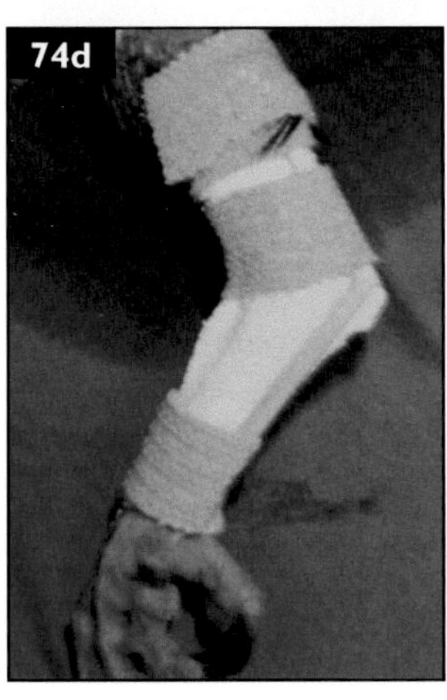

2 What alternative method may be used in smaller avian patients (<150 g)? In smaller birds (<150 g), a sandwich-type tape splint may be used to splint a tarsometatarsus. When constructed with cloth adhesive tape, the splint can be stiffened by coating with surgical cyanoacrylate glue, or a wooden stick added to provide additional support (**74d**). Such splints should extend over the full length of the tarsometatarsus; a padded aluminum splint may extend under the metatarsophalangeal joint.

3 If this patient was a falcon, what other action would you take during the recovery period? Falcons (even lightweight birds) are more prone to bumblefoot than hawks or owls. In any situation where an injury or treatment will result in excessive weight bearing (i.e. more than 50% of the bird's weight) on any foot, then prophylactic action should be taken to prevent excessive pressure on the good foot. In such cases, an interdigitating bandage, doughnut, or corn plaster-shaped foam support dressing should be attached with tape under the good foot, to prevent bumblefoot occurring.

Further reading

Redig PT, Cruz L (2008) Fractures. In: *Avian Medicine*, 2nd edn. (ed. J Samour) Mosby, St. Louis, pp. 215–248.

CASE 75

1 True or false? Because many parrot species are long-lived, the majority of parrots are relinquished because of changes in the owner's lifestyle (such as marriage, children, illness, death) after 15–20 years of ownership. False. Many birds are given up within a few years of being brought into their owner's homes. In many cases, birds are relinquished because owners had false expectations when they purchased the parrot or had not been properly educated and made aware of normal psittacine behavior.

2 In a 2002 survey in the USA, The National Parrot Relinquishment Research Project respondents were asked to indicate the reasons owners gave when relinquishing their parrots. What was the number one reason? Not enough time.

3 What preventive actions might reduce the number of birds relinquished to sanctuaries? Provide education for potential owners about the challenges associated with keeping parrots. Provide parrot owners with adequate instruction when obtaining a new parrot regarding the need for enrichment and training. During clinical appointments, veterinarians can ask about behavioral issues and provide guidance and resources to assist owners.

Further reading

Clubb SL (1998) Captive management of birds for a lifetime. *J Am Vet Med Assoc* **21**(8):1243–1245.

Engebretson M (2006) The welfare and suitability of parrots as companion animals: a review. *Anim Welf* **15**:263–276.

Hoppes S, Gray P (2010) Parrot rescue organizations and sanctuaries: a growing presence in 2010. *J Exot Pet Med* **19**(**2**):133–139.

Leonard AL (2005) *Companion Parrots and Their Owners: A Survey of United States Households*. M.S. Thesis, University of California, Davis.

Meechan CL (2004) National Parrot Relinquishing Research Project 2003/2004. http://www.thegabrielfoundation.org/documents/NPRRPReport.pdf.

CASE 76

1 What parameters would you use to evaluate dyslipidemia in birds? Cholesterol, triglycerides, high-density lipoprotein (HDL), low-density lipoprotein (LDL), and very low-density lipoprotein (VLDL).

2 What lifestyle and dietary changes would you recommend to correct this disorder? Lifestyle and dietary risk factors for dyslipidemia overall have not been well characterized and demonstrated by epidemiologic studies. However, some changes extrapolated from known risk factors of other lipid metabolism abnormalities in other species may be extrapolated to birds.

Lifestyle and dietary changes include increasing activity level, decreasing stress, and reducing reproductive stimulation in females. In Psittaciformes, feeding a diet with reduced saturated fatty acids (e.g. animal fat [eggs, chicken, meat, milk]), with an increase in the consumption of omega-3 fatty acids (e.g. flaxseeds), which is balanced (pelletized diet, fresh fruit and vegetables with added vitamin supplements) is recommended. It is noteworthy that seeds, while high in fat, do not contain cholesterol as it is purely an animal molecule. In birds of prey, because they are fed on a diet of predominantly day-old chicks (with yolk sac), which have a very high cholesterol content, it is advisable to decrease the consumption of day-old chicks or remove the yolk, especially in Falconidae and other species susceptible to atherosclerosis. An increase in the consumption of fish and insects may also be beneficial to omnivorous, piscivorous, or insectivorous birds of prey species (e.g. fish eagles, kites, kestrels). Kites and some small species of falcons in particular have been shown to be extremely susceptible to atherosclerosis.

3 What therapeutic options are available in birds? Medical interventions include the use of gonadotropin-releasing hormone (GnRH) agonists, statins, drugs reducing intestinal cholesterol, and fibrates. GnRH agonists may lower the synthesis of cholesterol and LDLs that are estrogen-induced in females. Drugs such as leuprolide acetate and deslorelin implants have been used successfully for this purpose. Several cholesterol lowering drugs may be prescribed. Overall, there is a lack of pharmacologic data on these drugs in birds. Statins are a class of hypocholesterolemic drugs acting at the level of cholesterol biosynthesis in the liver. Several statin drugs are available and need to be compounded in an oral suspension. A pharmacokinetic study on rosuvastatin did not lead to adequate plasma concentration in Hispaniolan Amazon parrots. Atorvastatin (10–15 mg/kg q12h) has been used in parrots with some success. The consumption of grapefruit interacts with the absorption of statins, so dietary grapefruit should be avoided. There are also pharmacologic interactions between statins and commonly used drugs in captive birds, such as triazole antifungals. Drugs reducing intestinal cholesterol absorption, such as ezetimibe, are unlikely to work in parrots due to the absence of cholesterol in their normal diet. However, it may be beneficial in the treatment of dyslipidemia in birds of prey. Fibrates are a class of hypolipidemic drugs stimulating the β-oxidation of fatty acids. There are no scientific or empirical data on their use in birds. Fibrates mainly cause a decrease in blood triglycerides.

Further reading

Beaufère H (2013) Avian atherosclerosis: parrots and beyond. *J Exot Pet Med* **22(4)**: 336–347.

Beaufère H, Papich MG, Brandão J *et al.* (2015) Plasma drug concentrations of orally administered rosuvastatin in Hispaniolan Amazon parrots (*Amazona ventralis*). *J Avian Med Surg* **29(1)**:18–24.

Petzinger C, Bauer J (2013) Dietary considerations for atherosclerosis in avian species commonly presented in clinical practice. *J Exot Pet Med* **22(4)**:358–365.

CASE 77

1 What is the most likely cause of such mortality? The most likely cause is clostridial enteritis caused by *Clostridium perfringens*.

2 What is the source of such organisms? Gastroenteritis resulting from anaerobic organisms, such as *Clostridium* spp., has been documented in psittacine birds, ratites, poultry, and waterfowl. In wild avian species such as swans, capercaillies, white storks, crows, geese, western bluebirds, lories, lorikeets, and bobwhite quail, *C. perfringens* type C has also been reported but seems to be uncommon. *Clostridium* species are large, anaerobic, gram-positive, spore-forming rods that normally inhabit soil and the gastrointestinal tract of many animals and can produce exotoxins. Raptors and birds that have well-developed ceca, such as Galliformes, Anseriformes, and ratites, may have clostridial organisms as part of the normal gastrointestinal flora; however, most psittacine birds lack ceca or have only vestigial remnants. Enteric *Clostridium* spp. found in psittacine birds are aberrant and are generally considered either pathogenic or transitory passengers. Pathogenic strains of these bacteria can be acquired in birds by ingestion, wound contamination, or overgrowth of normal gastrointestinal flora (most commonly after antibiotic medication, the feeding of frozen food, change onto a diet with much higher starch content, or the feeding of unwashed sprouted seeds or pulses). Fresh food was typically left with these birds for 24–48 hours; it is considered that infection most likely arose due to decomposition of fresh food.

3 What are the recommended treatment options? The most commonly recommended drugs for the treatment of *C. perfringens* infection in dogs are metronidazole and tylosin, although amoxicillin, tetracycline, erythromycin, and cephalexin have been used. Studies showed that most *C. perfringens* isolates were highly susceptible to metronidazole, but often resistant to macrolides and tetracyclines. In birds, reported therapy for *Clostridium* spp. infections includes clindamycin, piperacillin, amoxicillin, tylosin, and lincomycin. An *in-vitro* study of isolates from poultry demonstrated that penicillins and cefazolin had excellent activity and no resistance, while tetracycline and streptomycin were not recommended.

Further reading

Brandão J, Beaufrère H (2013) Clinical update and treatment of selected infectious gastrointestinal diseases in avian species. *J Exot Pet Med* **22**:101–117.

Ferrell ST, Tell L (2001) *Clostridium tertium* infection in a Rainbow Lorikeet (*Trichoglossus haematodus haematodus*) with enteritis. *J Avian Med Surg* **15**:204–208.

O'Toole D, Mills K, Ellis R *et al.* (1993) Clostridial enteritis in red lories (*Eos bornea*). *J Vet Diagn Invest* **5**:111–113.

Silva ROS, Lobato FCF (2015) *Clostridium perfringens*: a review of enteric diseases in dogs, cats and wild animals. *Anaerobe* **33**:14–17.

CASE 78

1 What are the cells indicated by the arrowheads? The arrowheads indicate immature erythrocytes. Because of the round shape and the cytoplasm that resembles the polychromatic erythrocytes, the majority of these cells are late polychromatic rubricytes. Their presence represents a marked erythrocytic regenerative response.

2 What is the significance of the cells depicted by the short arrows? The short arrows point to erythrocytes with intracytoplasmic inclusions. These inclusions resemble *Plasmodium* spp. gametocytes because they dramatically alter the position of the host cell nucleus, pushing it towards the edge of the cell and becoming eccentric.

3 What is the structure indicated by the long arrow? The long arrow indicates a *Leukocytozoon* gametocyte. The pale color indicates a microgametocyte.

Further reading

Campbell TW (2015) Peripheral bood of birds. In: *Exotic Animal Hematology and Cytology*, 4th edn. Wiley Blackwell, Ames, pp. 37–66.

CASE 79

1 What surgical devices can be used to ensure hemostasis during avian endosurgery? The most common method of hemostasis in avian endosurgery is radiosurgery. Plastic instrument handles feature radiosurgical connections, allowing various 3 mm endosurgical instruments to be used as monopolar devices. Bipolar 3 mm forceps that can be passed through the cannulae are also available. For larger birds (>5 kg), 5 mm ligasure devices and endoscopic vascular clip applicators can be used. Diode laser fibers are flexible and can be passed through the instrument channel of the 4.8 mm operating sheath or the cannulae. CO_2 lasers are less flexible, but a ceramic probe is available for the 4.8 mm operating sheath.

2 Name the instruments shown (79a), which are commonly used in avian diagnostic endoscopy. (1) 5-Fr grasping forceps; (2) 5-Fr biopsy forceps; (3) remote injection/aspiration needle; (4) 5-Fr single action scissors.

3 Name the two instruments shown (79b), which are most commonly used in avian endosurgery. (1) 3 mm short curved Kelly dissecting and grasping forceps; (2) 3 mm serrated, curved, double-action scissors.

Further reading

Divers SJ (2010) Endoscopy equipment and instrumentation for use in exotic animal medicine. *Vet Clin North Am Exot Anim Pract* **13(2)**:171–185.

CASE 80

1 What disease is most likely? Marek's disease is most likely in this case because of the age and the typical clinical signs observed. Clinical signs are generally seen in birds that are 10–20 weeks of age, but can be seen in birds as young as 3–4 weeks of age. The incubation period is typically 4–12 weeks. These chicks presented with typical clinical signs of the neurologic form with an asymmetric paralysis, or 'range paralysis', where they cannot stand because one leg is pointed forward while the other leg is pointed backward, but necropsy also revealed the visceral form. If the chicken was older than 14 weeks, another possible differential diagnosis presenting with similar clinical signs is lymphoid leukosis. The clinical signs and gross and histopathologic signs are sometimes difficult to differentiate from those of Marek's disease, but lymphoid leukosis does not occur before 14 weeks of age, whereas Marek's disease can occur at varied ages and usually occurs in birds less than 20 weeks of age.

2 What gross necropsy findings can be associated with this disease? There are several forms of Marek's disease. The more common neurologic form exhibits an enlarged ischiadic (sciatic) nerve at necropsy, while others present with the visceral form shown here with lymphoid tumors of the liver and spleen. Other less common forms include the ocular form, where the color of the iris gradually changes from brown to gray and the pupil becomes irregular in shape, and the cutaneous form where skin tumors are seen.

3 How do you prevent this disease? This highly contagious disease associated with a high morbidity and low mortality affects only chickens and is caused by a herpesvirus. Transmission is from virus shed in skin and feathers, secretions, and droppings. The virus can persist in the environment indefinitely (feathers and dander in poultry houses and yards). There is no treatment. Prevention is by administration of a polyvalent vaccine in the egg or after hatching at 1 day of age (vaccination after 3 days of age is not efficacious, due to prior infection). Marek's disease must be differentiated from lymphoid leukosis based on age at onset of clinical signs and gross and histopathologic lesions (ischiadic/sciatic nerve enlargement).

Further reading

Schat KA, Nair V (2013) Marek's disease. In: *Diseases of Poultry*, 13th edn. (eds. DE Swayne, JR Glisson, LR McDougald *et al.*) Wiley-Blackwell, Ames, pp. 513–675.

CASE 81

1 What are the most likely differentials in this case? Zinc intoxication. Pennies minted after 1982 contain a core of zinc.

2 Which organ do you sample in priority for histopathology? The pancreas (target organ). Primary microscopic lesions in acute cases are degranulation and vacuolization of acinar cells. Necrosis of individual cells may also be present. In chronic cases, pancreatic interstitial fibrosis may also be present.

3 During what time of the day do you take a blood sample from the remaining bird to improve the specificity of this test? What characteristic of the sampling tube do you check? Zinc plasma concentrations may be measured. Zinc concentrations are higher in the morning and lower in the evening; therefore, an elevated plasma zinc concentration would be more specific in the evening. You need to check that the syringe used to collect and the tube used for blood storage do not contain any zinc, specifically that there is no rubber in the cap and no soft plastic, which commonly contain zinc.

Further reading

Dumonceaux G, Harrison GJ (1994) Toxins. In: *Avian Medicine: Principles and Application.* (eds. BW Ritchie, GJ Harrison, LR Harrison) Wingers Publishing, Lake Worth, pp. 1030–1052.

Rosenthal KL, Johnston MS, Shofer FS *et al.* (2005) Psittacine plasma concentrations of elements: daily fluctuations and clinical implications. *J Vet Diagn Invest* **17**(3):239–244.

Schmidt RE, Reavill DR (2014) Lesions of the avian pancreas. *Vet Clin North Am Exot Anim Pract* **17**:1–11.

CASE 82

1 What is the most likely causative agent? Based on the clinical signs, affected species, and potential zoonotic transmission, *Chlamydia psittaci* infection should be considered as the likely causative agent.

2 What diagnostic tests should be performed? Postmortem examination of dead animals should be performed. The gross and histologic diagnosis of avian chlamydiosis requires demonstration of the pathogen by histochemical, immunohistochemical, or in situ hybridization techniques. Gimenez or Macchiavello stain should be used and may allow identification of Chlamydiaceae within macrophages in smears or tissues (e.g. liver, conjunctival, spleen, respiratory secretions). In live animals, the combination of culture, antibody detection, and antigen detection methods is recommended. Although other diagnostic test combinations can be used, PCR techniques from blood and combined conjuntival–choanal–cloacal swabs, combined indirect fluorescent assay for IgY, and elementary-body agglutination test for IgM antibodies or species-specific ELISA if available, provide an overall good assessment of a live bird.

3 What treatment should be implemented? The drugs of choice for the treatment of chlamydiosis include tetracyclines (doxycycline by choice) and azithromycin. The recommended treatment period for avian chlamydiosis has historically been 45 days, except in budgerigars where 30 days of treatment can be effective.

In cockatiels, a 21-day course of either oral doxycycline or oral azithromycin was effective in eliminating *C. psittaci* infection in experimentally inoculated birds. It has long been suggested that for the treatment of *C. psittaci* in flock conditions, medication in either water or food may be adequate. Although doxycycline medicated water has been shown to reach therapeutic levels (>1 µg/ml) in African grey parrots, Goffin's cockatoos, and cockatiels, this has not been shown in budgerigars. On the other hand, hulled seed containing 300 mg of doxycycline hyclate/kg can safely establish and maintain plasma doxycycline concentrations that are considered adequate for treatment of chlamydiosis in adult nonbreeding budgerigars for 42 days without notable adverse effects.

Further reading

Flammer K, Trogdon MM, Papich M (2003) Assessment of plasma concentrations of doxycycline in budgerigars fed medicated seed or water. *J Am Vet Med Assoc* **223(7):** 993–998.

Flammer K, Whitt-Smith D, Papich M (2001) Plasma concentrations of doxycycline in selected psittacine birds when administered in water for potential treatment of *Chlamydophila psittaci* infection. *J Avian Med Surg* **15(4):**276–282.

Guzman DS, Diaz-Figueroa O, Tully T Jr. *et al.* (2010) Evaluating 21-day doxycycline and azithromycin treatments for experimental *Chlamydophila psittaci* infection in cockatiels (*Nymphicus hollandicus*). *J Avian Med Surg* **24:**35–45.

Papich MG, Davidson GS, Fortier LA (2013) Doxycycline concentration over time after storage in a compounded veterinary preparation. *J Am Vet Med Assoc* **242:** 1674–1678.

Powers LV, Flammer K, Papich M (2000) Preliminary investigation of doxycycline plasma concentrations in cockatiels (*Nymphicus hollandicus*) after administration by injection or in water or feed. *J Avian Med Surg* **14:**23–30.

Smith KA, Campbell CT, Murphy J *et al.* (2011) Compendium of measures to control *Chlamydophila psittaci* infection among humans (psittacosis) and pet birds (avian chlamydiosis), 2010. National Association of State Public Health Veterinarians (NASPHV). *J Exot Pet Med* **20:**32–45.

CASE 83

1 What overall anatomic structure has been damaged, and what structure is arrowed as L? The bird's right propatagium has suffered major trauma. If not satisfactorily repaired, the bird will never fly again. The structure labeled L is the *ligamentum propatagialis pars longus*, which runs from the humeral crest proximally and inserts on the extensor process of the metacarpus.

2 In order for repair of this injury to be possible, what structures need to be repaired and how? The *ligamentum propatagialis pars longus* has collagen sections at either end, with an elasticated central section; therefore, unlike other tendons and ligaments, it can afford to lose a short section of its length through trauma and yet still be reattached and in time return to normal function. In this and similar cases, the contracted ligament end (in this case at L) is found and test stretched to the carpus, where the reciprocal damaged ligament end can be located.

3 What suture technique would be used to repair structure L? The ligament ends are cleaned, débrided, and reattached using a Bunnell, Kessler, or similar technique (**83b**), before covering the repair with the propatagium itself. Once healed this patient was given 3 months rest while it moulted (**83c**), free flighted in an aviary, and after a period of rehabilitation was flying normally again 4 months after the injury.

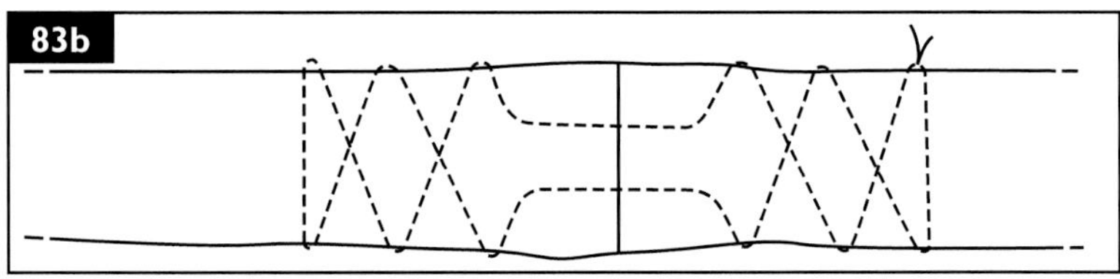
83b

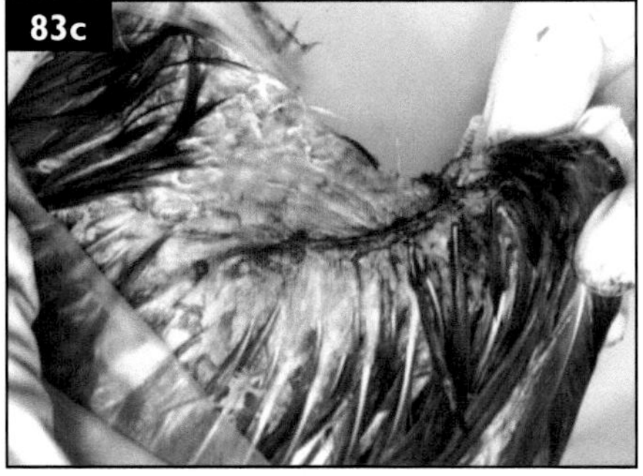
83c

Further reading

Forbes NA (2016) Soft tissue surgery. In: *Avian Medicine*, 3rd edn. (ed. J Samour) Mosby, St. Louis, pp. 294–331.

Harcourt-Brown NH (2000) Tendon repair in the pelvic limb of birds of prey. Part II: Surgical techniques. In: *Raptor Biomedicine III*. (eds. JT Lumeij, PT Redig, M Lierz *et al.*) Zoological Education Network, Palm Beach, pp. 217–238.

CASE 84

1 Describe your gross findings. The bird appears to be in poor body condition. There is also evidence of coelomic distension. The appearance of the dissected mass appears to be cystic in nature.

2 What are your primary differentials? Cystic ovary is the most likely differential. Ovarian neoplasms (granulosa cell tumor, adenocarcinoma, carcinoma, or other neoplasms) are also differentials, including oviductal neoplasia.
3 What are the treatment options for this condition? Aspiration of the cysts, salpingohysterectomy, and partial ovariectomy can be considered. GnRH analogs (leuprolide acetate, deslorelin) may be beneficial. Chemotherapy could be considered in the case of neoplasia but is associated with a guarded prognosis.

Further reading

Bowles H (2006) Evaluating and treating the reproductive system. In: *Clinical Avian Medicine*, Vol. 2. (eds. GJ Harrison, TL Lightfoot) Spix Publishing, Palm Beach, pp. 519–40.

CASE 85

1 What is the most likely diagnosis? Horner's syndrome caused by loss of sympathetic tone in the eye, and secondary to head trauma. The efferent sympathetic supply to the eye in birds, as in mammals, is composed of three levels of neurons: one upper motor neuron level and two levels of lower motor neurons. The upper motor neuron originates in the hypothalamus, whereas the preganglionic and postganglionic lower motor neurons originate in the thoracolumbar spinal cord and the cranial cervical ganglion, respectively. Lesions at any point on this route can result in Horner's syndrome. Ptosis, the prominent feature in birds, is caused by a loss of sympathetic supply to the smooth muscle of the eyelids. The erected feathers are caused by loss of adrenergic stimulation in the smooth muscles that control feather movement. The dominance of striated muscle fibers in the avian dilator muscle of the pupil has been suggested as the cause of the lesser degree of miosis in avian compared with mammalian cases of Horner's syndrome. The lack of clear enophthalmus and protrusion of the third eyelid in birds may be attributed to anatomic features of the avian eye, specifically the limited amount of retrobulbar space, lack of a retractor bulbi muscle, and the absence of smooth muscle in the third eyelid.
2 How would you confirm your diagnosis? Pharmacologic testing may be used to assist in the diagnosis of Horner's syndrome and to differentiate between pre- and postganglionic lesions. Topical application of catecholamine-releasing agents (e.g. hydroxyamphetamine) may ameliorate clinical signs in cases with preganglionic lesions, while topical adrenergic agonists (phenylephrine 0.25%) may ameliorate clinical signs in both pre- and postganglionic cases of Horner's syndrome and

thus do not differentiate between the two. Although testing for response to hydroxyamphetamine was not attempted in this bird, the history, involvement of feathers on the entire side of the neck and head, and the rapid response to phenylephrine treatment, suggest that the lesion was preganglionic, likely affecting the cervical paravertebral trunk at the base of the neck.
3 What is the treatment and prognosis for this condition? No specific treatment is needed for the clinical signs associated with Horner's syndrome. Because of the scarcity of Horner's syndrome reports in birds, there is little information regarding prognosis in these types of case. Based on the cases published, and on the information available for other species, prognosis appears to be good with partial to complete resolution of the clinical signs over time.

Further reading

Gancz AY, Malka S, Sandmeyer L *et al.* (2005) Horner's syndrome in a red-bellied parrot (*Poicephalus rufiventris*). *J Avian Med Surg* **19(1)**:30–34.

CASE 86

1 What are the four parasitic nematode worm species that can inhabit both partridges and pheasants? (1) Roundworms (ascarids), typically around 5 cm long and visible with the naked eye; these are most commonly found in the large intestine. (2) Hairworms (*Capillaria* spp. – as shown in **86**). Adults cause significant damage by burrowing into the villi lining; they are often found in the crops of birds. (3) Cecal worm (*Heterakis* spp.). Adults are mainly found in the ceca and may just be seen with the naked eye. This nematode acts as the intermediate host for *Histomonas meleagridis*, so 'blackhead' may be a significant clinical consequence. (4) Gapeworm (*Syngamus trachea*). Adults reside mainly in the trachea (**86**); pheasants are mainly affected.

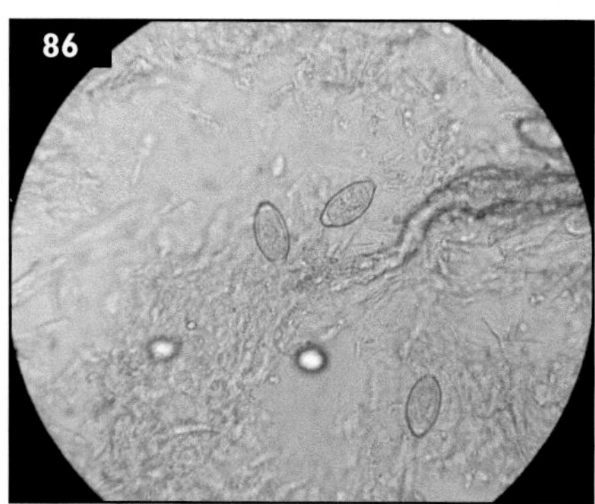

2 What are the clinical signs observed in *Capillaria* spp. and *Syngamus trachea* infections? *Capillaria* spp. are very good at burrowing into the villi of the gastrointestinal tract, especially the crop and esophagus of game birds. Partridges from around 10 weeks onwards are especially susceptible to this worm. The worm causes inflammation. In severe cases the bird is likely to stop eating and succumb to secondary infections such as *Hexamita*. *Syngamus trachea* (gapeworm) is mainly noticed by the 'snicking'

(coughing with a sneeze) sound. The gapeworms can grow both in size and numbers sufficient to result in physical obstruction of the bird's trachea to the point of death.

3 What are the treatments available for game bird species, and how often should these be administered? Flubenvet^{TM} (flubendazole) is the only licensed product to worm both pheasants and partridges in the UK. It is administered via feed and incorporated at the feed mills. The worming regimen should be for a 7-day treatment and this should be repeated every 2–3 weeks until such time that the worm burden is considered low, or close proximity to the start of the shooting season, in respect of required meat withdrawal interval. *Heterakis* spp., *Capillaria* spp., and *Syngamus trachea* all have both a direct life cycle (i.e. reinfection by eating food from contaminated soil) and an indirect life cycle via earthworms (i.e. reinfection after eating infected earthworms), therefore reinfection from contaminated substrate is inevitable unless birds can be effectively treated and then moved onto a clean grazing area.

Further reading

Fernando MA, Stockdale PHG, Remmler O (1971) The route of migration, development, and pathogenesis of *Syngamus trachea* (Montagu, 1811) Chapin, 1925, in pheasants. *J Parasitol* 57(1):107–116.

CASE 87

1 What is the cardiohepatic silhouette? On the ventrodorsal radiograph, the normal liver silhouettes with the heart to form an 'hourglass' shape and it does not extend laterally beyond a line drawn from the scapula to the acetabulum. The normal liver does not extend beyond the caudal aspect of the sternum on the lateral radiograph.

2 What can cause the cardiohepatic silhouette to appear widened with a loss of the 'cardiohepatic waist'? The cardiohepatic waist is the narrowest portion of the normal hourglass-shaped cardiohepatic silhouette in parrots. It represents the region where the caudal aspect of the heart is situated in between the cranial portion of the two hepatic lobes. Hepatomegaly, cardiomegaly, splenomegaly, proventricular enlargement (dilatation or neoplasia), pancreatic neoplasia, and enlargement of the reproductive tract can result in a widening of the cardiohepatic waist.

3 Is the cardiohepatic silhouette widened in this patient and, if so, what diagnostic testing would you recommend to further evaluate this abnormality? Yes, there is moderate widening of the caudal aspect of the cardiohepatic silhouette on the ventrodorsal projection and a heterogeneous soft tissue opaque mass, which is contiguous with the cardiac silhouette, on the right lateral projection.

The recommendation would be to investigate these findings with additional imaging studies including ultrasonography, gastrointestinal contrast radiography, and/or fluoroscopy.

Further reading

Lumeij JT (1994). Hepatology. In: *Avian Medicine: Principles and Application.* (eds. BW Ritchie, GJ Harrison, LR Harrison) Wingers Publishing, Lake Worth, pp. 640–672.

CASE 88

1 How would you correct respiratory arrest if it occurs? The prognosis for respiratory arrest, especially when caused by gaseous anesthesia overdose, is good. When faced with respiratory arrest, decrease the vaporizer setting or discontinue gas anesthesia while initiating positive pressure ventilation with oxygen until the patient starts breathing on its own again. Maintain end-tidal CO_2 between 30 and 45 mm Hg.

2 How would you address bradycardia and what appears to be hypotension? Bradycardia and hypotension (defined as systolic BP <90 mm Hg) develop secondary to several conditions during anesthesia, including cardiovascular depression caused by the anesthetic agent, hypothermia, vagal response due to severe pain, and hypovolemia related to dehydration or blood loss. The anesthetist must assess whether it represents a true emergency (e.g. continuing blood loss during a procedure) or is a transient response (e.g. vagal response due to pain during fracture manipulation). The level of inhalant anesthesia should be reduced if bradycardia and hypotension are thought to be caused by a high anesthetic plane. The administration of IV fluids is indicated if the bradycardia and hypotension are attributed to hypovolemia or for immediate correction of a hypotensive state. Anticholinergic agents such as atropine (fast acting, short lasting) or glycopyrrolate (slow acting, long lasting) can be used to increase the heart rate, but might result in sinus tachycardia and increase myocardial work and oxygen consumption. IV or IO administration of warmed crystalloid fluids (10 mL/kg/h or 10–15 mL as a bolus over 5–10 min) is indicated for hypovolemic birds and can be repeated if necessary to increase systolic BP to >90 mm Hg. Synthetic colloid solutions (i.e. hetastarch [5 mL/kg IV over 5–10 min]) may be used in hypoproteinemic birds or birds that have suffered acute blood loss during surgery. Blood transfusions (5 mL/kg/h) may also be indicated for acute blood loss. Dobutamine (5–15 μg/kg/min) and dopamine (5–10 μg/kg/min) have been shown to help correct severe hypotension in Hispaniolan Amazon parrots caused by anesthesia maintained with 2.5% isoflurane. A marked second-degree atrioventricular block occurred with dobutamine administration at a CRI of 15 μg/kg/min.

3 How would you treat cardiac arrest if it happens? If cardiopulmonary arrest does occur in an intubated anesthetized patient, gaseous anesthesia should be stopped immediately and positive-pressure ventilation with 100% oxygen initiated. Cardiac arrest carries a poor prognosis in avian species because direct compression of the heart is not possible because it is overlaid with the keel, although in the event of cardiac arrest attempts should be made to compress the sternum at a rate of 60–300 compressions per minute. Epinephrine (0.1 mg/kg 1:10,000 solution = 0.1 mg/mL) and atropine (0.02 mg/kg) can be given IV, IO, or via the endotracheal route (double dose used for IV administration) for two to three rounds. The use of vasopressin at a dosage of 0.8 U/kg IV, IO, or a double dosage IT in addition to instead of epinephrine has been suggested. However, there are currently no data available for avian species on the use of this drug. End-tidal CO_2 should be used to monitor cardiac output during CPR. A steady increase in end-tidal CO_2 during CPR is more likely to be associated with a successful outcome. When end-tidal CO_2 does not increase to >10 mm Hg after a resuscitation time of 15–20 minutes, the resuscitative effort may be ineffective.

Further reading

Acierno MJ, da Cunha A, Smith J *et al.* (2008) Agreement between direct and indirect blood pressure measurements obtained from anesthetized Hispaniolan Amazon parrots. *J Am Vet Med Assoc* **233(10)**:1587–1590.

Schnellbacher RW, da Cunha AF, Beaufrère H *et al.* (2012) Effects of dopamine and dobutamine on isoflurane-induced hypotension in Hispaniolan Amazon parrots (*Amazona ventralis*). *Am J Vet Res* 73(7):952–958.

Zehnder AM, Hawkins MG, Pascoe PJ *et al.* (2009) Evaluation of indirect blood pressure monitoring in awake and anesthetized red-tailed hawks (*Buteo jamaicensis*): effects of cuff size, cuff placement, and monitoring equipment. *Vet Anaesth Analg* 36(5):464–479.

CASE 89

1 When giving IM injections, which portion of the pectorals should be avoided, and why? Avoid the cranial (especially lateral) portion of the pectoral muscles to prevent inadvertent injection into vasculature located in this region.

2 Why are the leg muscles generally not recommended for IM injections in birds? Drugs injected into the leg muscles may be excreted by the kidneys through the renal portal system before reaching the systemic circulation. The injection of nephrotoxic drugs into the legs is particularly dangerous and contraindicated. There is also a greater risk of causing neural damage when injecting into poorly muscled legs, compared with the pectoral muscles.

3 Vascular access can be challenging in small and hypotense patients and in these cases IO access for fluid therapy may be necessary. Where are IO injections most commonly delivered? IO injections are most commonly delivered into the distal ulna or proximal tibia using a 22- to 25-gauge hypodermic or spinal needle in most species. Because of the presence of some pneumatized bones that communicate with the respiratory system in most species (e.g. femur and humerus), IO catheters should be avoided in these locations.

Further reading

Powers L (2006) Common procedures in psittacines. *Vet Clin North Am Exotic Anim Pract* **9(2)**:293–294, 287, 301–302.

CASE 90

1 Which laboratory diagnostic test offers the highest correlation with disease? The diagnostic test with the highest laboratory correlation with PBFD is the presence of high virus antigen titers shed from feathers, which is measurable by hemagglutination activity (HA). The diagnosis of PBFD requires the observation of clinical or histopathologic lesions, which includes feather dystrophy, feather loss, and basophilic intracytoplasmic inclusions. When clinical signs of feather disease are present, supportive diagnostic tests such as PCR assays are useful for assisting clinicians with making a diagnosis, but PCR tests may detect viral DNA in birds that are clinically normal, subclinically infected, and/or recovering from infection. The best sample for PCR testing is blood since this minimizes the potential for environmental contamination, a risk if feathers were collected for testing instead. Many clinically normal birds can be PCR positive for many months as they mount an effective immune response. While most birds with high serum antibody concentrations are free from the disease, some birds and individual bird species can also be antibody positive.

2 How many different genotypes of BFDV exist? All psittacine bird species are susceptible to BFDV, which is considered a single virus species with little if any antigenic variation. However, there is great genetic diversity with numerous studies demonstrating quasi-species genetic variation of BFDV within individually infected birds. This genetic variation has implications for the sensitivity and specificity of individual diagnostic PCR tests. Assay protocols should be targeted to the most conserved regions of the BFDV genome, but even then a very small percentage of BFDV genotypes may not be detected by an individual PCR test. PCR tests that target small regions of the genome tend to be the most sensitive for detecting viral DNA but with less discrimination of active viral replication. PCR tests that target larger sections of the genome have a stronger correlation with active virus replication and shedding.

3 Would genetic variation in BFDV interfere with diagnostic testing? Ideally, at least two methods of detection should be used to validate test results. This could be through combined viral DNA testing (PCR) and antigen detection or by targeting two regions of the virus genome with different PCR tests. BFDV is a single-stranded DNA virus that replicates autonomously in the nucleus of infected cells where it relies on host DNA replication machinery; it does not insert itself into the host genome.

Further reading

Khalesi B, Bonne NJ, Stewart M *et al.* (2005) A comparison of haemagglutination (HA), haemagglutination inhibition (HI) and PCR for the detection of psittacine beak and feather disease virus (BFDV) infection and a comparison of isolates obtained from Loriids. *J Gen Virol* **86**:3039–3046.

CASE 91

1 What species are these chicks? Are they precocial or altricial? These neonatal ratite chicks are cassowaries (*Casuarius* spp.). They are precocial, hatched with eyes open, feathers, and able to walk, run, forage, and hunt soon after hatch.

2 These chicks will be raised by their paternal parent. Why is this? These newly hatched ratite chicks will be raised by their paternal parent, as their maternal parent is polyandrous. Polyandrous cassowary females mate with up to four males per breeding season. Once the female cassowary lays her eggs she is chased away from her nest by her mate. She then goes off to find another mate. The paternal parent incubates the eggs and raises the chicks.

3 How and what does their paternal parent feed them? The paternal cassowary parent feeds the chicks by teaching them to forage for fruit (berries) and hunt for small prey (small insects and eventually reptiles, rodents, carrion and fish) and by coprophagia. Precocial cassowary chicks are omnivores and predominately frugivores.

Further reading

Romagnano A, Glenn Hood R, Snedeker S *et al.* (2012) Cassowary pediatrics. *Vet Clin North Am Exot Anim Pract* **15(2)**:215–231.

CASE 92

1 Which bone is repaired first? The radius.

2 What additional method of surgical stabilization could be added to reduce the oblique ulnar fracture and increase resistance to the distractive force of the triceps muscle? Hemicerclage wire could be used to tie down the oblique

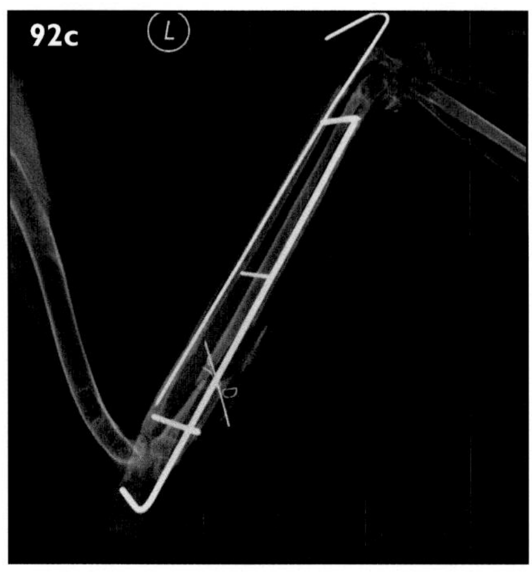

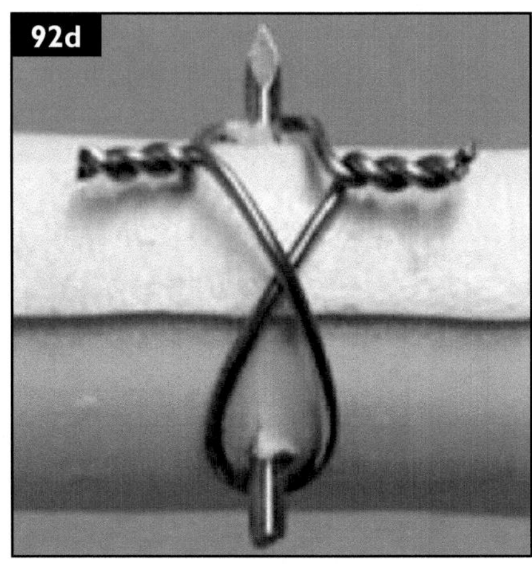

ends of the fracture; in this case a k-wire/figure-of-eight wire combo was used (**92c**). During open surgery, a k-wire pin (0.035 in) was driven perpendicularly through the oblique bone fragments. Cerclage wire was then wrapped in a figure-of-eight pattern around the pin and tightened (**92d**). The ends of the k-wire were then cut prior to closure of the skin and soft tissues. Cerclage should only be used in conjunction with other fixation methods and never by itself when repairing fractures. Circumferential cerclage can cause tissue necrosis and other complications in avian patients, and therefore should be used cautiously.

Further reading

Redig PT, Ponder J (2016) Orthopedic surgery. In: *Avian Medicine*, 3rd edn. (ed. J Samour) Mosby, St. Louis, pp. 312–350.

CASE 93

1 How would you describe this gross lesion, and what is the most likely cause for it? The brachiocephalic arterial wall is thickened with yellowish discoloration and apparent decreased luminal diameter. This gross lesion is typical for atherosclerosis.

2 What are the histopathologic hallmarks of these types of lesions, and what are the different lesion types that have been described? Histopathology is characterized by the infiltration of fat, foamy macrophages, necrotic materials, and increased extracellular matrix in the subintimal and medial layers of the artery, causing the formation of a necrotic atheromatous core. The atheromatous lesion is frequently calcified with chondroid formation. The lesions may also contain a large amount of collagen (fibrosis). The dense collagen material covering a fibroatheromatous lesion is called the fibrous cap. Lesions may be complicated by hemorrhage, thrombosis, and fissures, but these are uncommon in birds. Advanced lesions tend to cause drastic disruption in arterial anatomy with significant arterial luminal stenosis. In birds, clinical signs are more often attributed to 'flow-limiting stenosis' rather than atherothrombosis and emboli, as seen in humans. Atheromatous lesions are classified in seven lesion types: pre-atheromatous lesions (I: scattered foamy macrophages with mild increase in extracellular matrix; II: sheets of foamy macrophages and small pools of extracellular lipid); intermediate lesions (III: larger coalescent fatty deposition starting to disrupt arterial architecture); advanced lesions (IV: large lipid area forming a lipidonecrotic core = atheroma; V: increased presence of fibromuscular tissue forming a fibrous cap over the lipid core = fibroatheromas); complicated lesions (VI: hematoma, emboli, and fissures); and predominantly calcific lesions (VII).

3 What risk factors associated with the development of these types of lesions were present in this bird? This bird had several risk factors, namely its species, gender, and advanced age. Psittacine species predisposed to atherosclerosis are African grey parrots (*Psittacus erithacus*), Amazon parrots (*Amazona* spp.), cockatiels (*Nymphicus hollandicus*), and quaker parrots (*Myiopsitta monachus*). In contrast to mammals, female birds are more prone to atherosclerosis than males. Age is also a significant risk factor; psittacine birds aged over 20–30 have a probability >30% of having a severe atherosclerotic lesion. Chronic reproductive activity is another risk factor that was identified in an epidemiologic survey. While it has not been conclusively demonstrated, other risk factors are expected to occur and include dyslipidemia (e.g. high blood cholesterol), inadequate diet, and lack of activity.

Further reading

Beaufrère H (2013) Avian atherosclerosis: parrots and beyond. *J Exot Pet Med* **22(4)**:336–347.

Beaufrère H, Ammersbach M, Reavill DR *et al.* (2013) Prevalence of and risk factors associated with atherosclerosis in psittacine birds. *J Am Vet Med Assoc* **242(12)**:1696–1704.

Beaufrère H, Nevarez JG, Holder K *et al.* (2011) Characterization and classification of psittacine atherosclerotic lesions by histopathology, digital image analysis, transmission and scanning electron microscopy. *Avian Pathol* **40(5)**:531–544.

Beaufrère H, Pariaut R, Rodriguez D *et al.* (2010) Avian vascular imaging: a review. *J Avian Med Surg* **24(3)**:174–184.

Beaufrère H, Rodriguez D, Pariaut R *et al.* (2011) Estimation of intrathoracic arterial diameter by means of computed tomographic angiography in Hispaniolan Amazon parrots. *Am J Vet Res* **72(2)**:210–218.

CASE 94

1 What are the treatment options? Masterly inactivity and hope for the best; however, the natural method of feeding by a raptor (i.e. holding food between the talons and pulling at it with the beak) would be anticipated to result in further instability and spinal cord damage. Alternatively, one could consider external splinting, but if this were a padded neck support, the cranial extremity would be close to the fracture site and actually increase the risk.

2 If external support is to be provided, how can this be achieved? Effective external support of the fracture can only be provided if the head can also be immobilized. This can be achieved with a transfrontal sinus pin, linked to the external cervical support (**94b**).

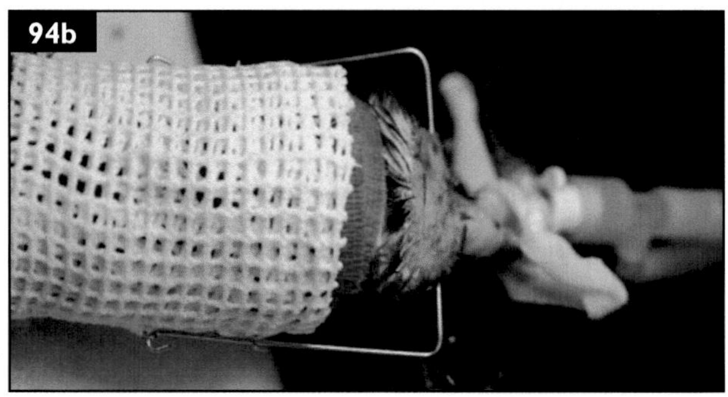
94b

3 If an external support is provided, how should the bird be fed? Feeding during recovery can be achieved using an esophagostomy feeding tube, placed via the proximal crop into the proventriculus and administering a carnivore critical care diet that will pass via such a tube. The support and pin were removed from this case after 3 weeks and the bird made an uneventful and full recovery.

Further reading

Forbes NA (2015) Recent advances in raptor orthopaedic surgery. In: *Proceedings British Veterinary Zoological Society Spring Meeting*, Loughborough.

Huynh M, Sabater M, Brandão J *et al.* (2014) Use of an esophagostomy tube as a method of nutritional management in raptors: a case series. *J Avian Med Surg* **28(1)**:24–30.

CASE 95

1 What surgical procedure would you perform to resolve this condition? Tracheal resection and anastomosis.

2 How would you perform this procedure? Tracheal surgery requires prior air sac intubation to maintain anesthesia. The bird is positioned in dorsal recumbency.

The skin is incised along the ventral midline of the neck or just lateral to the crop. The subcutaneous tissues are dissected to reveal the paired sternothyroideus muscles. The recurrent nerves are identified and avoided. A tracheal ring cranial and caudal to the affected segment is bisected circumferentially with a No. 11 scalpel blade. The tracheal ends are approximated by preplacing simple interrupted sutures of 4-0 to 6-0 polydioxanone on a tapered needle. The sutures are tightened individually with extraluminal knots to appose the tracheal ends. The sternohyoid muscles are apposed over the ventral aspect of the trachea. The thoracic inlet must be closed (air tight) by reattaching the crop/esophagus. The skin closure is routine. In any avian patient it is possible to safely remove six tracheal rings, while in some additional rings may also be removed. In cases with extended areas of damage, an alternative treatment option is the placement of a Teflon stent within the tracheal lumen. Such stents are commercially available for diameters of 4 mm and upwards.
3 What postoperative complications might occur? Damage to the recurrent nerves might result from surgical manipulation or radical resection. The recurrent nerve does not innervate the larynx in birds but instead innervates the esophagus, crop and the tracheal and syringeal muscles; thus, damage to the recurrent nerves will not cause laryngeal paralysis but might instead cause a change in voice. The larynx in birds is innervated by the glossopharyngeal nerve. Postsurgical tracheal stenosis is another possible postoperative complication and efforts should be made to minimize anastomotic stenosis by near-perfect apposition of the anastomosis site, minimally reactive suture material, applying appropriate suture technique, and reducing tension at the surgical site if needed with tension-relieving sutures, each encircling a tracheal cartilage proximal and distal to the anastomosis site.

Further reading

Guzman DS, Mitchell M, Hedlund CS *et al.* (2007) Tracheal resection and anastomosis in a mallard duck (*Anas platyrhynchos*) with traumatic segmental tracheal collapse. *J Avian Med Surg* **21(2)**:150–157.

CASE 96

1 What are your differential diagnoses? Differential diagnoses would include fungal infection, trauma, neoplasia, and psittacine beak and feather disease (PBFD) caused by psittacine circovirus. The bird is suffering from a fungal infection of the keratin layer, which over time has resulted in a severe malformation and deviation with cracking of the beak.
2 What diagnostic tests would you carry out to confirm your diagnosis? Hematology and biochemistry panel may be useful to exclude any other metabolic diseases. Radiographs would provide some information on the extent of a possible infection to rule out involvement of the mandible. Biopsy for histopathology

and bacterial and fungal culture of flaky beak material is essential. PBFD, while unlikely, could be tested by PCR for circovirus from a blood sample or feather pulp material.

3 What treatment would you recommend, and for how long should it be maintained? Systemic and possibly topical antifungal therapy is essential and will need to be maintained for at least 2 weeks after the beak appears normal, which might require 8–12 weeks.

Further reading

Cooper JE, Harrison GJ (1994) Dermatology. In: *Avian Medicine: Principles and Applications*. (eds. BW Ritchie, GJ Harrison, LJ Harrison) Winger's Publications, Lake Worth, pp. 607–639.

CASE 97

1 How does end-tidal partial pressure of carbon dioxide ($PETCO_2$) correlate with partial arterial pressure of carbon dioxide ($PaCO_2$) in psittacine birds? Results of studies in African grey parrots indicate that $PETCO_2$ reliably estimates $PaCO_2$ in isoflurane anesthetized birds receiving intermittent positive-pressure ventilation (IPPV) and suggest that IPPV combined with capnography is a viable option for anesthetic maintenance in avian patients. $PETCO_2$ overestimated $PaCO_2$ by approximately 5 mmHg, which is the opposite of what is seen in mammals. $PETCO_2$ exceeds $PaCO_2$ in birds secondary to the parabronchial cross-current gas exchange mechanism. $PaCO_2$ in awake birds ranges from approximately 25 to 40 mm Hg. $PETCO_2$ of 30–45 mm Hg is considered appropriate for isoflurane anesthetized patients.

2 How do pulse oximetry values correlate with heart rates and arterial oxygen saturation (SaO_2)? Pulse oximetry is accurate in estimating heart rates. However, the pulse oximeter underestimates the actual SaO_2 in birds. Despite the poor accuracy of reported values, trends in oxygenation are apparent and valuable. Motion artifact and the fact that calibration uses the human hemoglobin dissociation curve are the most important factors that interfere with the accuracy of avian measurements. With inhalant anesthesia, arterial partial pressure of oxygen is high because of the high fraction of inspired oxygen delivered; furthermore, respiratory problems are difficult to detect without assessing the arterial blood gases.

3 Doppler has been used in avian anesthesia for indirect blood pressure measurements. What were the conclusions of those studies? Studies showed blood pressure measurements varied significantly between cuff placements on the same limb from the same bird and between individual birds. The precision of these indirect blood pressure measurements was poor. From these results, the meaning and value of Doppler derived indirect blood pressure measurements obtained in psittacine birds remains questionable and should be interpreted as a trend but without relying on the absolute value. Indirect blood pressure (Doppler) measurements were closer to mean arterial pressure measurements than to systolic arterial pressure measurements.

Further reading

Edling TM, Degernes LA, Flammer K *et al.* (2001) Capnographic monitoring of anesthetized African grey parrots receiving intermittent positive pressure ventilation. *J Am Vet Med Assoc* **219(12)**:1714–1718.

Johnston MS, Daviddowski LA, Rao S *et al.* (2011) Precision of repeated, Doppler-derived indirect blood pressure measurements in conscious psittacine birds. *J Avian Med Surg* **25(2)**:83–90.

Paré M, Ludders JW, Erb HN (2013) Association of partial pressure of carbon dioxide in expired gas and arterial blood at three different ventilation states in apneic chickens (*Gallus domesticus*) during air sac insufflation anesthesia. *Vet Anaesth Analg* **40(3)**: 245–256.

Schmitt PM, Göbel T, Trautvetter E (1998) Evaluation of pulse oximetry as a monitoring method in avian anesthesia. *J Avian Med Surg* **12(2)**:91–99.

Zehnder AM, Hawkins MG, Pascoe PJ *et al.* (2009) Evaluation of indirect blood pressure monitoring in awake and anesthetized red-tailed hawks (*Buteo jamaicensis*): effects of cuff size, cuff placement, and monitoring equipment. *Vet Anaesth Anal* **36(5)**:464–479.

CASE 98

1 What are common options for creating an ESF construct or external connecting bar for birds? The common options for creating an ESF construct or external connecting bar for birds are:

- Positive profile threaded ESF half-pins connected with an acrylic bar using:
  - Commercial methacrylate based composite (e.g. Acrylx® IMEX).
  - Horse hoof acrylic using a Penrose drain or straw as a mold.
- Positive profile threaded half-pins with a FESSA tubular fixator (shown in **98**).
- Positive profile threaded ESF half-pins connected with a traditional bar and clamp system.

2 What advantages and disadvantages should be considered for each of these constructs? Fixator constructs based on ESF models vary in weight, cost, flexibility, and ease of use. General considerations are that any system used must by extremely versatile, lightweight, removable, effective, and well tolerated. The system with an acrylic bar can be inexpensive, can be countered (curved) as needed, being extremely versatile, and can be made to the exact length. Main drawbacks are the excessive odor during acrylic curing time, and that once it is set, it cannot be adjusted. The FESSA tubular fixator can be used as a guide during transvers pin placement and is more easily adjusted postoperatively than others. It allows easy addition or removal of pins for extra stabilization or dynamic destabilization, as well as advancing or pulling back transverse pins if needed. The connecting bar is rigid and has fixed length (3, 4.5, 6, 10, 15, 20 cm). The size of the half-pins that can be used with the different sized bars is also limited. The cost of this construct is significantly higher, but it can be re-used. The traditional bar and clamp system is adjustable, requires exact pin placement, and is quite heavy relative to other systems. It is often used as a temporary fixation to stabilize the fracture site prior to surgery to complete an ESF-IM tie-in.

3 What are the advantages and disadvantages of plate fixation in birds compared with these constructs? In birds, an advantage of bone plates is excellent patient tolerance, because plates are completely internal and provide rigid fixation with less callus formation. This might be particularly useful in some species, such as large psittacines and aquatic birds. Disadvantages of bone plating are high costs for instrumentation and implants, specialized training in placing the plates, prolonged anesthesia times, soft tissue disruption, lack of soft tissue in many areas to cover the plate, and potential thermal conduction. One complication associated with bone plating in birds is plate bending. It has been suggested that long bone fractures in birds need to be repaired with longer plates than similar canine and feline fractures. A combination of an IM pin and a bone plate reduces internal plate stress and thereby increases fatigue life of the plate. In general, plates are not removed unless they cause a problem. This should be a consideration in wild birds as ideally all fixation is removed prior to release back to the wild.

CASE 99

1 What are the abnormal radiographic findings? There is an approximately 1.2 cm × 0.7 cm irregular, ovoid, mildy heterogeneous mineral opacity in the mid-caudal coelomic cavity between the ends of the pubic bones.

2 What is the most likely diagnosis? How would you confirm your diagnosis? A cloacolith. Cloacoliths in birds are composed of urates. Uric acid, the main end product of nitrogen catabolism, is excreted with urine by the renal tubules, forming a colloid suspension stabilized by mucopolysaccharides and glycoproteins. These form microspheres that prevent precipitation of urates within the ureters, cloaca, and lower gastrointestinal tract. In supersaturated urine, changes in the solubility and chemistry of the uric acid mucopolysaccharide microspheres may predispose to cloacoliths. Shifts in bacterial flora composition in the distal rectal and coprodeal environment or an improper diet could be considered contributors. Dehydration and infection are likely the most common causes. Nutritional deficiencies might also alter the composition of the protein part of the urine microspheres. A cloacal examination under deep sedation or a cloacoscopy procedure under general anesthesia would confirm the diagnosis.

3 How would you treat this condition? The cloacolith is gently broken down inside the cloaca with or without the aid of an endoscope. The fragments are then removed and the cloaca is lavaged with warm saline. Systemic antibiotics, since the cloacal mucosa is likely to suffer damage, and analgesia with opioids and local anesthetics are essential.

Further reading

Beaufrère H, Nevarez J, Tully TN Jr (2010) Cloacolith in a blue-fronted Amazon parrot (*Amazona aestiva*). *J Avian Med Surg* **24(2)**:142–145.

CASE 100

1 What species are these chicks? These neonatal chicks are umbrella cockatoos (*Cacatua alba*).

2 Are they precocial or altricial? They are altricial, hatched with eyes closed, down is minimal to absent, and mobility is limited. Nourishment, warmth (93–98°F [33.9–36.7°C]), and a safe place must be provided for altricial chicks.

3 What is wrong with the beak of the chick that is sitting up? This chick has a prognathic beak malformation (**100b**). Cockatoos are prone to prognathism or pug beak. The cause of this beak malformation is unclear but genetics, nutrition, and incubation are suspect. This maxilla beak malformation is characterized by a shorter maxilla (upper beak) that grows into the normal sized mandible (lower beak). If detected, early firm bilateral physical therapy helps to uncurl and pull the upper beak out and over the lower beak. If done several times daily during postnatal development, before beak calcification, it is correctable. If presented later, a rhinotheca extension is attached, so that each time the beak is closed, the rhinotheca is pulled forward. The prosthesis often does not stay on for more than 10 days, but by then the beak will have corrected, so long as this is done while the beak is still soft and not fully developed.

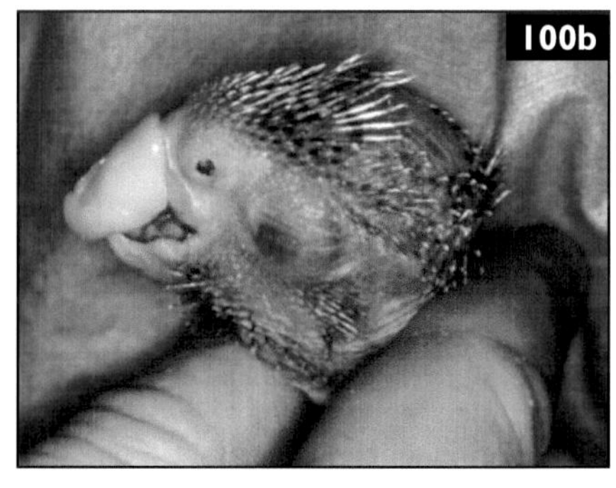
100b

Further reading

Romagnano A (2012) Psittacine pediatrics. *Vet Clin North Am Exot Anim Pract* **15(2)**: 163–182.

CASE 101

1 The presence of megathrombocytes (enlarged thrombocytes) in avian blood films has been associated with which pathologic process? Chronic inflammatory process. This is commonly observed in species kept in confinement with the tendency to crash repeatedly on the walls or ceiling of the enclosure or cage. A common clinical finding is chronic inflammation of the carpal joint after repeated injuries sustained in captivity.

2 Thrombocyte counts in avian hematology samples are commonly achieved using which quantitative method? Counting directly from the blood film during the differential cell count.

3 What are the main differential morphologic characteristics of thrombocytes in birds? Rectangular shaped cell with basophilic cytoplasm with numerous vacuoles and a rectangular shaped nucleus.

Further reading

Samour J (2016) Hematology analysis. In: *Avian Medicine*. (ed. J Samour) Elsevier, St. Louis, pp. 35–52.

CASE 102

1 What are the four key bones involved in elevating and lowering the upper bill? Quadrate, jugal, pterygoid, and palatine.

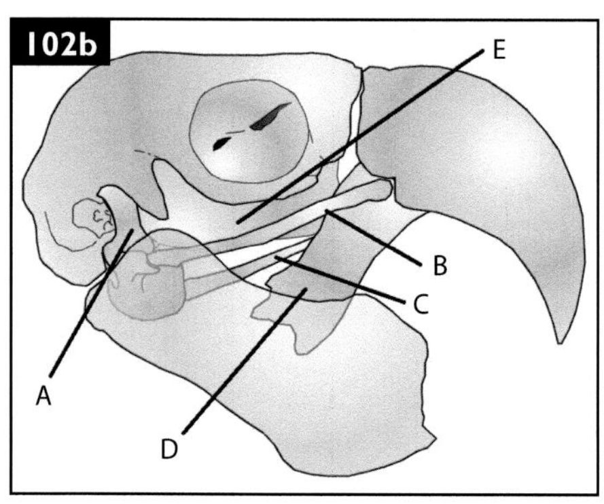

2 Explain the role of each of these bones in the kinesis of the psittacine beak. Rotation of the quadrate bones (A) rostrally pushes on the jugals (B) and pterygoids (C), moving them rostrally and resulting in an upward push being applied to the palatine bone (D), causing it to slide rostrally on the central boney ridge of the ventral brain case (os mesethmoidale) (E) and forcing the upper jaw to swing upward at the craniofacial hinge (protraction) (**102b**). Rotation of the quadrate bones caudally causes the upper jaw to swing downwards (retraction).

3 How many synovial joints are involved in prokinetic motion of the upper bill, and what bones are they associated with? Fifteen.

- Jugal: two bones, synovial joints at both ends (4).
- Pterygoid: two bones, synovial joints at both ends (4).

- Palatine: one fused pair, rostral points of articulation (2).
- Quadrate: two bones, dual articulation at braincase (neurocranium) (4), jugal, pterygoid (already counted).
- Craniofacial hinge (nasofrontal hinge) (ginglymus) (1).

(The articulation of the palatine and the os mesethmoidale is a syndesmoidal joint and is not synovial.)

Further reading

King AS, McLelland J (1984) Skeletomuscular system. In: *Birds: Their Structure and Function*, 2nd edn. (eds. AS King, J McLelland) Baillière-Tindall, Philadelphia, pp. 43–51.

CASE 103

1 **Which two important behavioral events take place in the life of a juvenile parrot (i.e. in the period from hatching to weaning)?** (1) (Sexual) *imprinting*, which is the process by which animals learn the characteristics of appropriate mates by learning the characteristics of their parents or siblings; and (2) *socialization*, which is the process by which the bird adopts the behavior patterns appropriate to the social environment in which it lives, allowing it to co-exist and interact with other individuals.

2 **Provide at least three examples of medical issues that may arise following hand-rearing of psittacine chicks.** (1) Reduced growth rate; (2) beak trauma and/or deformities (e.g. scissors beak, prognathism); (3) crop stasis, overstretching, impaction, and/or trauma (including crop burn and esophageal perforation), with potential secondary infections; (4) aspiration of food, resulting in pneumonia or asphyxiation; (5) hepatic lipidosis (resulting from feeding excessive amounts of high-energy diets); (6) intoxications, particularly of vitamin D (which can result in renal failure and gout); (7) nutritional deficiencies (e.g. hypocalcemia and hypovitaminosis D), which result in metabolic bone disease and bone and joint abnormalities.

3 **Provide at least three examples of behavioral problems that may arise following hand-rearing.** (1) Delayed weaning and continued begging and whining for food; (2) inappropriate reproductive behavior (e.g. impaired copulatory behavior, floor laying of eggs) resulting in decreased chances of successful reproduction; (3) disrupted social bonds with conspecifics; (4) overbonding to humans; (5) display of inappropriate sexual behavior towards humans (e.g. regurgitation, courtship behavior); (6) (territorial) aggression; (7) fears and phobias; (8) excessive vocalizations; (9) feather damaging behavior and other stereotypies.

Further reading

Flammer K, Clubb SL (1994) Neonatology. In: *Avian Medicine: Principles and Application.* (eds. BW Ritchie, GJ Harrison, LR Harrison) Wingers Publishing, Inc., Lake Worth, pp. 805–838.

Fox R (2006) Hand-rearing: behavioral impacts and implications for captive parrot welfare. In: *Manual of Parrot Behavior.* (ed. A Luescher) Blackwell Publishing, Ames, pp. 83–92.

CASE 104

1 What type of organism is infesting these canaries? The organism seen is a feather louse. Based on the broad-based head, this is likely a chewing louse and not a sucking louse.

2 What is the clinical significance of this finding? Lice infestation can lead to irritation, excessive preening, and feather abnormalities in affected canaries. In addition, lice may act as intermediate hosts for parasites such as microfilarids and act as mechanical vectors for avipox virus.

3 What treatment options are available for this flock of 60 birds? Given the large number of individuals in this flock, treatment options that require individual dosing are less than ideal, but include dusting with either a permethrin or carboryl powder product or with fipronil spray (spray on hands and then rub onto feathers). Treatment of the flock may be done by using an aqueous-based ivermectin product in the water. It is important for the client to understand that because the birds live outdoors, they will continuously come into contact with wild birds who can transmit this parasite to his flock.

Further reading

Macwhirter P (1994) Passeriformes. In: *Avian Medicine: Principles and Application.* (eds. BW Ritchie, GJ Harrison, LR Harrison) Wingers Publishing, Lake Worth, pp. 1172–1199.

CASE 105

1 What is the most likely diagnosis for this mass? Oropharyngeal angiofibroma. Angiofibromas are rare, benign tumors comprised of aggregates of abnormal blood vessels surrounded by connective tissue stroma. This presentation has been described in cockatiels involving the oropharyngeal cavity.

2 How would you confirm your diagnosis? Diagnosis of angiofibromas in man and dogs relies on histopathology and advanced imaging. For resectable cases, such as this one, complete surgical removal remains the treatment of choice. In this case, surgical removal of the angiofibroma was easily achieved by ligation of the 'stalk-like' base with two ligatures with 5-0 PDS without hemorrhage. If clear margins are not achieved, follow-up radiation treatment or intralesional chemotherapy should be considered.

3 What is the prognosis? There is limited information on long-term follow up of excised angiofibromas in birds. In this case and another case published, there was no recurrence a few months after surgery. Recurrence rates in the human literature are variable, with some reports as high as 22.6%.

Further reading

Doss GA, Miller JA, Steinberg H *et al.* (2015) Angiofibroma in a cockatiel (*Nymphicus hollandicus*). *J Comp Pathol* **152**(2–3):274–277.

CASE 106

1 What diagnostic test can be performed antemortem to confirm the diagnosis? Oropharyngeal and cloacal swab samples are used routinely for antemortem diagnosis of WNV infection by detection of infectious particles or viral RNA. Serum samples tested by real time-PCR for WNV could result in a false-negative result despite the high sensitivity of this test due to clearance of the virus from the blood. Different avian species have been shown to be viremic for differing periods of time and with different levels of viremia, with peak viremia occurring approximately 2–4 days post inoculation in most species followed by a decrease or clearance of the virus from the blood. Serology is most useful when applied to paired (acute and convalescent) samples. Plaque reduction neutralization test is the gold standard for anti-WNV antibody detection and titer determination, although cross-reactivity to other flaviviruses (e.g. St. Louis encephalitis virus) is possible. Other antibody tests, such as blocking ELISAs, have been used for high-throughput screening. Virus isolation in Vero cell plaque assay is the gold standard for the confirmation of acute WNV infection.

2 What is the prognosis? What lesions would you expect on postmortem examination? The prognosis for recovery, with severe clinical signs like seizures, is guarded to poor. On gross postmortem examination, no significant lesions except for mild to moderate enlargement of liver and spleen are likely. On histopathology, lymphoplasmacytic and histiocytic hepatitis, interstitial nephritis, myocarditis, splenitis, enteritis, pancreatitis, and encephalitis might be seen. For postmortem diagnosis, virus isolation or RT-PCR testing of homogenized tissue (e.g. kidney, spleen, heart, and brain) might be useful. Detection in tissues is rare more than 2–3 weeks after the infection.

3 What treatment and preventive measures would you recommend? Treatment of WNV infection in birds consists of supportive care, such as fluid electrolyte therapy, supplemental heat or cold, antibiotic or antifungal agents to treat or prevent secondary infections, assisted feeding or nutritional supplementation, NSAIDs, and anticonvulsants if needed. Because there is no specific treatment for WNV infection in birds, minimizing mosquito contact to lessen the likelihood of infection is crucial. Smaller scale strategies include eliminating standing water, covering upright containers, and filling holes or depressions. For captive birds housed outdoors, mosquito nets or screens may be used to cover caging. Alternately, bird-safe mosquito repellents (e.g. geraniol, Fasst Products) aerosolized around caging have been shown to deter mosquitoes. Although no WNV vaccinations are currently approved for use in birds, several commercially available equine vaccines (e.g. killed and recombinant canarypox-vectored vaccines) have been tested in birds. Seroconversion rates are generally low following vaccination and may vary by species and vaccine construction. Few data are available regarding vaccine-induced protection against virus challenge.

Further reading

Stockman J, Hawkins MG, Burns RE *et al.* (2010) West Nile virus infection in a green-winged macaw (*Ara chloropterus*). *Avian Dis* **54(1)**:164–169.

CASE 107

1 **What are the effects of oiling on individual birds?** Individual birds may be directly contaminated by external oiling, ingestion of oil, respiration of volatile components, or by contamination of embryos through the egg shell. External contamination is the most important, resulting in high mortality due to the bird's inability to repel water, thermoregulate, and fly. Ingestion may lead to disruption in nutrient absorption and subsequent diarrhea, anorexia, regurgitation, and hemorrhage. Polycyclic aromatic hydrocarbons can damage directly the respiratory system and result in systemic toxicity. Oxidative damage to red blood cells may lead to hemolytic anemia. Immunosuppression and reproductive impairment are also known direct effects.

2 **What are the different steps in the process of caring for oiled birds?** Recovery of oiled birds from the environment and transport to a rehabilitation center or field stabilization site, processing and intake, stabilization, cleaning, pre-release conditioning, and release back to the wild. The washing and rinsing procedures are the most stressful steps in the rehabilitation process. Birds that have not been stabilized prior to washing often die. The stabilization process usually requires 48 hours of indoor care before washing. The bird should meet minimum health criteria (e.g. adequate packed cell volume, total plasma protein concentration, blood glucose concentration, and absence of infectious disease) before being washed. The exception to stabilization before washing is in cases of highly volatile products. The birds are washed initially to remove the bulk of the toxic material quickly, but not to restore waterproofing. A second bath and rinse procedure is required after stabilization.

3 **How would you prevent secondary diseases in this process?** Prophylactic antifungals and 10–15 air changes per hour to prevent respiratory aspergillosis. Net-bottomed cages to prevent pododermatitis and keel 'donuts' over the keel to prevent pressure sores are some of the common considerations for these problems.

Further reading

Mazet JAK, Newman S, Gilardi KVK *et al.* (2002) Advances in oiled bird emergency medicine and management. *J Avian Med Surg* **16(2)**:146–149.

CASE 108

1 What is the most likely diagnosis? Renal neoplasia (e.g. adenocarcinoma, adenoma). Renal masses occur more frequently in young to middle-aged male budgerigars and are often located in the anterior division of the affected kidney. This clinical sign results from tumor compression of the ischiadic nerve as it passes through the kidney or from tumor growth adjacent to the synsacrum and ilium. Although these tumors rarely metastasize, local infiltration of the spine, as seen in this case, has been reported. Some cases may also have other clinical signs such as lethargy, loss of body condition, coelomic distension, dyspnea due to the intracoelomic pressure or organ displacement.

2 What diagnostic test would you perform to confirm your diagnosis? CBC, plasma biochemistry panel, survey and contrast gastrointestinal radiographs, and ultrasound of the coelomic cavity. In the cases reported, uric acid does not seem to be a sensitive indicator of renal neoplasia unless affecting both kidneys. On plain radiographs, the position of the grit-filled ventriculus relative to the kidneys can be used as a landmark for changes in renal size. Also, normal sized kidneys do not extend ventral to an imaginary horizontal line parallel to the spine that passes through the ventral border of the acetabulum. In contrast radiographs, lateral displacement of the proventriculus and caudal displacement of the ventriculus on the VD view, and ventral displacement of the intestines and ventriculus in the laterolateral view might be present depending on the size and location of the mass. High-frequency transducers with a small contact surface are necessary to obtain diagnostic ultrasonographic images in these cases.

3 What are the treatment options and prognosis? Therapeutic options for renal neoplasia in budgerigars are limited due to the bird's small size and the location of the tumor. There are no reports of successful surgical treatment. The short distance of their artery to the aorta makes ligation and hemostasis difficult or impossible with the current techniques. There are anecdotal reports of chemotherapy treatment. The platinum analog carboplatin (5 mg/kg diluted 1:10 with sterile water IV once a month for 3 months) has been reported in one case, which seemed to alleviate signs for a few weeks. Analgesics (e.g. tramadol) and NSAIDs (e.g. meloxicam) have been used anecdotally to alleviate pain associated with the growing mass. More information is needed on chemotherapeutic agents in budgerigars before further recommendations are made.

Further reading

Simova-Curd S, Nitzl D, Mayer J *et al.* (2006) Clinical approach to renal neoplasia in budgerigars (*Melopsittacus undulatus*). *J Small Anim Pract* **47**:504–511.

CASE 109

1 What is the most likely cause of the lesions noted around the joints? Articular gout is caused by deposition of uric acid crystals in the synovial capsules and tendon sheaths of joints. This is secondary to hyperuricemia likely related to renal disease and inability to clear the uric acid from circulation. To confirm the diagnosis, a fine needle aspirate and cytology (do not fix with alcohol as it will dissolve the uric acid crystals) or a murexide test should be performed. To perform a murexide test: a drop of nitric acid is mixed with a small amount of suspected material on a slide and dried by evaporation in a Bunsen flame. After cooling, one drop of concentrated ammonia is added. In the presence of urates, a mauve (pale purple) color will develop. Alternatively, a polarizing microscope can be used to identify urate crystals.

2 What medications can be used to help this patient? Analgesics (e.g. opioids or opioid-like) can be used to provide palliative relief since these lesions are typically painful. Surgery to remove the uric acid crystal deposits will not be feasible in most cases. To slow progression of the disease, allopurinol can be administered orally. This medication is a competitive xanthine oxidase inhibitor that blocks the conversion of xanthine into uric acid. As allopurinol is contraindicated in some birds of prey, urate oxidase may be used in these species as well as pigeons. Urate oxidase catalyzes the conversion of urate and oxygen into allantoin and hydrogen peroxide. Additionally, colchicine reversibly inhibits xanthine dehydrogenase and has been used anecdotally in some avian species. None of these medications will decrease the crystals that are already present in the joints. Probencid, a uricosuric drug used in people that acts mostly by reducing the absorption of uric acid in the tubuli, appears to be contraindicated in birds. Birds lack the reabsorptive mechanism of uric acid and probencid could further reduce the active secretion of uric acid into the tubuli. A low protein diet could potentially slow down the progression of the disease, although this has not been clinically evaluated in birds.

3 What other systems may be affected by this disease? Visceral gout can also occur. This occurs when excessive plasma uric acid levels are present and these crystals precipitate on various organs such as the liver, spleen, and pericardium, as well as in the kidneys.

Further reading

Burgos-Rodríguez, Armando G (2010) Avian renal system: clinical implications. *Vet Clin North Am Exot Anim Pract* **13**(3):393–411.

Fudge AM (2000) Laboratory reference ranges for selected avian, mammalian, and reptilian species. In: *Laboratory Medicine Avian and Exotic Pets.* (ed. AM Fudge) WB Saunders, Philadelphia, pp. 375–400.

Poffers J, Lumeij JT, Redig PT (2002) Investigations into the uricolytic properties of urate oxidase in a granivorous (*Columba livia domestica*) and in a carnivorous (*Buteo jamaicensis*) avian species. *Avian Pathol* **31(2)**:573–579.

CASE 110

1 What are the differential diagnoses for 'swollen head syndrome' in pheasants and/or partridges (110)? The so called 'swollen head syndrome' can be caused by one type of virus or bacteria or, most commonly, by a mixed viral and bacterial infection. The top four possible differentials would be: *Mycoplasma gallisepticum* (Mg), avian rhinotracheitis (ART) caused by pneumovirus, infectious bronchitis (IB) caused by coronavirus, and various secondary bacteria such as *E. coli*, *Pasturella* spp., and *Ornithobacterium rhinotracheale* (ORT).

2 What are the most appropriate tests available to diagnose the cause of this syndrome? Although in theory serologic testing would give an indication as to exposure, it does not help identify the current causative organisms. The best diagnostic procedures would be to take multiple swabs of the trachea/sinuses and cloaca for PCR techniques. These swabs can be sent off to a laboratory to identify if ART/Mg/IB or ORT are present. Swab samples should also be taken of the trachea and sinuses and placed in a charcoal-based medium for laboratory culturing and antibiotic sensitivity testing; this type of swab will identify the most likely secondary bacterial infections such as *E. coli* or *Pasturella* spp.

3 What are the most appropriate treatment methods available for flocks of pheasants and partridges? This syndrome can often be difficult to treat and resolve due to the nature of the disease involved, as both ART and IB, if found, are caused by viruses and there is no current treatment available. *Mycoplasma* is a bacterium that will likely infect the bird for life and although antibiotics will reduce the clinical signs, they will often return when the bird becomes stressed again. In the UK, Aivlosin™ (tylvalosin) is the only licensed antibiotic for *Mycoplasma* in pheasants. This product is administered in the drinking water for 3 days. If other bacteria are identified, then the use of an off-license product may be applicable, but since withdrawal periods are unknown in these cases, the choices for animals that might enter the food chain are limited.

Further reading

Bradbury JM, Yavari CA, Dare CM (2001) Mycoplasmas and respiratory disease in pheasants and partridges. *Avian Pathol* **30:4**:391–396.

CASE 111

1 Describe the anatomic entry points for a double-entry orchidectomy. The first entry point is made caudal to the last rib, cranial to the pubis bone, and ventral to flexor cruris medialis muscle, identical to that used for single-entry diagnostic coelioscopy (**111b**, black arrow). Following insertion of a telescope, a second port is created under endoscopic guidance, caudal to the pubic bone (**11b**, white arrow) and ventral to the flexor cruris medialis muscle (**111b**, m).

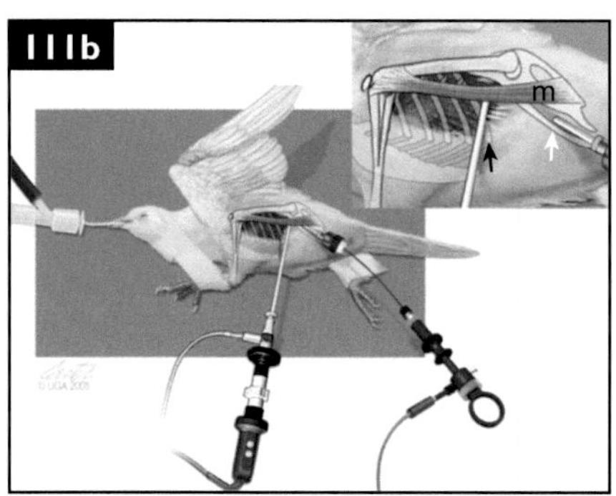

Courtesy of Educational Resources, UGA

2 Name the structures labeled (2), (3), and (4) in image 111a that are closely associated with the left avian testis (1) and need to be avoided during orchidectomy. Avian testes are located very close to the left adrenal gland (4), the cranial division of the left kidney (2), and the common iliac vein converging into the caudal vena cava (3), and are suspended by a short mesorchium. This makes inadvertent entrapment of or coagulative damage to these structures, including severe hemorrhage, important considerations during orchidectomy.

3 What are the possible complications of a single-entry vasectomy technique in birds? Ureter perforation and hemorrhage are the most commonly reported complications of an endoscopic vasectomy.

Further reading

Heiderich E, Schildger B, Lierz M (2015) Endoscopic vasectomy of male feral pigeons (*Columba livia*) as a possible method of population control. *J Avian Med Surg* **29(1)**: 9–17.

Hernandez-Divers SJ, Stahl S, Wilson GH *et al.* (2007) Endoscopic orchidectomy and salpingohysterectomy of pigeons (*Columba livia*): an avian model for minimally invasive endosurgery. *J Avian Med Surg* **21(1)**:22–37.

CASE 112

1 What is the most likely date of death? From the maggot size, the estimate is December 3rd.

2 What do you believe the bird's normal flying weight would be? The bird's P8 length (368.5 mm) is three SDs (3 × 11.5) less than the average of 403 mm. This means that the bird is very small for its species and so one would expect its 'fat weight' to be three SDs (3 × 123.6 g) less than the species average weight (1,105 g) (i.e. 734.2 g).

As the bird was in the middle of a flying season (hence at flying weight), he would ordinarily be expected to be some way below 'fat weight'. The flying weight of a nonimprint falcon would normally be 5–10% less than its fat weight (i.e. 36–72 g less than this bird's fat weight). In this bird its flying weight would therefore be expected to be 734.2 g less 36–72 g = 662–698 g.

3 How long do you think it could have been starved for? The postmortem weight was 645 g. The bird had not been fed the previous evening (as the gastrointestinal tract was empty). It was also dehydrated and had had no water available. This was winter time (i.e. cold) and an unfed bird would lose weight fast. Considering the bird's likely flying weight, its postmortem weight, and the findings of diarrhea and dehydration, one would not have expected this bird to have been ill for more than 1–2 days prior to death (i.e. not prior to November 30th). The client was hospitalized before the bird became ill.

Further reading

Amendt J, Krettek R, Zehner R (2004) Forensic entomology. *Naturwissenschaften* **91**:51–65.

CASE 113

1 What abnormality is seen to be affecting which eye in this sparrow hawk? Right eye hyphema and uveitis.

2 What is the most common cause for this disorder in birds? Blunt or sharp trauma in birds can cause anterior and/or posterior uveitis, frequently associated with hyphema. Other differential diagnoses for uveitis in birds include infections, immune-mediated inflammation, and neoplasia. Clotting disorders tend to manifest bilaterally and systemically.

3 What ophthalmologic tests should be conducted? After completing a full physical examination including assessment of the periocular structures, additional ophthalmologic diagnostic tests can be used to evaluate the consequences of trauma within the eye. Anatomic particularities of the raptor eye mean they respond differently to blunt trauma compared with mammals. The shape of the eye is normally maintained by the scleral ossicles even in cases of severe blunt trauma. If asymmetries are suspected, radiographs, CT or MRI may be of value in diagnosing periocular and intraocular disorders. The avian cornea is larger and less protected by periocular bones compared with those of mammals, which, in combination with the longitudinal shape of the globe in some species, means that blunt trauma typically results in lesions of greater severity within the posterior rather than the anterior segment. Direct and indirect ophthalmoscopy and slit lamp microscopy permit examination of the anterior and posterior chambers and should be used in all avian trauma cases, even when there is no external indication of ocular damage. Tonometry measures the intraocular pressure. Fluorescein dye test allows assessment of the integrity of the cornea. Ocular ultrasonography may aid in the diagnosis of some disorders in the posterior segment of the eye, whereas electroretinography is useful to assess the retinal function.

Further reading

Seruca C, Molina-López R, Peña T *et al.* (2012) Ocular consequences of blunt trauma in two species of nocturnal raptors (*Athene noctua* and *Otus scops*). *Vet Ophthalmol* **15**(4):236–244.

CASE 114

1 What is your top differential diagnosis for the cause of death in these ducklings? Based on the clinical history of this disease within the flock, it is highly suspicious that these ducklings died as the result of duck hepatitis virus (DHV) type 1. DHV-1 is an *Avihepatovirus* in the family Picornaviridae, is internationally widespread, and is highly virulent in young ducklings.

2 What pathologic changes do you expect to see on gross necropsy? Typical lesions associated with DHV-1 include hepatomegaly with hemorrhagic foci, splenomegaly, and swelling of the kidneys with congestion of the renal vasculature.

3 In addition to necropsy, what diagnostic tests should be performed to confirm the cause of this die-off? Virus isolation from the liver tissue of affected ducklings is the most common confirmatory test performed for DHV-1. Virus neutralization and PCR testing are also available but less widely used.

Further reading

Woolcock PR (2015) Duck viral hepatitis. *OIE Manual of Diagnostic Tests and Vaccines for Terrestrial Animals.* Accessed online at: http://www.oie.int/international-standard-setting/terrestrial-manual/access-online/

CASE 115

1 What gross lesions are shown in the image? The presence of white material throughout the serosa of visceral organs and within the kidneys is characteristic of visceral gout (**115b**).

2 What is the histologic lesion? The tophi are deposits of uric acid in the parenchyma of the organ. Tissues should be harvested into alcohol (not formalin), as urates dissolve in the latter. Histopathology of the affected organ will confirm the presence of uric acid crystals in the organs.

3 What is the pathophysiology of this disease? Uric acid is the primary non-nitrogenous waste product of avian kidneys. When avian kidneys are in end-stage renal disease, they are unable to actively secrete uric acid. The resulting hyperuricemia causes precipitation of this nonsoluble product on the serosal surface of many visceral organs; this tends to be an acute/peracute end-stage presentation. Articular gout (precipitation of uric acid in joint spaces) can also develop following chronic kidney disease (CKD), and the combination of visceral and articular gout is often observed in birds with CKD; however, this swan only had visceral gout, and all of the examined joints were grossly normal. The underlying cause for renal disease in this swan was never determined. In other waterfowl, lead toxicosis, nutritional (i.e. excess dietary protein, hypovitaminosis A), and other toxin exposure (oil exposure, mycotoxins) have been associated with development of CKD.

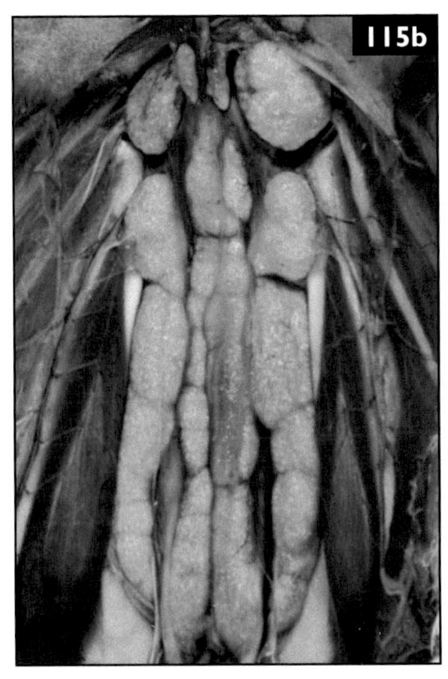
115b

Further reading

Speer BL (1997) Urogenital disorders. In: *Avian Medicine and Surgery*. (eds. R Altman, S Clubb, G Dorrestein, K Quesenberry) WB Saunders, Philadelphia, pp. 625–644.

CASE 116

1 What surgical procedure would you perform to resolve this condition? Salpingohysterectomy, as the oviduct and not the ovary is removed. Ovariectomies in birds are technically difficult and carry a high risk of hemorrhage or incomplete resection.

2 How would you perform this procedure? The bird is positioned in right lateral recumbency and the left leg may be retracted cranially to increase exposure of the cranial and caudal coelom, respectively. The skin is incised over the left paralumbar region from the last rib to the caudal aspect of the pubic bone. The abdominal muscles are incised and the superficial medial femoral artery and vein over the lumbar fossa should be cauterized. The last two ribs might be transected to provide adequate exposure of the cranial coelomic cavity. The ventral ligament is dissected to allow the oviduct to be released and positioned in a linear fashion. The fimbria of the infundibulum lies caudal to the ovary and may be elevated to expose the dorsal ligament. A small blood vessel can be identified coursing from the ovary through the infundibulum and should be coagulated and dissected. The remainder of the dorsal suspensory ligament may then be dissected, from craniad to caudal, with hemostasis of the vasculature with radiosurgery or hemoclips. The oviduct is retracted ventrally and caudally as it is released. It is ligated at its junction with the vagina a short distance from the cloaca. Closure is in 2–3 layers and is routine with 3-0 to 5-0 monofilament absorbable suture.

3 What intra- and postoperative complications might occur? Intraoperative complications include hemorrhage if there is inadequate hemostasis during dissection of the dorsal ligament of the oviduct, and damage to the ureters during caudal dissection of the oviduct before entering the cloaca. If the oviduct is friable, contamination of the field is likely without careful manipulation of the tissue. Postoperative complications include peritonitis, airsacculitis, and pneumonia if there was contamination of the peritoneum or air sacs during the procedure, and internal ovulation and egg yolk peritonitis if the bird continues ovulating in the future. Administration of GnRH agonists (e.g. deslorelin acetate implants) is recommended to avoid the latter.

Further reading

Guzman DS (2016) Avian soft tissue surgery. *Vet Clin North Am Exot Anim Pract* **19(1):** 133–157.

CASE 117

1 What major structure will be revealed if the kidneys of this yellow-crowned Amazon parrot (*Amazona ochrecephala*) are dissected away? The kidneys lie in the renal fossa formed by the pelvis, which is fused to the synsacrum. Between the fossa and the kidney is the lumbosacral plexus forming the femoral nerve (F), obturator nerve (O) and the ilioischiadic nerve (I) (**117b:** 1 = cranial division; 2 = intermediate division; 3 = caudal division; 4 = lumbosacral plexus).

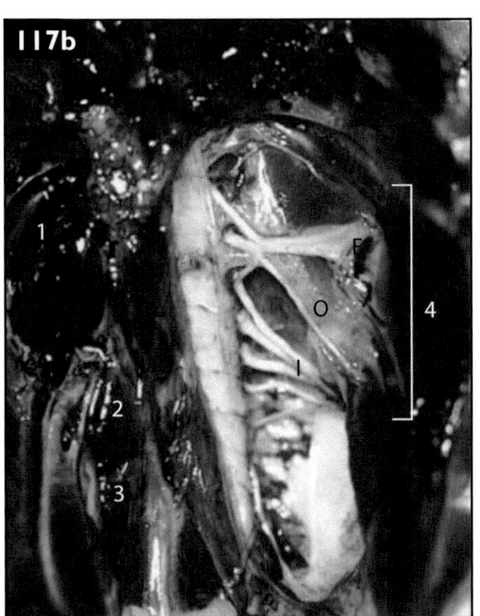

2 How can disease in this area cause paralysis of the legs? Because of the close proximity of the nerves to the kidneys, nephritis can frequently cause neuritis; likewise, renal neoplasia will cause pressure on the nerves. In both cases the legs can become paralyzed.

CASE 118

1 What is the correct terminology for the behavior modification techniques that can be used to decrease the conditioned fear response? Also explain briefly how these techniques work. The most commonly used technique to reduce fear and phobias is *systematic desensitization*, which involves the gradual and systematic exposure to a stimulus until the conditioned response to the stimulus is extinguished. To boost its effects, the procedure is combined with *counterconditioning*, during which a positive stimulus is noncontingently paired with the aversive stimulus to change the value of the conditioned stimulus. *Flooding* (also referred to as response blocking) is another technique that can be used, but due to its negative side-effects (e.g. promotion of *learned helplessness* due to depriving the animal of the ability to choose) veterinarians are discouraged from using this technique.

2 What are the key factors that need to be taken into consideration for the successful implementation of the above mentioned procedure? Key to a successful implementation of systematic desensitization are the following: the owner needs to be able to recognize what calm behavior looks like in their parrot by assessing the parrot's activities as well as its plumage, eyes, and the position of its head, body, and legs; the fear-eliciting stimulus can be identified, reproduced, and controlled (in terms of distance, intensity, or duration, but also in terms of its occurrence outside of the behavior modification sessions); the stimulus is initially presented at a low enough duration, intensity, or far enough distance to prevent eliciting a fear response; the incremental steps are sufficiently small to prevent the triggering of a fearful response; and advancement of the next step only occurs if the animal remains calm in the presence of the stimulus at that level.

3 In case of extreme fear or patients being refractory to behavior modification therapy, pharmacologic intervention may be considered. What drug classes may be used to reduce anxiety? Pharmacologic treatment options for fear or phobias include: benzodiazepines (e.g. diazepam, midazolam, lorazepam); tricyclic antidepressants (e.g. amitriptyline, doxepin, clomipramine); (selective) serotonin reuptake inhibitors (e.g. fluoxetine, paroxetine); and azapirone derivatives (e.g. buspirone).

Further reading

Martin KM (2006) Psittacine behavioral pharmacotherapy. In: *Manual of Parrot Behavior.* (ed. A Luescher) Blackwell Publishing, Ames, pp. 267–279.

van Zeeland YRA, Friedman SG, Bergman L (2016) Behavior. In: *Current Therapy in Avian Medicine and Surgery.* (ed. BL Speer) Elsevier, St. Louis, pp. 177–251.

Wilson L, Luescher AU (2006) Parrots and fear. In: *Manual of Parrot Behavior.* (ed. A Luescher) Blackwell Publishing, Ames, pp. 225–231.

CASE 119

1 Which crop shape corresponds to the following bird species: budgerigar, cormorant, pigeon, chicken, vulture? (a) Cormorant; (b) vulture; (c) chicken; (d) pigeon; (e) budgerigar. The simplest form is merely a spindle-shaped enlargement of the cervical esophagus, which is also present in ducks, geese, and a number of songbirds. Parrots have well-developed crops that lie at the caudal cervical esophagus. A prominent right pouch and a small left pouch typify parrots. Pigeon crops have a more complicated structure. Both right and left lateral pouches or diverticulae are well developed.

2 Which bird species lack a true crop? A common misconception is that all birds have a crop, but it is absent in many groups including owls, toucans, gulls, and penguins.

3 Which bird species are known to produce secretions in the crop or esophagus that are used to feed the chicks? Pigeons secrete nutrients into the crop. In pigeons the epithelium of the crop thickens by the 13th day of egg incubation. The epithelial cells accumulate protein and fat, which are subsequently shed into the lumen. This holocrine secretion is referred to as crop milk. It contains 12.4% protein, 8.6% lipids, 1.37% ash, and 74% water. It is predominantly a protein and fatty acid source for their chicks, and is devoid of carbohydrate and calcium. Both parents produce crop milk. The pituitary hormone that controls the secretion of nutrients into the crop is prolactin, which is produced in the cephalic lobe of the adenohypophysis. Male emperor penguins (*Aptenodytes forsteri*) produce a similar holocrine secretion into the esophagus that also consists of desquamated epithelial cells. Greater flamingos (*Phoenicopterus roseus*) also secrete nutrients into the esophagus. Esophageal mucous glands produce a merocrine secretion that is fed to the young.

Further reading

Klasing KC (1998) Anatomy and physiology of the digestive system. In: *Comparative Avian Nutrition*. CAB International, Wallingford, pp. 20–21.

Lumeij JT (1994) Gastroenterology and endocrinology. In: *Avian Medicine: Principles and Application*. (eds. BW Ritchie, GJ Harrison, LR Harrison) Wingers Publishing, Inc., Lake Worth, pp. 490 and 584.

CASE 120

1 Based on the history and physical examination findings, what are your differential diagnoses? Lead toxicosis, West Nile virus infection, avian influenza infection, inanition due to extreme weather condition, trauma, advanced aspergillosis.

2 What diagnostic test would you perform to confirm the diagnosis? Hematology and blood chemistry; blood sample for measuring lead concentrations; blood sample for serology for virology; oropharyngeal and/or cloacal PCR for virology.

3 The falcon appeared to be suffering from lead toxicosis. How is it possible to have such a high lead level? Which is the ideal therapeutic agent for treatment? Serology for West Nile virus and influenza infection was negative. No lead pellets or particles were observed in the gastrointestinal tract. Lead level was 6.52 µmol/L (135 µg/dL) (reference interval <0.966 µmol/L [<20 µg/dL]). Lead is quickly absorbed from the gastrointestinal tract as soon as the lead particles reach the ventriculus, causing characteristic clinical signs as seen in this case. The severity of clinical signs is associated with the amount of lead ingested. Lead pellets and lead fragments are sometimes cast out together with casting material (especially in birds >1 kg in weight), hence the absence of metallic particles in the gastrointestinal tract as seen in this particular case. Primary therapy: $CaNa_2EDTA$ (50–100 mg/kg IM or SC q12h for one week) and retest. Continue therapy until lead level is below 0.966 µmol/L (20 µg/dL). Provide supportive therapy with Ringer's lactate, vitamins B_1 and B_{12}, and nutritional support by gavage feeding two or three times a day until willing to eat on its own.

Further reading

Samour J, Naldo J (2002) Diagnosis and therapeutic management of lead toxicosis in falcons in Saudi Arabia. *J Avian Med Surg* 16(1):16–20.

CASE 121

1 What are the 'abnormal feathers' noted by the client and seen in this image? The feathers are pin feathers, or developing feathers.

2 What process is occurring in this bird, and how would you explain this process to a client? This bird is actively molting. Molting is a normal process of feather replacement, where a new feather starts to grow, pushing out the old feather from its follicle to be replaced by the new feather, which is growing from the same follicle.

3 The client would like to know how frequently this process will occur, and asks what physiologic factors control this process? Most birds molt annually, some twice a year, while some large psittacine birds molt every other year. Control of molt is a complex process that is controlled by light cycles experienced by the bird and hormonal influences; however, nutrition, stress, life stage, and local (feather follicle) factors also play a role.

Further reading

Cooper JE, Harrison GJ (1994) Dermatology. In: *Avian Medicine: Principles and Application*. (eds. BW Ritchie, GJ Harrison, LR Harrison) Wingers Publishing, Lake Worth, p. 607.

CASE 122

1 What is the most likely diagnosis? This is superficial chronic ulcerative dermatitis. In raptors the condition appears most commonly in birds kept in damp, cold, or poorly ventilated accommodation.

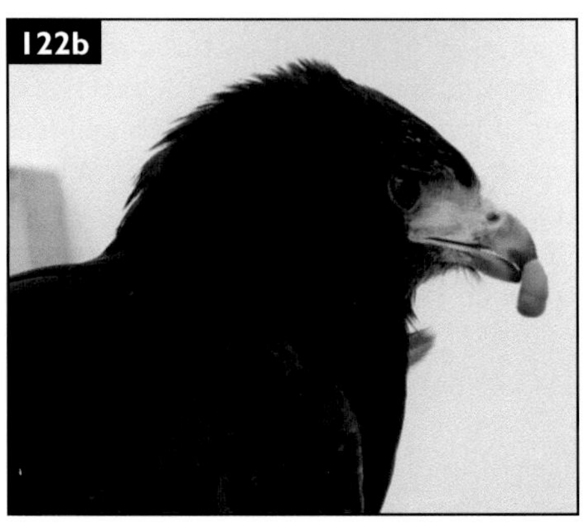
122b

2 How is the disease best managed? Improving ventilation or moving the bird. Preventing ongoing self-trauma is an important part of the therapy. While in parrots a collar might be applied, in a raptor, a dental acrylic 'blob' may be attached to the end of the beak (**122b**). Bacterial and fungal culture and sensitivity testing is indicated, and some cases have been shown to be associated with methicillin-resistant *Staphylococcus aureus*. Topical (not oily) and systemic antimicrobial medication is indicated and should be maintained until at least 2 weeks after the lesion has totally resolved, which typically requires 6–8 weeks.

3 How it might progress if left untreated? In Harris' hawks and peregrine falcons these lesions have been reported to undergo neoplastic transformation, resulting in squamous cell carcinoma at this site. Lesions respond well to excision. Squamous cell carcinoma in this site is considered to be locally invasive (hence can reoccur if not totally removed), but does not tend to distally metastasize.

Further reading

Forbes NA, Cooper JE, Higgins R (2000) Neoplasms of birds of prey. In: *Raptor Biomedicine III*. (eds. JT Lumeij, JD Remple, PT Redig *et al.*) Zoological Education Network, Palm Beach, pp. 127–146.

Smith SP, Forbes NA (2007) Treatment of pyotraumatic dermatitis infected with methicillin-resistant *Staphylococcus aureus* in three pet psittacines. *Proc Europ Comm Assoc Avian Vet Conf*, Zurich, pp. 177–184.

Smith SP, Forbes NA (2009) A novel technique for prevention of self-mutilation in three Harris' hawks (*Parabuteo unicinctus*). *J Avian Med Surg* **23(1)**:49–52.

CASE 123

1 What are your differential diagnoses for the radiographic intestinal findings? An irregular and marginated intestinal mucosa may be due to infiltrative disease such as mycobacteriosis, inflammatory bowel disease, or neoplasia (e.g. lymphoma). The bird in this case had diffuse intestinal lymphoma. Lymphoma is the most commonly reported lymphoid neoplasia in psittacines and has been reported in many species. The onset of lymphoma is highly variable, being reported in birds of all ages. Clinical signs are variable as well, depending on the distribution and severity of the disease, and range from nonspecific signs such as lethargy, anorexia, and weight loss to periorbital or cutaneous swelling, coelomic distension, lameness, and diarrhea. Anemia is a common clinical pathologic finding, but a leukemic blood profile is uncommon in psittacines with lymphoma.

2 What are the intra- and postoperative risks associated with this procedure? The surgical approach varies with the location of the intestinal loop of interest. The coelomic cavity should be packed with moist laparotomy pads or gauze to prevent contamination. Following enterotomy and intestinal biopsy, the intestinal wall is sutured using a 5-0 to 8-0 absorbable monofilament suture on a one-fourth-circle atraumatic needle. The surgical site is tested for leakage carefully with a 26-gauge needle catheter or smaller and saline solution. If the tissue is diseased, the risk of dehiscence and peritonitis is high and a serosal patch could be used to prevent this. Birds do not have omentum, and the risk of peritonitis is higher than in mammals with gastrointestinal surgery. A partial luminal stricture could occur if too much tissue is removed or the intestinal wall is not closed carefully.

3 How would you treat lymphoma in this bird? What is the prognosis? Numerous chemotherapy protocols for the treatment of lymphoma in birds have been described, but no protocols specific for diffuse intestinal lymphoma in birds are available. Most chemotherapy protocols include a combination of therapeutics such as prednisone, vincristine, cyclophosphamide, asparaginase, chlorambucil, and doxorubicin. Most of these chemotherapeutic agents require IV administration, and the placement of an IV catheter or vascular access port is needed. There is limited information regarding the adverse effects of these chemotherapeutic agents in birds, and close monitoring, including CBC, is needed to evaluate immunosuppression, thrombocytopenia, and other adverse effects. There are few reports in the literature on intestinal lymphoma and further information is needed to provide an accurate prognosis, but it is generally considered guarded to poor.

Further reading

Souza MJ, Newman SJ, Greenacre CB *et al.* (2008) Diffuse intestinal T-cell lymphosarcoma in a yellow naped Amazon parrot (*Amazona ochrocephala auropalliata*). *J Vet Diagn Invest* 20(5):656–660.

CASE 124

1 At what age is septicemia usually seen in game bird chicks? Septicemia usually starts at between 2 and 15 days.

2 What are the main causes of septicemia in chicks? Weakened chicks due to early abnormal environmental temperatures. Poor gastrointestinal health leading to bacteria gaining entry to the blood. High water contamination leads to a high burden of bacteria. Yolk sac infection, which progresses and develops into septicemia (**124a, b**). Poor environmental conditions, leading to an increased bacterial load.

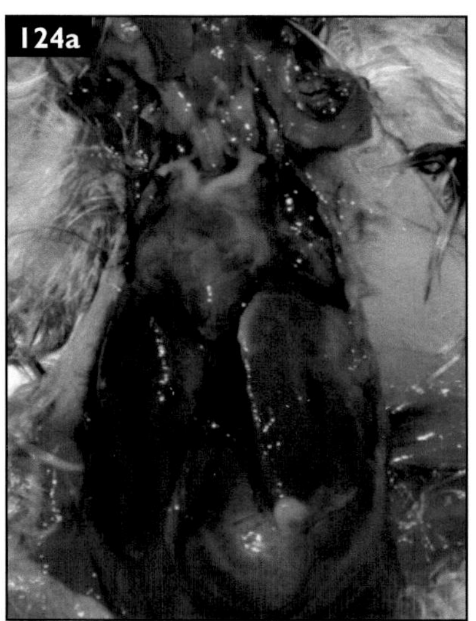
124a

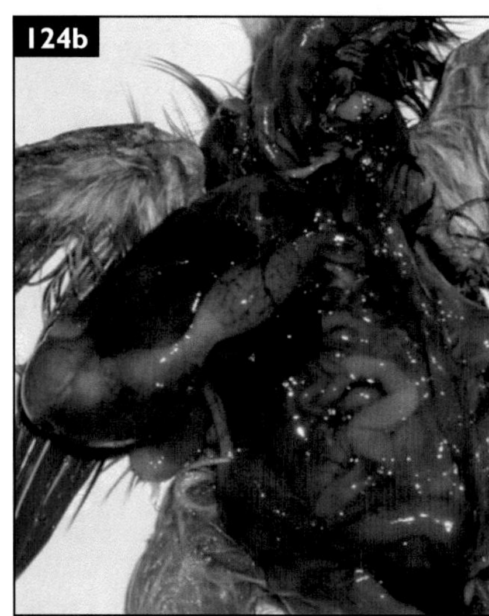
124b

3 What is the recommended course of action when birds show clinical signs suggestive of septicemia? Clinical signs usually manifest as high mortality and dull depressed birds. The bacteria usually found in the blood are *E. coli* or *Pseudomonas* spp. However, there are several common bacteria that can all take advantage of a weakened chick. The recommended course of action is to take several samples using a cotton swab and transport them in charcoal-based media to a laboratory for culture and sensitivity to assess which antibiotic would be most appropriate to use. Tetracyclines usually have good sensitivities in these situations.

CASE 125

1 Describe the abnormality and list the most common differential diagnoses for this finding. There is a red proliferative mass arising from the right cloacal wall and obscuring the right uroproctadeal fold. Differential diagnoses include neoplasia (e.g. carcinoma, leiomyosarcoma, fibrosarcoma) and papilloma.

2 Describe the technique for obtaining a biopsy of this structure in order to confirm a diagnosis. What is a possible complication of this procedure? Proliferative lesions can be biopsied under endoscopic guidance. Performing cloacoscopy with saline infusion will allow superior visualization and therefore more accurate biopsy. Cloacal wall perforation can occur if full-thickness biopsy of the cloacal wall is inadvertently obtained.

3 What treatment modalities are possible, using the 2.7-mm endoscope system, that may be applicable to this case? Cloacal papillomas and neoplasias can be ablated using radiosurgical or diode laser probes, which can be passed through the instrument channel of the operating sheath. Further treatment may be indicated, depending on the disease process diagnosed.

Further reading

Antinoff N, Hoefer HL, Rosenthal KL *et al.* (1997) Smooth muscle neoplasia of suspected oviductal origin in the cloaca of a blue-fronted Amazon parrot (*Amazona aestiva*). *J Avian Med Surg* **11(4)**:268–272.

Divers SJ (2010) Avian diagnostic endoscopy. *Vet Clin North Am Exot Anim Pract* **13(2)**:187–202.

Hernandez-Divers SJ, Wilson H, Lester VK *et al.* (2006) Evaluation of coelioscopic splenic biopsy and cloacoscopic bursa of fabricius biopsy techniques in pigeons (*Columba livia*). *J Avian Med Surg* **20(4)**:234–241.

Palmieri C, Cusinato I, Avallone G *et al.* (2011) Cloacal fibrosarcoma in a canary (*Serinus canaria*). *J Avian Med Surg* **25(4)**:277–280.

Reavill DR (2004) Tumors of pet birds. *Vet Clin North Am Exot Anim Pract* **7(3)**:537–560.

CASE 126

1 What common factors are considered to be involved? This is a complex subject; the following factors should be considered:

- Calcium, phosphorus, vitamin D_3 content of the diet, most importantly not what is offered, but what is consumed. Also access to UV light is a relevant factor.
- Rate of growth. If protein levels in the diet are increased or if total daily food intake is increased, the growth rate may be excessive, the outcome being inadequate mineralization of bones. This will result in bones that are unable to sustain what in other ways would be normal forces and thus cause bony abnormalities.
- Smooth rearing substrate, as this might result in an improper stance that will cause abnormal bone pressures during growth.
- Exercise during growth should be encourage in precocial species (e.g. cranes), while it might need to be limited together with weight supporting in altricial species (e.g. psittacines).

2 How is bone growth different in birds compared with mammals? What are the implications when evaluating birds radiographically? Birds do not have a calcified epiphysis until the end of the growth period. In birds, as the femur grows it does not undergo endochondral ossification as it does in mammals, instead the epiphyseal cartilage persists as a wide basophilic hyaline zone covered by a narrow eosinophilic articular cartilage. The elongation of this cartilage model is achieved by interstitial growth of chrondocytes. It is only when the growth cartilage becomes exhausted that the invading marrow tissue enters the epiphyseal cartilage. Individual chondrocytes undergo hypertrophy, allowing final endochondral ossification of the epiphyseal cartilage. Mammalian bones in contrast show endochondral ossification; in other words they ossify as they increase in length.

3 Why might young raptors changing from whole day-old chicks to quartered rabbit or pigeon carcases develop metabolic bone disease? It is not the Ca:P ratio of what is offered, but the Ca:P ratio of what is consumed. Unless pigeon and rabbit carcases are minced up finely prior to feeding, the bones will be too large for young chicks (5–25 days when bone growth is most important) to ingest, resulting in an increased rate of metabolic bone disease.

Further reading

Dellman HD (1971) *Veterinary Histology: An Outline Text-Atlas*. Lea & Febiger, Philadelphia.

Forbes NA (2010) Managing pelvic limb developmental condition in birds. In: *Proceedings British Veterinary Zoological Society Autumn Meeting*, Dudley, pp. 62–64.

Pratt CWM (1961) The effect of age on the arrangements of fibres in the bone matrix of the femur of domestic fowl. *J Anat* **95**:110–122.

CASE 127

1 What factors cause death of eggs in each of the first, second, and third trimesters? First trimester: contaminated eggs; poor egg handling or storage; poor incubation (temperature; humidity; lack of turning); genetic abnormalities (inbreeding); breached integrity of the eggshell; transovarian or postlaying infection of the egg; drug or pesticide effects on the egg.

Second trimester: genetic abnormalities (inbreeding); parental nutritional deficiencies or imbalances; infections (bacterial, viral, or fungal); poor incubation (temperature, humidity, lack of turning); poor egg handling in the first trimester.

Third trimester: incubation faults (temperature, humidity, lack of turning); brooder faults (temperature; humidity; lack of turning); infections; malpositioning prior to hatching; parental nutritional deficiencies; genetic abnormalities; poor hatchery hygiene.

2 What levels of fertility and hatchability should be strived for? Fertility and hatchability levels vary greatly between species and individuals. Fertility tends to be lower in inbred, older, or younger birds, and at the beginning and end of each breeding season. The breeder should try to achieve 85–95% fertility. Hatchability is also variable with respect to the species and the above factors; the breeder should aim for 80–85%.

3 How often should eggs be turned during incubation? Most eggs are positioned on their side with the round (air sac) end slightly elevated. Eggs should be turned 6–12 times daily, each turn being between 30 and 45° or the eggs may be turned along the longitudinal axis. The first trimester is the most crucial period for egg turning; failure to turn in this period will usually lead to disaster. If a chick appears to be developing slowly, increasing the turns is thought to be of assistance in some cases.

Further reading

Joyner KL (1994) Theriogenology. In: *Avian Medicine and Surgery: Principles and Techniques*. (eds. BW Ritchie, GJ Harrison, LR Harrison) Wingers Publishing, Lake Worth, pp. 748–804.

CASE 128

1 What abnormal radiographic findings are seen in the radiographs at this point (128a, b)? The radiolucent halo surrounding the proximal transverse pin indicates that the pin is loose (**128c, d**, circled areas). From these two images, it is not certain if the proximal pin traversed fully through both cortices; this may be the cause of the problem. A small sequestrum has also formed (**128c**, arrow). The proximal humeral cortex also appears to have overridden the distal fragment, which will have resulted in a shortening of the humerus.

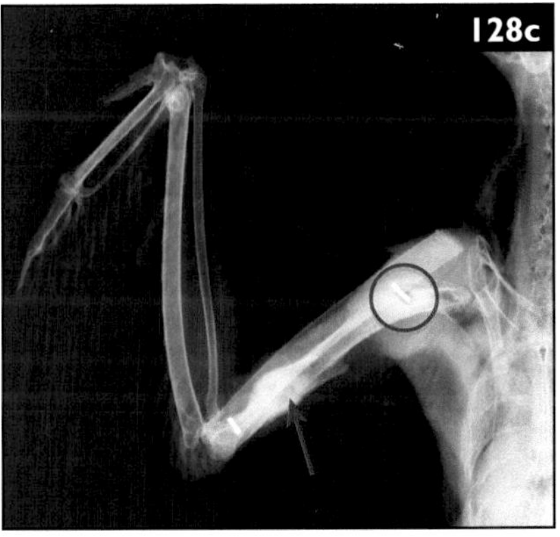
128c

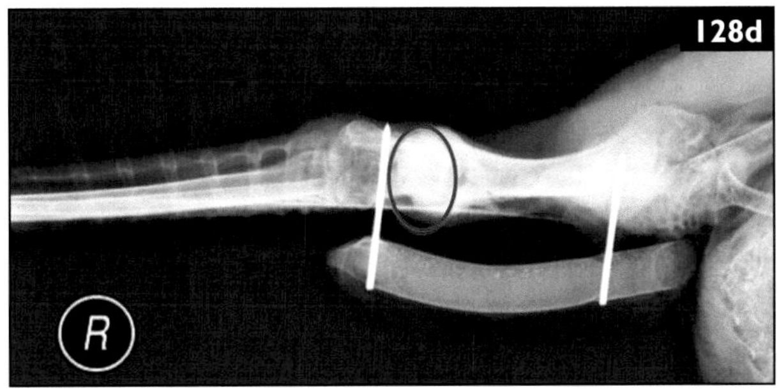

128d

2 What is the clinical significance? The sequestrum is a piece or area of devitalized bone that lost its blood supply either at the time of injury or during surgical repair from rough tissue handling; these areas are frequently associated with open fractures. Pin loosening may result from poor insertion technique such as excessive motion when using a hand drill, leading to a slightly larger hole than necessary or failure to engage two cortices (as is the case in this patient), or infection.

3 What is the recommended course of action? Loose pins should be removed as they do not contribute to fixation rigidity and they may lead to complications. If a fracture is not healed enough to be managed conservatively without fixation, new ESF pins should be placed in a different location from the loose pins and incorporated into a new fixator. The sequestrum should be surgically explored, débrided, and any infected or dead tissue removed.

Further reading

Redig PT, Ponder J (2016) Orthopedic surgery. In: *Avian Medicine*, 3rd edn. (ed. J Samour) Mosby, St. Louis, pp. 312–350.

CASE 129

1 What is the most likely diagnosis, and how can this diagnosis be confirmed? The most likely diagnosis is an infection with *Salmonella typhimurium* var. Copenhagen. The bacterium is officially named *Salmonella enterica* subsp. *enterica* serovar Typhimurium variant Copenhagen. Confirmation of the diagnosis can be made by culturing a pooled fecal sample from the pigeon loft. In the past serology has been used to test pigeons, but this test was found to be unreliable as it does not identify carriers, which constitute the majority of the infected pigeons.

2 What treatment and preventive options are available? Although antibiotics (e.g. trimethoprim/sulfamethoxazole) may be used to combat the bacterial infection, it is important to realize that despite treatment, many carriers will remain in the flock. Optimizing housing conditions, thereby limiting reinfections and decreasing the amount of stress by the avoidance of overcrowding, is very important. Euthanasia of (less valuable) birds that display clinical signs may be considered to decrease the infection load. Valuable birds may be best isolated and treated individually to ensure that an accurate dose of antibiotics is given to the patient. In addition, a vaccine can be used after an outbreak of pigeon salmonellosis. This vaccine, however, is not 100% protective against infection.

3 Does the disease pose a health risk for the pigeon fancier? Explain how and why. Research has shown that strains of *Salmonella typhimurium* var. Copenhagen are of low virulence to humans and therefore do not pose a significant risk for the pigeon fancier. If the pigeon fancier is immunocompromised, extra precautions to prevent transmission are advised.

Further reading

Hooimeijer J, Dorrestein GM (1997) Pigeons and doves. In: *Avian Medicine and Surgery*. (ed. R Altman) WB Saunders, Philadelphia, pp. 886–909.

Pasmans F, van Immerseel F, Hermans K *et al.* (2004) Assessment of virulence of pigeon isolates of *Salmonella enterica* subsp. *enterica* serovar Typhimurium variant Copenhagen for humans. *J Clin Microbiol* **42**:2000–2002.

CASE 130

1 What structures were entered as the trephination procedure was performed? Lateral rhinotheca (keratin), dermis, maxilla (bone), maxillary diverticulum of the infraorbital sinus.

2 How would you manage the trephination site postoperatively? The trephination sites were left open and covered with a tape bandage, allowing the topical application of antimicrobials, which were selected based on sensitivity of the prior *Pseudomonas aeruginosa* isolate while histopathology and microbiology were pending. In this case, amikacin was used. Complete healing of the surgical wounds was accomplished in 2 weeks.

3 How would the trephination affect the growth of the rhinotheca? There were no adverse effects noted on rhinothecal regrowth, and the trephination site was indiscernible within 1–2 months postoperatively.

Further reading

Baumel JJ, Raikow RJ (1993) Arthrologia. In: *Handbook of Avian Anatomy: Nomina Anatomica Avium*, 2nd edn. (eds. JJ Baumel, AS Kings, JE Breazile) Nuttall Ornithological Club, Cambridge, pp. 264–265.

King AS, McLelland J (1984) Integument. In: *Birds: Their Structure and Function*, 2nd edn. (eds. AS King, J McLelland) Baillière-Tindall, Philadelphia, pp. 24–26.

King AS, McLelland J (1984) Skeletomuscular system. In: *Birds: Their Structure and Function*, 2nd edn. (eds. AS King, J McLelland) Baillière-Tindall, Philadelphia, pp. 43–51.

King AS, McLelland J (1984) Respiratory system. In: *Birds: Their Structure and Function*, 2nd edn. (eds. AS King, J McLelland) Baillière-Tindall, Philadelphia, p. 112.

CASE 131

1 Birds have a small functional residual capacity (FRC). True. Although birds have a greater respiratory volume (per kg body weight) compared with mammals, only 10% of this volume is located within the gas exchange system (parabronchi and air capillaries). With a small FRC, gas exchange does not occur without airflow. Periods of apnea rapidly decompensate the acid–base balance and may become life-threatening.

2 Oxygen absorption in avian lungs is more efficient compared with mammalian lungs. True. Oxygen absorption in the avian lung is 10 times more efficient compared with mammals due to several adaptations. Air capillaries are much smaller than mammalian alveoli (diameter less than one-third). The valves in the tertiary bronchi together with the bellows mechanism of the air sacs enable continuous unidirectional air flow across the gas exchange area throughout inspiration and expiration. There is a thinner blood–gas barrier across the air capillaries in the lungs and the rigid lungs allow 20% greater gas exchange area compared with mammals. The cross-current exchange system (blood flowing at right angles to the unidirectional airflow) enables an oxygen gradient to form between oxygenated blood and deoxygenated air, so that more oxygen is absorbed from the air into the blood.

3 **Birds are more sensitive to hypercapnia.** True. Birds are more sensitive to hypercapnia than mammals. Gas flow rates during anesthesia should therefore be higher, at least three times the normal minute volume (which is approximately 800 mL/min/kg). As the flowmeter on most anesthetic machines is inaccurate, a minimum of 1 L/min should be used with small birds (increasing appropriately in larger birds).

Further reading

Longley L, Fiddes M, O'Brien M (2008) Section 2: Avian anaesthesia. In: *Anaesthesia of Exotic Pets*. (ed. L Longley) Saunders Elsevier, Edinburgh, pp. 129–182.

CASE 132

1 **What is the structure and function of the tunnel arrowed?** The bony tunnel is formed by the supratendinal bridge that runs over the tendon of insertion of the long digital extensor (LDE) muscle and keeps the tendon close to the surface of the bone as it runs over the joint.

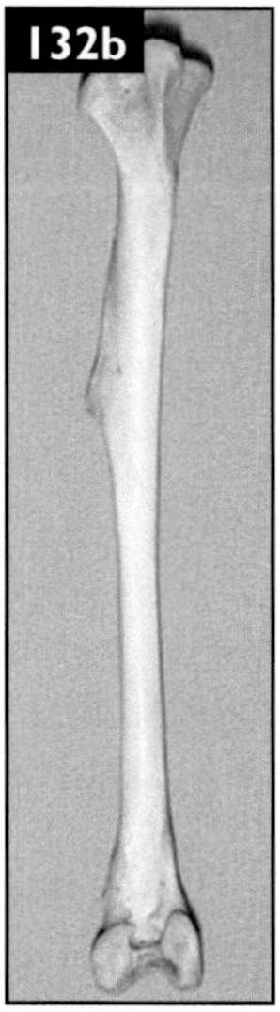

132b

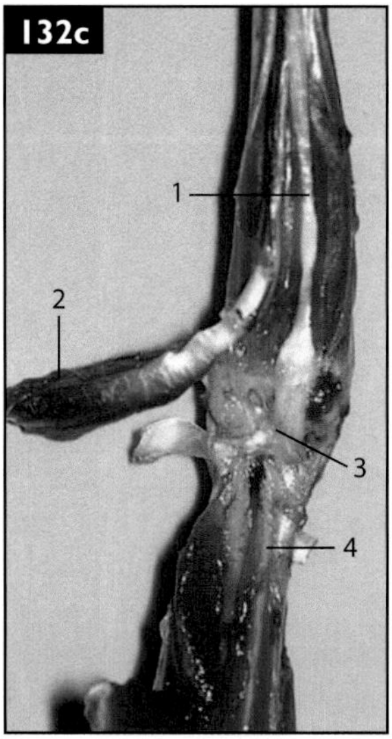

132c

2 **What difference is there in this region in Psittaciformes?** The supratendinal bridge in parrots (e.g. red-fronted macaw [*Ara rubrogenys*] is fibrous not bony (**132b, c:** 1 = LDE tendon; 2 = *M. tibialis oranialis*; 3 = supratendinal bridge; 4 = LDE muscle).

3 **What complications might occur with distal tibiotarsus fracture repair?** If fractures in this region are repaired by immobilization of the intertarsal joint, the tendon's free running will be compromised and this joint, and those of the toes, will be prevented from extending.

CASE 133

1 What are the medical and nonmedical differential diagnoses that should be considered in parrots presented with this behavior? Medical differentials that have been implicated in the development and maintenance of feather damaging behavior include: endoparasitism (particularly giardiasis in cockatiels); ectoparasitism; bacterial or fungal dermatitis or folliculitis; infectious disease (e.g. circovirus, polyomavirus, chlamydiosis); systemic disease (e.g. hepatopathy, nephropathy, reproductive disease); malnutrition (e.g. hypovitaminosis A); intoxications (e.g. lead, zinc); neoplasia; allergies; endocrine disease (e.g. hypothyroidism); and pain.

Nonmedical factors include: boredom, frustration, anxiety, hand-rearing and imprinting on humans, socialization deficits, neurochemical abnormalities, temperamental traits, genetic factors, hormonal influences, socio-environmental factors (e.g. overcrowding, social isolation, sleep deprivation, lack of ability to perform species-specific behaviors, exposure to aversive stimuli), and learning factors (reinforced behavior).

2 Describe the different aspects that need to be considered when designing an initial treatment plan for a parrot with feather damaging behavior. A treatment plan should always be tailored to the individual bird, based on the results of a thorough history, physical examination, behavioral assessment, and other diagnostic tests. Treatment should aim at correcting any nutritional deficiencies and environmental factors that may be involved. If any medical issues are encountered or suspected to contribute to the behaviour, these should be appropriately addressed. Promoting a more stimulating environment (e.g. by foraging enrichment, means of social contact, chewing toys, and other types of enrichment) is also an important part – if not the primary focus – of any treatment regimen for feather damaging behavior. In addition, behavior modification techniques may help to replace the behavior of the bird with other, more desirable behaviors. Restraint options (e.g. collars, jackets) are only recommended as a temporary measure to stop birds from self-mutilating or temporarily stop the cycle of habitual feather damaging behavior, as these primarily serve to prevent clinical signs rather than eliminate the underlying cause.

3 In birds that do not respond to the initial treatment plan, pharmacologic intervention may be considered. What categories of pharmacologic agents may be considered for treatment of refractory feather damaging behavior? Pharmacologic interventions that may be considered include: benzodiazepines (e.g. diazepam); dopamine antagonists (e.g. haloperidol); tricyclic antidepressants (e.g. clomipramine); (selective) serotoninergic reuptake inhibitors (e.g. paroxetine, fluoxetine); and opioid antagonists (e.g. naltrexone).

Further reading

Seibert L (2006) Feather picking disorder in pet birds. In: *Manual of Parrot Behavior*. (ed. A Luescher) Blackwell Publishing, Ames, pp. 255–265.

van Zeeland YRA, Friedman SG, Bergman L (2016) Behavior. In: *Current Therapy in Avian Medicine and Surgery*. (ed. BL Speer) Elsevier, St. Louis, pp. 177–251.

CASE 134

1 At what age does coccidiosis typically affect partridges? Recent studies of game bird coccidiosis have identified that levels of coccidial oocysts do not get high enough to cause clinical signs until around 6–8 weeks of age.

2 How is coccidiosis commonly diagnosed in partridges? There are two main methods of diagnosing coccidiosis. The first is fecal oocyst counts, whereby feces from a selection of birds are combined and an overall OPG (oocysts per gram) count is measured (**134**). The disadvantage of this technique is that it can take several days for results and it will only provide the concentration of end-stage oocysts that are being secreted rather than what is clinically affecting the birds. The second option is to perform a postmortem examination on several birds, to conduct intestinal scrapes, and to assess the concentration of coccidial infection and whether there is any secondary bacterial disease that also requires treatment.

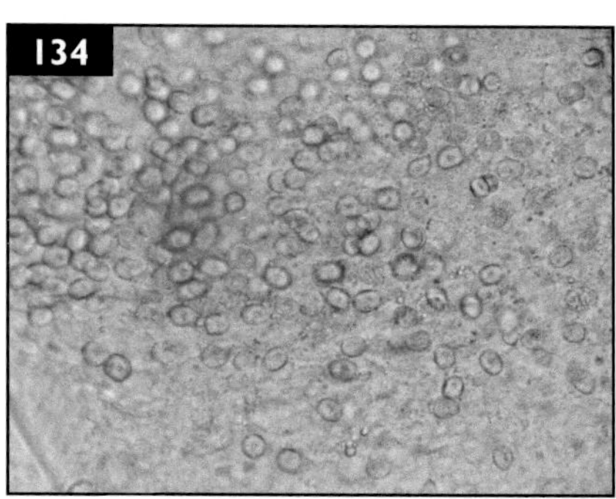

3 What are the treatment options for coccidiosis in partridges? Currently, the only licensed anticoccidial product for partridges in the UK is Avatec™ (lasalocid sodium) in feed; this is used as a preventive treatment during the rearing period and, unfortunately, will not treat a high burden of coccidia. Off-licence products include toltrazuril and amprolium, which should only be used under the guidance of a veterinarian following an in-depth evaluation of the disease burden on the site. Prevention should include cleaning the sheds with a disinfectant that kills the final coccidial oocyst stage as well as management of the land and improved hygiene around feed and water stations.

Further reading

Naciri M, Repérant JM, Fort G *et al.* (2011) *Eimeria* involved in a field case of coccidiosis in red-legged partridges (*Alectoris rufa*) in France: oocyst isolation and gross lesion description after experimental infection. *Avian Pathol* **40**(5):515–524.

CASE 135

1 What is the most likely etiology? What would be the most likely postmortem findings? Duck plague, otherwise known as duck viral enteritis (DVE), is a highly seasonal and rapidly fatal disease affecting only ducks, geese, and swans, caused by Anatid herpesvirus 1. Typically, birds are not found alive. The virus attacks the vascular system, causing areas of hemorrhage in the esophagus, proventriculus, intestine, and cloaca. The virus induces vascular damage, especially in smaller blood vessels, venules, and capillaries. This results in the development of generalized hemorrhages and progressive degenerative changes of parenchymatous organs. Recently, it has been proposed that apoptosis and necrosis of lymphocytes induced by this virus may result in lymphoid depletion and possibly immunosuppression, which may also explain the presence of secondary infections.

2 How should the disease outbreak be managed? In the face of a disease outbreak, the best option is depopulation, cleaning, and disinfection, and then repopulation with vaccinated stock. There is marked interspecies susceptibility to DVE with Muscovy ducklings (*Cairina moschata domesticus*) being more susceptible than white Pekin ducklings. Where a disease outbreak occurs, mortality typically reaches 90–95%. While any surviving birds are likely to have a solid immunity, they will be lifelong herpesvirus carriers and seasonal shedders of virus, creating a risk to any in-contact unvaccinated birds.

3 How can future outbreaks of disease be prevented? Disease occurs where one free living or captive bird is a virus carrier, shedding virus and triggering an outbreak of clinical disease and mortality. In an area where this has occurred, it will typically reoccur in subsequent years. It is advised that all susceptible waterfowl are vaccinated annually, in the 2 months prior to the seasonal risk period. Only live attenuated vaccines are efficacious. A chicken embryo-adapted, modified live virus vaccine has been approved in the USA to immunize domestic ducks in zoological aviaries and those kept by private aviculturists. A 0.5 mL dose is administered SC or IM to domestic ducklings >2 weeks old. An inactivated vaccine, which appears to be as efficacious as the modified live vaccine, has not been tested on a large scale and is not currently licensed.

Further reading

Banda A (2013) Overview of duck viral enteritis. *The Merck Veterinary Manual* (last full review/revision August 2013). www.merckvetmanual.com/poultry/duck-viral-enteritis/overview-of-duck-viral-enteritis

Campagnolo ER, Banerjee M, Panigrahy B *et al.* (2001) An outbreak of duck viral enteritis (duck plague) in domestic Muscovy ducks (*Cairina moschata domesticus*) in Illinois. *Avian Dis* **45**(**2**):522–528.

CASE 136

1 What is the most likely etiology of the observed clinical signs? Anticoagulant rodenticide toxicity is a common cause of coagulopathy in birds of prey. Any prey that has ingested a rodenticide bait could potentially be a source of secondary exposure for a hawk, including rodents and invertebrates. Other coagulopathies, for instance from hepatic insufficiency, can be considered. The coelomic distension could be due to a hemocoelom associated with a compression of the air sac, causing increased respiratory efforts.

2 How would you confirm your presumptive diagnosis? The presumptive diagnosis can be confirmed by measuring blood concentrations of a panel of anticoagulant rodenticides including brodifacoum, which has been reported as the most common anticoagulant found in birds of prey in various states of the USA. Alternatively, the same panel can be performed on a liver sample post mortem. Routine blood tests may also show anemia, hypoproteinemia, and prolonged whole blood clotting time.

3 How would you treat this bird? Vitamin K_1 is administered at 2.5 mg/kg IM or SC q4–12h, then at 2.5 mg/kg PO q24h when the bird is able to eat. The duration of treatment depends on the generation of anticoagulant rodenticide, with a 3–4-week long treatment recommended for second generation anticoagulants. The hematocrit may be evaluated a few days after discontinuing vitamin K_1 administration. Whole blood transfusions may also be administered as needed. Vision should be evaluated to assess releasability in this case.

Further reading

Murray M (2011) Anticoagulant rodenticide exposure and toxicosis in four species of birds of prey presented to a wildlife clinic in Massachusetts, 2006–2010. *J Zoo Wildl Med* **42(1)**:88–97.

Murray M, Tseng F (2008) Diagnosis and treatment of secondary anticoagulant rodenticide toxicosis in a red-tailed hawk (*Buteo jamaicensis*). *J Avian Med Surg* **22(1)**:41–46. (Treatment doses in Part 3.)

Redig PT, Arent LR (2008) Raptor toxicology. *Vet Clin North Am Exot Anim Pract* **11(2)**:261–282.

Stansley WI, Cummings M, Vudathala D *et al.* (2014) Anticoagulant rodenticides in red-tailed hawks, *Buteo jamaicensis*, and great horned owls, *Bubo virginianus*, from New Jersey, USA, 2008–2010. *Bull Environ Contam Toxicol* 92(1):6–9.

Thomas PJ, Mineau P, Shore RF *et al.* (2011) Second generation anticoagulant rodenticides in predatory birds: probabilistic characterization of toxic liver concentrations and implications for predatory bird populations in Canada. *Environ Int* **37**:914–920.

Wenick (2013) Comparison of fluid types for resuscitation in acute hemorrhagic shock and evaluation of gastric luminal and transcutaneous PCO_2 in leghorn chickens. *J Avian Med Surg* **27(2)**:109–119. (End of answer Part 3.)

CASE 137

1 What is the function of the foramen formed by the union of the scapula, coracoid, and clavicle? Does it have any clinical significance? The tendon of the supracoracoid muscle runs through the triosseal canal, which acts as a pulley, allowing the wing to be raised by the ventrally placed muscle found underlying the pectoral muscle (**137b**; 1 = coracoid; 2 = tendon of supracoid muscle; 3 = acrocoracoid ligament; 4 = humerus; 5 = ribs; 6 = supracoracoid muscle entering triosseal canal; 8 = supracoracoid muscle; 9 = cut edge of removed pectoral muscle). The supracoracoid tendon can be ruptured as a result of trauma and the bird is then unable to lift its wing; the tendon must be repaired in order to allow the bird to fly again. Fractures of this region are often seen after a wild bird flies head on into a window. Fractures are sometimes treated by immobilizing the wing, although this will allow callus around the triosseal canal to adhere to the supracoracoid tendon, causing permanent dysfunction of the wing. Multiple fractures in this region may be treated successfully with rest in a restricted area and no immobilization.

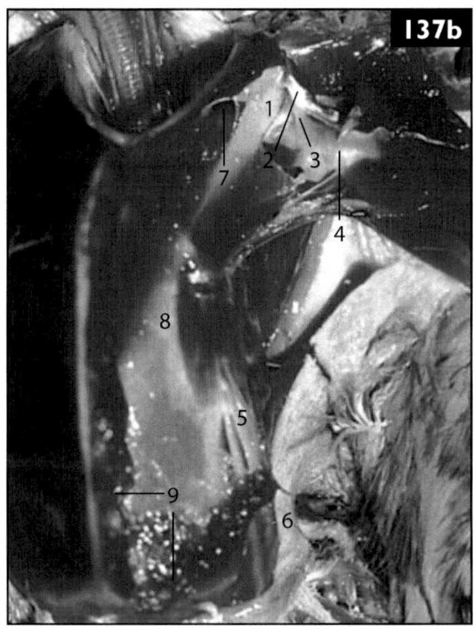

CASE 138

1 Briefly explain the theory behind the two imaging modalities. CT is a diagnostic imaging technique that uses x-rays to obtain cross-sectional images of the body, thereby overcoming the issue of superimposition of tissues and structures as seen in conventional radiography. With the help of special software, the obtained images can furthermore be digitally processed to obtain 3D views and/or reconstruct the data into alternate planes.

MRI, in contrast, uses a powerful magnetic field in combination with high-frequency radio waves to align and spin protons (hydrogen atoms) in the body and obtain signals resulting from the spinning protons. As most hydrogen atoms are trapped in water molecules, an MR image is mainly a representation of the different types, distributions, and volumes of water in the various tissues.

2 What are the main applications for both imaging modalities in birds? CT imaging is mainly performed to assess known or suspected abnormalities in the skeletal structures and respiratory tract. In birds, CT has been proven particularly helpful in diagnosing lower respiratory tract disease, but is also considered superior to radiographs for evaluating the nasal cavity, conchae, and sinuses as well as skeletal tissues with significant superimposition of overlying soft tissue structures such as the spine, shoulder joint, pelvis, and skull (in particular the hyoid bone and beak apparatus). Enlargement of various intracoelomic organs, such as liver, kidney, and spleen, may also be detected with CT imaging, especially when contrast medium is used. The gastrointestinal tract can also be visualized, although recognition of pathology is often more difficult without the use of an intraluminal contrast medium such as barium sulfate. The central nervous system, unless the lesions are severe (e.g. severe hydrocephalus), is best evaluated with MRI. CT angiography enables evaluation of the larger vessels, facilitating diagnosis of cardiovascular diseases.

MRI is used primarily to diagnose soft tissue changes. In birds, MRI has mainly been used for diagnosing neurologic disease (e.g. brain and spinal cord abnormalities such as hydrocephalus, ischemic strokes, and spinal cord trauma). MRI is also considered an excellent tool for evaluating the eye, orbit, and sinuses and may also have value when evaluating internal organs such as the gastrointestinal tract, liver, spleen, and urogenital tract. In contrast, MRI is less useful for imaging the heart and lungs because of the artifacts created by the cardiac motion, which hinder proper visualization of the heart and lungs.

3 What are the main limitations of both techniques with regard to their use in avian medicine? In practice, limitations of CT are mainly dependent on the spatial resolution of the CT scanner and size of the patient. Particularly in smaller sized birds, the resolution of most CT scanners may be poor, limiting its diagnostic value for evaluating organs and structures. Additionally, factors such as differences in density between the object of interest and its surrounding structures and the size of the object may play a role in the visualization of abnormalities.

The use of MRI in avian medicine is limited, predominantly because of the prolonged time needed to perform the MRI scan, resulting in a prolonged anesthesia, which may carry additional risks for the patient, especially since there is limited access to the patient during the procedure. Additionally, the relatively low spatial resolution of some systems (<0.5 Tesla) limits the diagnostic value of MRI in avian patients. Quality of imaging is further hindered by the high respiratory and heart rates and by artifacts created due to the presence of air sacs and/or a microtransponder. Finally, cost may also be an issue as MRI is usually more expensive than CT imaging.

Further reading

van Zeeland YRA, Schoemaker NJ, Hsu E (2016) Advances in diagnostic imaging. In: *Current Therapy in Avian Medicine and Surgery*. (ed. BL Speer) Elsevier, St. Louis, pp. 531–549.

CASE 139

1 What is the most likely etiologic agent? The most common cause of neural larval migrans in ratites in North America is *Baylisascaris procyonis*, the raccoon (*Procyon lotor*) roundworm. This condition can occur wherever raccoons (and their ascarid) have been introduced. Avian species are paratenic hosts for this parasite. Infectious embryonated L3 larvae are ingested, hatch in the digestive tract, and undergo systemic migration. Larvae appear to have a predilection for the brain and spinal cord, particularly the cerebellar white matter and brainstem. The paired lateral alae in the cross section of the parasite are a characteristic feature.

2 Describe the clinical signs that the affected bird was most likely to have shown. The most frequent clinical signs shown by ratites with neural larval migrans are ataxia and loss of balance. Birds frequently hock sit and will stagger backwards when disturbed. They are often bright and will continue to eat if food is provided nearby. Differential diagnoses include trauma, neurotropic migration with *Chandlerella quiscali* (whose natural host is the common grackle *Quiscalus quiscula*), and infection with Western equine encephalitis virus.

3 What management steps should be taken to prevent the occurrence of the same disease in other birds in the flock? The most important method of prevention is to restrict the access of raccoons to animal feed supplies and barns, and to identify and remove raccoon latrine sites on the farm. Eggs of *B. procyonis* are extremely hardy and survive for long periods of time in the environment. On farms where raccoon control is problematic, treatment of animals with ivermectin or other parasiticides at regular intervals can interrupt the migration of the larvae to the brain.

Further reading

Kwiecien JM, Smith DA, Key DW *et al.* (1993) Encephalitis attributed to larval migration of *Baylisascaris* sp. in emus. *Can Vet J* **34**(3):176–178.

CASE 140

1 Name the three haemosporidian genera known to affect avian species. *Haemoproteus* spp. (**140a**), *Leucocytozoon* spp. (**140b**), and *Plasmodium* spp. (**140c**).

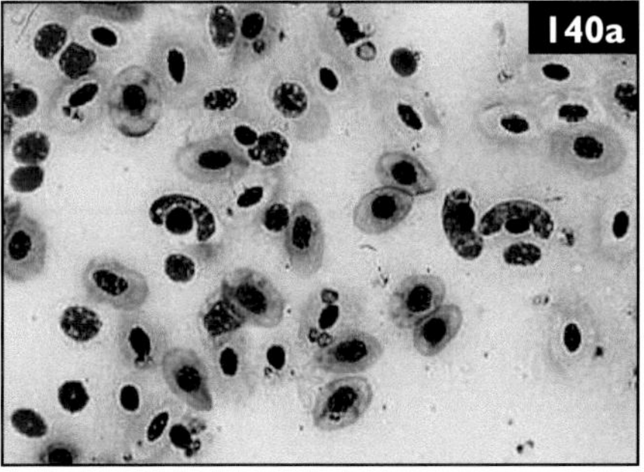
140a

2 Name the invertebrate hosts involved in their life cycle. *Haemoproteus* spp. are transmitted primarily by biting midges (Ceratopogonidae) and

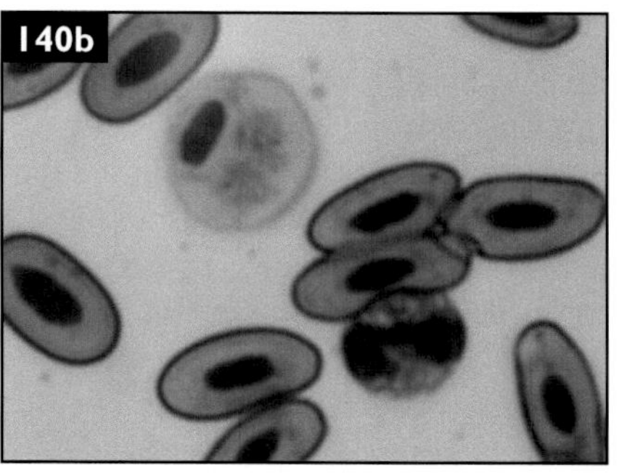

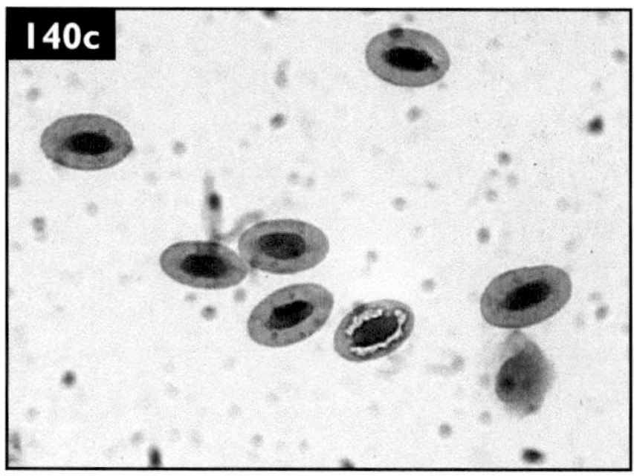

louse flies (*Hypoboscidae*), *Leucocytoozoon* spp. by blackflies (Simuliidae), and *Plasmodium* spp. by mosquitoes (Culicidae).

3 What is the importance of these parasites in captive and wild avian populations? *Haemoproteus* spp. are considered relatively benign while *Leucocytozoon* spp. and *Plasmodium* spp. are considered pathogenic. *Plasmodium* spp. have been reported to have severe effects in island naïve species such as honeycreepers in Hawaii and penguins in the Galapagos. Episodes of local mortality have been associated with *Leucocytozoon* spp. in waterfowl and multiple reports exist in captive avian species.

Further reading

Levin II, Parker PG (2012) Haemosporidian parasites: impacts on avian hosts. In: *Zoo and Wildlife Animal Medicine Current Therapy*, Vol. 7. (eds. RE Miller, ME Fowler) Elsevier Saunders, St. Louis, pp. 356–363.

CASE 141

1 What species is this chick? This neonatal chick is a caninde macaw (*Ara glaucogularis*).

2 Is it precocial or altricial? Caninde macaws are altricial, hatched with eyes closed, down is minimal to absent, and mobility is limited. Nourishment, warmth (93–98°F [33.9–36.7°C]), and a safe place must be provided for altricial chicks.

3 What is wrong with its beak? This chick has a lateral deviation of the maxilla beak malformation. Macaws are prone to lateral deviation of the maxilla or scissor beak. Scissor beak usually occurs post hatch secondary to handfeeding. However, nutrition and incubation are also suspected. The upper beak is pushed to one side, usually the bird's left. Caught early, physical therapy helps to push the upper beak back into proper alignment. If done several times daily during prenatal development (before beak calcification), it is correctable. If presented later, but before the maxilla is completely ossified, an acrylic ramp may be placed on the side to which the beak is deviating, so that as the beak is closed, the rhinotheca is pushed back to a normal central position. A small ramp may be required on the other side to ensure it does not go too far (**141c**).

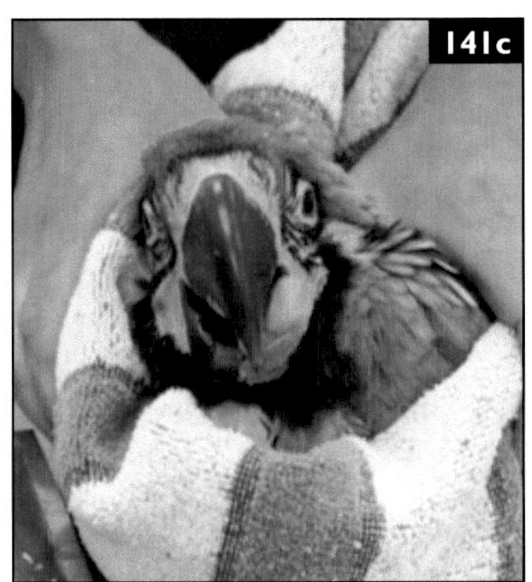
141c

Further reading

Romagnano A (2012) Psittacine pediatrics. *Vet Clin North Am Exot Anim Pract* **15(2)**: 163–182.

CASE 142

1 List some of the common soft tissue retractors used. The soft tissue retractors recommended are the smallest sized Balfour and Gelpi retractors for larger patients and the Bennett avian retractor and the Doolen avian retractor (Sontec Instruments) for smaller patients. The Lone Star Retractor (Lone Star Medical Products) is available in a variety of configurations but the rectangle is probably the most versatile retractor used in avian surgery.

2 What are the ideal characteristics of surgical loupes? The ideal surgical loupe system would be comfortable; provide magnification of ×3–5; have lenses with a large depth of field so more than one plane is in focus; and have a focal distance appropriate to the surgeon's working distance, minimizing stresses on the neck and back (ergonomic) and allowing the surgeon to look around the lenses to accomplish tasks that do not need magnification. Illumination with a focal light source is recommended. Head or lens-mounted lights direct the light to where it is needed by the surgeon, keeping it in the field of view when the head is moved, but focal lights are also available separate from loupes.

3 What are the key features of microsurgical instruments? They should be a standard length (usually 15–17 cm), have rounded handles, and have small working tips. Many microsurgical instruments are also counter balanced and shaped to fit the notch between the base of the thumb and the index finger. When performing surgery, the hands rest firmly on the operating table. Both hands are positioned in the same manner as when writing, and the instruments are manipulated with the fingers only. The most important instruments in addition to the standard surgical instruments are the microforceps, microscissors, and microneedle holders. Other instruments can be added to the set, such as microhemostats and vascular clamps. DeBakey thumb forceps are atraumatic vascular forceps that can be used to handle delicate tissues.

Further reading

Guzman DS (2016) Avian soft tissue surgery. *Vet Clin North Am Exot Anim Pract* **19(1)**: 133–157.

CASE 143

1 What is the most likely diagnosis? A coracoid injury (e.g. fracture or luxation) is most likely. Other differentials for this type of presentation without neurologic deficits would include a compression fracture of the cranial sternum or soft tissue damage (e.g. supracoracoideus muscle and tendon).

2 What are the expected physical examination findings with this type of injury? Diagnosing a coracoid luxation can be difficult on physical examination, because birds may only have a slight wing droop or may hold the wing in a normal position. Crepitus might be palpated with manipulation of the shoulder, and in larger birds the medial aspect of the coracoid might be able to be palpated deep in the thoracic inlet. Birds with a coracoid injury usually cannot fly or are only capable of flying minimal distances.

3 What diagnostic test would you perform to confirm your diagnosis? Radiographs are required to confirm a coracoid injury. In addition to ventrodorsal (**143b**) and laterolateral views of the pectoral girdle, a caudoventral–craniodorsal oblique radiographic view made at 45° to the frontal plane (H view, **143c**) would increase the sensitivity for detection of these type of injuries. With the H view, tilting the radiographic tube 45° avoids superimposition of the scapula, clavicle, and coracoid. This bird did not have a coracoid injury, as shown in the radiographs, and the wing droop resolved after cage rest (4 weeks) and NSAID administration.

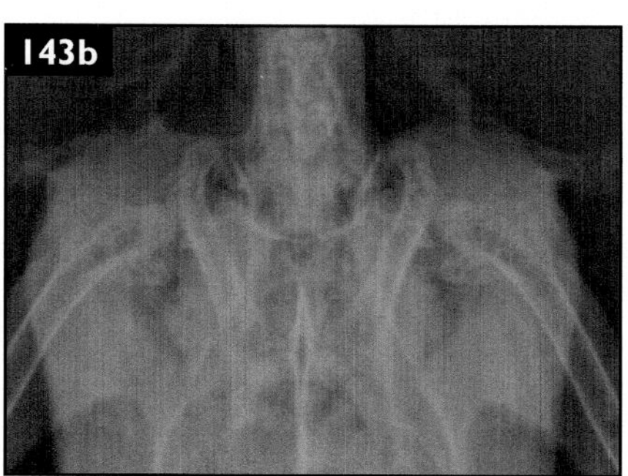

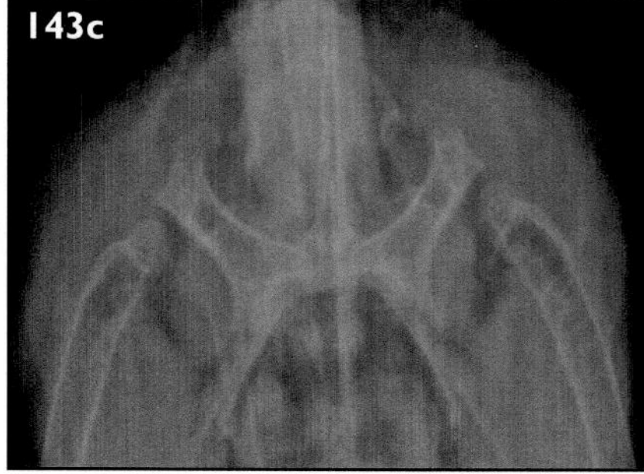

Further reading

Visser M, Hespel AM, de Swarte M *et al.* (2015) Use of a caudoventral-craniodorsal oblique radiographic view made at 45° to the frontal plane to evaluate the pectoral girdle in raptors. *J Am Vet Med Assoc* **247(9)**:1037–1041.

CASE 144

1 What is the most likely cause of this disease outbreak? The most likely cause is type C botulism.

2 What treatment should be implemented in the live animals? Treatment options for botulism toxicities depend on the number and types of avian species involved. Affected wild waterfowl that are still able to walk can usually be treated effectively with supportive care, access to fresh water, and shelter from inclement weather and predation. Smaller numbers of birds or more valuable birds from zoos or privately owned collections, which can be handled, will benefit from fluid therapy and activated charcoal by mouth together with nutritional support. Administration of type C botulism antitoxin may be advantageous. Recovery rates of 75–90% and higher may be achieved. Mink type C toxoid vaccine (Botumink®) did not provided adequate protection levels in a study in green-winged teal (*Anas carolinensis*).

3 What measures should be implemented to curtail further cases? Land–water interfaces should be surveyed and dead birds and other vertebrates removed as soon as possible; however, studies have shown that actual detection and removal of carcases has a low success rate, although annual staff training immediately prior to the risk period and cutting the vegetation short at the land–water interface have proven advantageous in some collections. Most outbreaks occur during the summer and autumn/fall, when ambient temperatures are higher and the bacteria are multiplying fast. Furthermore, water oxygen levels are lower and decaying leaves in the water predispose to anaerobic conditions. *Clostridium botulinum* spores in the soil are activated, and bacteria are consumed by invertebrates and fish, which are killed by bacterial toxins. Dead carcases attract blow flies (maggot laying); the maggots are then eaten by wildfowl, the latter then suffering disease. The water body becomes toxin contaminated. Preventive measures are to maintain water flow, keep the land–water interface clear, observation for and removal of any carcases, and capture and relocation of treated or unaffected birds to an uncontaminated site. The use of bird scarers or netting to prevent birds from having access to the water and maintaining stable water levels during the hot summer months to minimize invertebrate die-offs are recommended. If possible, the water body can be flooded or drained, or otherwise simply wait for the winter floods to wash the toxins away.

Further reading

Degernes LA (2008) Waterfowl toxicology. A review. *Vet Clin North Am Exot Anim Pract* **11:**283–300, vi.

Friend M, Franson JC (1999) *Field Manual of Wildlife Diseases: General Field Procedures and Diseases of Birds*. US Geological Survey, Biological Resources Division, Washington DC.

Rocke TE, Bollinger TK (2007) Avian botulism. In: *Infectious Diseases of Wild Birds.* (eds. NJ Thomas, DB Hunter, CT Atkinson) Blackwell Publishing, Ames, pp. 377–416.
Rocke TE, Samuel MD, Swift PK *et al.* (2000). Efficacy of a type C botulism vaccine in green-winged teal. *J Wildl Dis* **36**:489–493.

CASE 145

1 List the potentially zoonotic diseases that can be encountered in pet birds. The main diseases to consider with avian zoonoses are chlamydiosis, salmonellosis, mycobacteriosis, Newcastle disease, influenza, and West Nile virus. In addition, other bacterial diseases (including mycoplasmosis, campylobacteriosis, and pasteurellosis), fungal diseases (such as aspergillosis and candidiasis), and parasitic diseases (including giardiasis, cryptosporidiosis, and mite infestations) have the potential to cause infection in humans, but evidence of direct disease transmission is not yet published.

2 For each of the diseases you have listed, give the common clinical signs seen in birds.

- Chlamydiosis. Lethargy, decreased appetite, weight loss, ruffled feathers, respiratory signs (dyspnea, increased respiratory rate, nasal discharge), ocular signs (conjunctivitis, ocular discharge), lime-green diarrhea or green discolored urates (from liver disease). Birds can also be asymptomatic.
- Salmonellosis. Enteritis/diarrhea, lethargy, dehydration, crop stasis, weight loss, reduced egg production, swollen joints, neurologic signs, and sudden death. At postmortem, granulomas may be seen in the liver, spleen, and ceca.
- Mycobacteriosis. Depends widely on the *Mycobacterium* spp., species of bird, severity of infection, and organ or system affected. Weight loss is the most common sign, followed by respiratory signs, diarrhea, coelomic distension, and poor feathering.
- Newcastle disease. Respiratory, gastrointestinal, and central nervous system signs, more commonly seen in pigeons and poultry but can be seen in companion parrots.
- Influenza. Mild to severe respiratory signs, depression, anorexia, diarrhea, neurologic signs, decreased egg production, and sudden death of large groups of birds with no premonitory signs.
- West Nile virus. Varying degrees of neurologic compromise including recumbency and paralysis of pelvic and thoracic limbs.

3 For each of the diseases you have listed, give the common clinical signs seen in humans.

- Chlamydiosis. Flu-like symptoms such as fever, chills, headache, muscle aches, dry cough, dyspnea, confusion, and abnormal liver tests. There can be more severe signs including renal disease, hepatitis, pancreatitis, reactive arthritis, meningoencephalitis, seizures, endocarditis, myocarditis, and pericarditis.

- Salmonellosis. Symptoms for 4–7 days. Abdominal cramps, headache, fever, nausea, vomiting, and copious watery diarrhea. More serious manifestations can include arthritis, hepatitis, and neuritis.
- Mycobacteriosis. More likely to affect immunocompromised individuals. Fever, weight loss, abdominal pain, fatigue, chronic diarrhea, and anemia. Localized disease can also occur causing central nervous system infection, nodules, lymphadenitis, and endocarditis.
- Newcastle disease. Mild flu-like symptoms, conjunctivitis, laryngitis, and photophobia.
- Influenza. Conjunctivitis, fever, respiratory infection, cough, and gastrointestinal upset and, if highly pathogenic, death.
- Western Nile virus. 80% show no symptoms. Others show fever, headache, nausea, vomiting, and rash. Severe signs can rarely include high fever, neck stiffness, disorientation, seizures, loss of vision, and paralysis.

Further reading

Evans EE (2011) Zoonotic diseases of common pet birds: psittacine, passerine, and columbiform species. *Vet Clin North Am Exot Anim Pract* **14**:457–476.

CASE 146

1 **Describe the patient preparation required for this procedure.** Birds undergoing upper gastrointestinal tract endoscopy must be intubated and placed at an incline with the head elevated to reduce the risk of aspiration. The upper gastrointestinal tract, including the crop and proventriculus, should be flushed with warmed sterile saline prior to endoscopy, particularly if the patient is on a seed diet, as a large amount of debris can impede visualization. A temporary ingluviotomy is required in larger patients with long necks, such as cockatoos, in order to access the upper gastrointestinal tract using a 2.7 mm × 18 cm rigid endoscope. Alternatively, a small flexible endoscope can be used via the oral cavity.

2 **What are the advantages and disadvantages of using saline irrigation versus air insufflation for a gastroscopy?** Saline irrigation provides better visualization and helps dilate the lumen; however, there is a risk of aspiration with overzealous irrigation. Saline used for irrigation must be of body temperature, otherwise a marked hypothermia can occur. Air insufflation reduces the risk of aspiration, but provides poorer visual detail and makes lumen distension more difficult.

3 **Describe the abnormalities seen in the proventriculus of this umbrella cockatoo. What is the appropriate next diagnostic step?** There are numerous

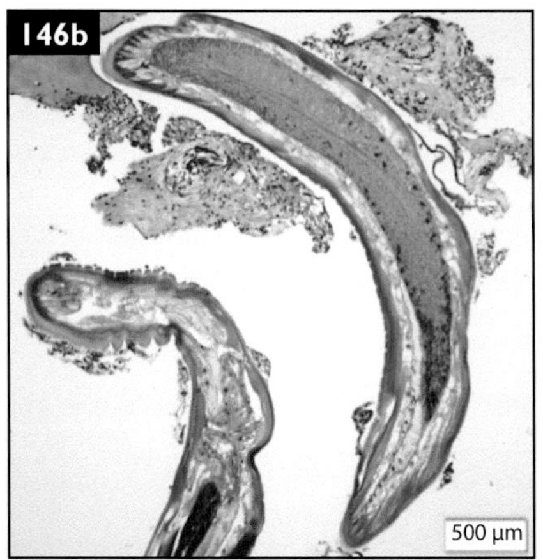

Courtesy of Dr. Stephen Divers, UGA

vesicle-like structures originating from the proventricular mucosa. A biopsy of these structures is indicated. In this case proventricular nematodiasis was diagnosed on histopathology (**146b**).

Further reading

Divers SJ (2010) Avian diagnostic endoscopy. *Vet Clin North Am Exot Anim Pract* **13**(**2**):187–202.

Mejia-Fava J, Divers SJ, Jimenez DA *et al.* (2013) Diagnosis and treatment of proventricular nematodiasis in an umbrella cockatoo (*Cacatua alba*). *J Am Vet Med Assoc* **242**(**8**): 1122–1126.

CASE 147

1 What is the reliability of an oscillometric unit or a sphygmomanometer and a Doppler flow unit in birds for the evaluation of blood pressure? Multiple studies have shown that the oscillometric technique is unreliable in the avian species investigated. Indirect blood pressure measurement using a Doppler unit and a cuff also appears to be grossly inaccurate in small to medium sized birds. However, measurements are closer to the mean arterial blood pressure in larger birds of prey (>1 kg), which shows that it may be of use in these larger species.

2 What are the main sources of variability in the measurement of indirect blood pressure in parrots using a sphygmomanometer and a Doppler flow unit? What are the clinical implications? A study in psittacines showed that the main sources of variability were cuff placement and individual birds, whereas the limb used was not a significant source of variability. As a result, monitoring trends in indirect blood pressure measurement following a single cuff placement event, such as during anesthetic monitoring, may be useful.

3 Which sites and arteries are used for direct blood pressure measurement in birds? In medium to large sized birds, invasive blood pressure measurements through arterial catheterization may be obtained to improve anesthetic monitoring.

The most accessible arteries for catheterization are the superficial ulnar artery, the deep radial artery, the external carotid artery (requires a cut-down procedure), and the cranial tibial artery. In smaller birds, significant bleeding may be encountered during catheter removal and fatal bleedings have been experienced in research birds up to 24 hours following arterial catheter removal.

Further reading

Acierno MJ, da Cunha A, Smith J *et al.* (2008) Agreement between direct and indirect blood pressure measurements obtained from anesthetized Hispaniolan Amazon parrots. *J Am Vet Med Assoc* **233(10)**:1587–1590.

Johnston MS, Davidowski LA, Rao S *et al.* (2011) Precision of repeated, Doppler-derived indirect blood pressure measurements in conscious psittacine birds. *J Avian Med Surg* **25(2)**:83–90.

Schnellbacher R, da Cunha, Olson EE *et al.* (2014) Arterial catheterization, interpretation, and treatment of arterial blood pressures and blood gases in birds. *J Exot Pet Med* 23(2):129–141.

Zehnder AM, Hawkins MG, Pascoe PJ *et al.* (2009) Evaluation of indirect blood pressure monitoring in awake and anesthetized red-tailed hawks (*Buteo jamaicensis*): effects of cuff size, cuff placement, and monitoring equipment. *Vet Anesth Analg* **36(5)**:464–479.

CASE 148

1 Review the image shown and name the structures identified with the black and green arrows. Black arrow = thyroid gland; green arrow = parathyroid gland and ultimobranchial gland.

2 List at least two histologic or physiologic features of these structures that are similar and two that are different from those described in mammals. Similar: (1) thyroid gland formed by follicles lined by a single layer of epithelial cells and filled with colloid (thyroglobulin); (2) the mechanism of synthesis and release of T_4 and T_3, with T_3 production being mostly extrathyroidal; and (3) calcium metabolism is regulated by parathyroid hormone, calcitonin, and 1,25-dihydroxy vitamin D_3. Different: (1) calcitonin secreting cells (parafollicular cells in mammals) are not within the avian thyroid gland, but form a separate gland, the ultimobrachial gland, which is located caudal to the parathyroid glands; (2) the avian thyroid gland produces relatively more T_4 than T_3, although avian plasma contains less T_4 and similar concentrations of T_3 compared with mammals; (3) avian thyroid-stimulating hormone (TSH) has a different structure than mammalian TSH; (4) calcium metabolism adjustments in birds occur faster than in mammals; (5) the number of parathyroid glands in birds varies between two and four depending on the species; (6) the parathyroid gland consists primarily of chief cells – it does not contain the oxyphil cells found in mammalian parathyroid glands; and (7) birds have high circulating levels of calcitonin.

3 Which disease processes have been described relating to these two structures in avian species? Diseases of the thyroid gland include goiter, hyperthyroidism, and hypothyroidism.

4 Which specific assays can be used to investigate the function of these structures in birds? Assays for evaluation of the thyroid gland include measurement of T_4 blood levels pre- and post-TSH administration and measurement of free T_4. Low blood levels of T_4 and response to L-thyroxine supplementation may be suggestive of hypothyroidism, but measuring T_4 blood levels pre- and post-TSH administration is required for an accurate diagnosis.

Diseases of the parathyroid gland include nutritional secondary hyperparathyroidism and adenoma. Primary hypoparathyroidism or hyperparathyroidism, renal secondary hyperparathyroidism, tertiary hyperparathyroidism and pseudohypoparathyroidism have not been reported in avian species.

Assays for evaluation of the parathyroid gland function include evaluation of total calcium and ionized blood calcium levels, determination of blood levels of parathyroid hormone, and determination of blood levels of vitamin D_3.

Further reading

Brandao J, Manickam B, Blas-Machado U *et al.* (2012) Productive thyroid follicular carcinoma in a wild barred owl (*Strix varia*). *J Vet Diagn Invest* **24(6)**:1145–1150.

de Matos R (2008) Calcium metabolism in birds. *Vet Clin North Am Exot Anim Pract* **11**:59–82.

Hudelson KS, Hudelson PM (2006) Endocrine considerations. In: *Clinical Avian Medicine.* (eds. GJ Harrison, TL Lightfoot) Spix Publishing, Palm Beach, pp. 541–557.

King AS, McLelland J (1984) Endocrine system. In: *Birds, Their Structure and Function*, 2nd edn. Baillière Tindall, Eastbourne, pp. 200–213.

McNabb FM, Darras VM (2015) Thyroids. In: *Sturkie's Avian Physiology*, 6th edn. (ed. CG Scanes) Academic Press, Waltham, pp. 535–547.

Schmidt RE, Reavill DR, Phalen DN (2015) Endocrine system. In: *Pathology of Pet and Aviary Birds*, 2nd edn. Iowa State Press, Ames, pp. 161–174.

CASE 149

1 What condition is the bird suffering from, and what investigations should be carried out on the other youngsters? This bird is suffering from a 'crop burn'. Excessively hot food has been fed to the bird; this occurs most commonly when food has been heated in a microwave and not adequately mixed prior to feeding, resulting in hot spots within the bowl of food. It is not uncommon for only one or two chicks fed from the same bowl to be affected.

In respect of the other two birds, careful examination of the crop is required. It is not uncommon for partial-thickness burns to occur, so no leakage is detected. Any chick with delayed emptying should be checked, by way of a crop swab, for abnormal bacterial or fungal (*Candida* spp.) infection. If a partial-thickness burn is present, antibiotics and/or antifungals, as indicated by cytology or culture, should be maintained until the lesion has healed and resolved or matured and leakage is visually apparent.

2 How should this bird be treated? Correction of a crop burn cannot be undertaken until all necrotic or devitalized tissue has recovered or died, so that vital tissue can be surgically separated from dead tissue. The bird should have an empty crop at the time of planned surgery. By this stage, adhesions will have formed between the crop wall and the overlying skin. Following induction of anesthesia, intubation, fluid therapy, analgesia, and antimicrobials as required, the overlying skin is plucked and surgically prepared. A skin incision is extended longitudinally above and below the orifice, without incising into the crop. The adhesions between the skin and crop wall are surgically resected, and the crop defect is closed using a double inversion pattern, using an absorbable monofilament suture material (due to risk of infection tracking from within the crop to the subcuticular space). The tissue is flushed copiously and the skin is closed separately. Care is taken not to permit excessive crop stretching for a few days following surgery.

3 How can the condition be avoided? The condition is easily avoided by not heating food in a microwave or mixing well after heating and measuring the temperature of the food before feeding the birds.

Further reading

Forbes NA (2016) Soft tissue surgery. In: *Avian Medicine*, 3rd edn. (ed. J Samour) Mosby, St. Louis, pp. 294–311.

CASE 150

1 Name four drugs used to treat PDD and describe their mode of action. (1) Celecoxib: NSAID, selective COX-2 inhibitor. Most commonly used drug to treat PDD. Has been shown in limited studies to reverse clinical signs as well as pathologic lesions. (2) Tepoxalin: NSAID, combined COX-1, COX-2, and 5-lipoxygenase inhibitor. Based on a single limited study may be more effective than celecoxib in reversing clinical signs as well as pathologic lesions. (3) Cyclosporine: specific T-cell inhibitor. Very limited data show this drug to reverse clinical signs in PDD patients and to improve pathologic lesions. (4) Amantadine hydrochloride: antiviral, induces release of dopamine and norepinephrine in the brain. Has been reported to alleviate clinical signs in PDD patients with severe neurologic signs, but to be ineffective in reducing virus shedding and/or clearing the infection.

2 Name two groups of drugs commonly used as supportive therapy for patients suffering from PDD. (1) Gastrointestinal motility modifiers to enhance gastrointestinal motility. (2) Antibiotics and antifungals to treat secondary infections.

3 Is PDD a lethal disease? Not necessarily. Long-term clinical remissions and resolution of the lesions have been reported with NSAIDs and, in some cases, cyclosporine therapy, especially if treatment was initiated at an early stage of the disease. Titrating medical doses and frequency of administration based on post-barium contrast fluoroscopic assessment has been found to be far more effective than basing the latter on physical assessment or owner observations. Meloxicam has been shown to be ineffective at the dosages evaluated.

Further reading

Gancz AY, Clubb S, Shivaprasad HL (2010) Advanced diagnostic approaches and current management of proventricular dilatation disease. *Vet Clin North Am Exot Anim Pract* 13(3):471–494.

CASE 151

1 What would be the most likely differential diagnoses for this case? In any cockatiel, or similar size bird, presented with acute-onset respiratory distress, an important differential is tracheal obstruction following the inhalation of a millet seed. Patients with nonobstructive upper respiratory disease (e.g. rhinitis, sinusitis) or lower respiratory disease (pneumonia, coelomic fluid or masses, airsacculitis) present with variable respiratory rate and effort and a more progressive onset of clinical signs. Many have a palpably enlarged coelomic cavity and sometimes low body condition.

2 What initial emergency treatment and diagnostic plan would you pursue? This bird is presented with acute respiratory distress and requires immediate attention. The degree of distress will dictate the urgency of intervention. The bird should be placed immediately in an oxygen chamber. Stress must be decreased to avoid increasing the oxygen demand. The bird is premedicated with midazolam (0.5 mg/kg) and butorphanol (1 mg/kg) IM and anesthesia is induced and maintained with isoflurane or sevoflurane with 100% O_2. Air sac cannula placement with a 2.0 endotracheal tube is performed as an emergency procedure. This can provide the bird with an alternative airway until the tracheal compromise is relieved. Radiographs would be required to rule out other respiratory and nonrespiratory diseases responsible for the clinical signs; however, an inhaled millet seed is not always apparent radiographically. If the feathers on the cranial neck are parted, and the trachea is transilluminated, the seed might be visualized in the cranial portion of the trachea. Alternatively, once the air sac breathing tube is in place, endoscopy with a 1.9 mm telescope will allow visualization of the tracheal lumen and bifurcation to confirm the diagnosis.

3 What treatment would be required? Treatment of tracheal obstruction by a foreign body (e.g. millet) in the cockatiel is challenging due to small patient size and limited access to the proximal trachea and syrinx. Treatment options include:

- Inserting a 25- or 27-gauge needle carefully between tracheal rings just caudal to the seed, inserting a fine hypodermic needle attached to a 3 mL syringe just below the seed, then air is blown from the syringe and the seed will often pass craniad, typically lodging in the glottis, from where it may be removed with fine forceps. The procedure is repeated as needed until the millet is propelled out of the glottis. The bird should be monitored carefully during this procedure.
- Inserting a 25- or 27-gauge needle carefully between tracheal rings just caudal to the seed, then passing per glottis a fine soft rubber feeding tube (e.g. 4 Fr), which in turn is attached to a suction unit. Pass the tube via the glottis into the trachea, turn on the suction, and advance the tube. The seed will often become attached to the end of the tube and may then be withdrawn from the trachea.
- Removal of a millet seed from the syrinx via tracheotomy using magnification and microsurgical techniques.

CASE 152

1 List four noninvasive methods of evaluating eggs and avian embryos during incubation? (1) Candling; (2) floating eggs; (3) radiographs; (4) digital cardiac egg monitor (Buddy, Vetronic Services). The Buddy digital egg monitor shown (**152**) has a chicken egg in the egg holder end and the tracing of the heart rate at 269 beats per minute on the readout screen.

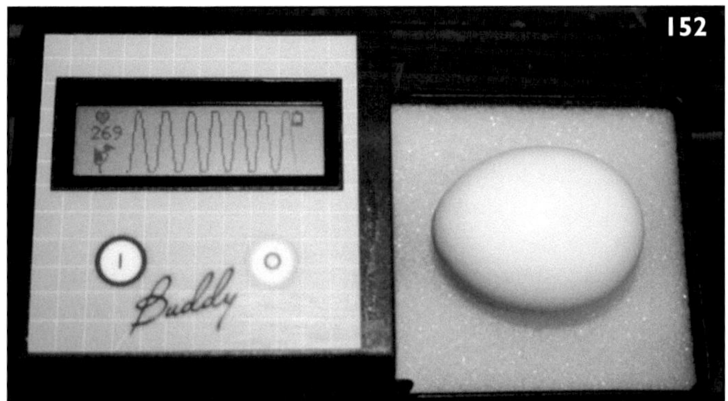

2 At what stages of incubation are the above noninvasive methods most useful? Candling is most useful to monitor fertility and early embryonic development, but not as useful for later embryonic development when the embryo fills the egg. Floating eggs is most useful in the last days of incubation when small movements of the embryo in the egg can be detected and are visible as small ripples on the water in the floatation container. Radiographs are useful in very late-term embryo development to help evaluate bony structures and determine the position of the embryo within the egg. The Buddy digital egg monitor is useful for detecting embryonic heart beats, starting about 25% of the way through incubation.

3 Which of the above methods may be useful in determining if and when to assist a weak or malpositioned embryo in hatching, and why is each useful? All four methods can be useful. Candling can be used to locate and determine if the air cell is in the normal location in the blunt end of the egg, and to visualize the bill after it enters the air cell (internal pip). Floating eggs can be used to determine how weak or strong the embryo appears to be by its movement, but this is a very subjective measurement. Radiographs are useful to determine embryonic positioning. The Buddy digital egg monitor is useful for assessing the heart rate of the embryo. One study reported that the heart rate starts dropping as much as 24 hours before late-term embryonic death. The heart rate can be used to determine if the embryo is healthy and slow to hatch or weak and in need of assistance to hatch.

Further reading

Lierz M, Gooss O, Hafez HM (2006) Noninvasive heart rate measurement using a digital egg monitor in chicken and turkey embryos. *J Avian Med Surg* 20(3):141–146.

CASE 153

1 What is the organ protruding from the vent? The tissue is a prolapsed phallus. In Anseriformes the resting phallus is a long blind-ending tube that lies coiled in a sac with peritoneum along the ventrolateral wall of the cloaca, like an invaginated finger of a glove. The tip of this phallus shows erythema, mucosal erosions, and swelling secondary to trauma.

2 How would you initially treat this condition? The phallus may be viable, despite the swelling and mild trauma, but the duration of the prolapse makes recurrence quite likely. The presence of potential sexual partners for the drake also makes recurrence likely as soon as the bird is returned to the flock. If the owners are willing to attempt replacement, or the bird is required for breeding, the exposed tissue is cleaned, débrided, and returned to the cloaca. Two transverse simple interrupted sutures are placed on both sides of the vent to hold the phallus *in situ*, without compromising defecation. Depending on the degree of damage and potential scarring, breeding may still be compromised. Supportive treatment, including analgesics and antibiotics, should be administered as needed.

3 How would you treat this condition if it recurs? Chronic phallus prolapse in male ducks may require amputation. The phallus is penetrated with absorbable 3-0 to 5-0 suture material between the fossa ejaculatoria and the sulcus phalli, and sutured with a transfixion suture pattern. The phallus is transected distal to the ligature, and the stump is reintroduced into the cloaca. Since the phallus is only a copulatory organ separated from the urinary tract, urination will not be affected.

Further reading

Guzman DS (2016) Avian soft tissue surgery. *Vet Clin North Am Exot Anim Pract* 19(1):133–157.

CASE 154

1 Name the condition. A synostosis (bridging callus) has formed between the radius and ulna. This bony bridge prevents the normal rotational motion and extension of the wing. It is most likely to occur in fractures of the distal radius and ulna.

2 How is it prevented? Synostosis occurs more commonly when radius/ulna fractures are managed with coaptation rather than with surgical fixation. Because restricted movement encourages callus formation between the bones, physical therapy should be performed every 2–3 days during coaptation. Physiotherapy should consist of passive range of motion exercises using gentle extension for each joint and holding for 30–45 seconds. Anesthesia should be used during physical therapy as necessary. Surgical fixation of radius and ulna fractures is the preferred method to avoid formation of synostosis. If despite surgical repair of both bones there is deemed to be a risk of synostosis occurring, then a fat pad (harvested fresh into saline [sterile], prior to the orthopedic surgery, from a subcutaneous site in the mid line over the old yolk sac attachment) is placed between the ulna and radius at the site of risk. The bird is medicated with NSAIDs postoperatively and wing movements are encouraged from 48 hours post surgery.

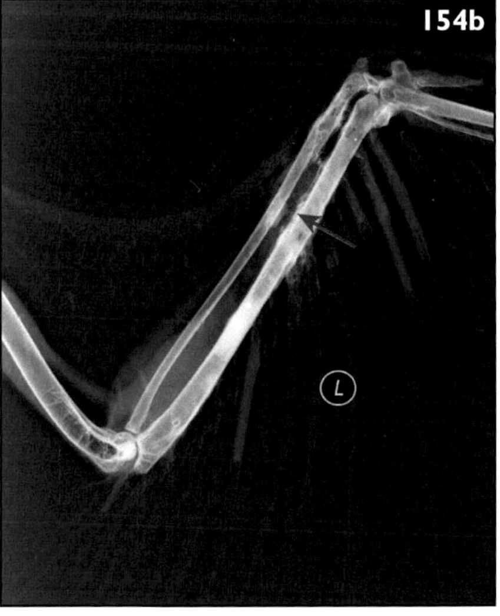

3 How is it treated? If range of motion is limited by the presence of a synostosis, surgical intervention is necessary to return normal function. The site is approached from the dorsal aspect. The bony bridge may be removed using a compressed air dental drill or, in larger patients, an osteotome or rongeurs. Polypropylene mesh or a harvested fat pad from the abdominal area may be placed in the resulting channel (**154b**)

to discourage recurrence of the synostosis. As movement is essential to preventing recurrence, surgical separation should only be performed once a bird is healthy enough to be moved to a flight enclosure or flown frequently after a few days of postsurgical wound care.

Further reading

Redig PT, Ponder J (2016) Management of orthopedic issues in birds. In: *Avian Medicine*, 3rd edn. (ed. J Samour). Mosby, St. Louis, pp. 312–350.

CASE 155

1 What are the main changes present in the erythrocytes? The blood smear shows evidence of erythrocytes with polarized nuclei and a proportional increase in anucleate erythrocytes (erythroplastids). Avian erythrocytes are typically nucleated, but in many birds a very small proportion of erythroplastids may be encountered in the peripheral blood during routine hematology; in rare cases of disease these may comprise >40% of the circulating erythrocytes. However, there are no strong relationships between the concentration of erythroplastids and the hematocrit or with regenerative responses.

2 What are the main cytologic features used to assess signs of a regenerative response in avian blood smears? The main cytologic feature that is used to assess a regenerative response in avian blood smears is the degree of erythrocyte polychromasia, with a percentage of polychromatophilic erythrocytes counted for each blood smear.

3 What is the best anticoagulant to use to preserve avian blood for routine hematologic evaluation? While dipotassium ethylenediaminetetraacetic acid (K2EDTA) is the preferred anticoagulant for preserving cellular morphology for the majority of avian species, the blood of some bird groups such as corvids, some exotic waterfowl, ostriches (*Struthio camelus*), black curassows (*Crax alector*), black crowned cranes (*Balearica pavonina*), gray crowned cranes (*Balearica regulorum*), hornbills (*Tockus alboterminatus*), and brush turkeys (*Alectura lathami*) will hemolyze in K2EDTA. In those species where this occurs, heparin is the preferred anticoagulant. It is important to remember that heparin will not prevent thrombocyte aggregation, but clumping of thrombocytes alone does not affect the WBC count. For routine avian hematology, it is always best to make fresh blood smears at the time of collection, especially when blood is being collected from smaller birds or when the volume for analysis is limited.

Further reading

Clark P, Hume A, Raidal SR (2013) Erythroplastidcytosis in a Major Mitchell cockatoo. *Comp Clin Pathol* **22**(3):539–542.

CASE 156

1 Which nematodes would you consider as the most likely differential diagnoses? Capillarid nematodes such as *Eucoleus dispar, Eucoleus contortus*, *Baruscapillaria falconis*, and *Capillaria tenuissima*.

2 How would you confirm the presence of the parasite? Fecal sample or mucosal scraping examination allows detection of eggs or adult worms.

3 What treatment would you suggest in this case? Fenbendazole (20 mg/kg PO q24h for 5 days), febantel (30 mg/kg PO once), levamisole (10 mg/kg PO q24h for 2 days), and ivermectin (0.2 mg/kg PO, SC, IM, two dosages 10–14 days apart) have been proven effective in treating capillarid nematodes. *Capillaria* spp. commonly demonstrate multiple anthelmintic resistance. Post-treatment fecal examination is always recommended. Nutritional support is likely to be required if the upper gastrointestinal tract lesions are severe and lead to anorexia and regurgitation, as in this case. *Capillaria* spp. have a direct and indirect life cycle, with earthworms as an intermediate host. Apart from treating the infection, exclusion of the intermediate host from the environment (e.g. impervious aviary floors) or suspended flights are required.

Further reading

Yabsley MJ (2014) Capillarid nematodes. In: *Parasitic Diseases of Wild Birds*. (eds. CT Atkinson, NJ Thomas, DB Hunter) Wiley-Blackwell, Ames, pp. 463–497.

CASE 157

1 What four factors, whether using natural or artificial incubation, are important to the microenvironment surrounding an egg? The four factors important to the egg environment in the nest and, especially, in incubators are: (1) temperature of the air surrounding the egg and the temperature of anything in contact with the egg, such as the brood patch of the incubating adult bird; (2) the humidity of the air around the egg; (3) movement or rotation and orientation of the egg in the nest or in the incubator; and (4) ventilation or air movement around the egg.

2 Why change the air in incubators? Why is the incubator and room ventilation important? Does an egg need ventilation during the entire course of incubation? Initially the ventilation requirements for an egg are minimal. Early in embryonic development, the primary energy source in the developing embryo is a lactic acid pathway not involving a need for oxygen. For chicken eggs, this changes around day 4–5 of a 21-day incubation as the embryonic heart develops and there is a change to an energy pathway involving intake of oxygen and production of carbon dioxide waste gas. For most avian species this occurs about 20–25% of the way through incubation.

3 How much oxygen does a developing embryo (chicken) need in an egg during incubation? How much carbon dioxide does the developing embryo produce during incubation? During the normal 21-day incubation of a chicken egg, the developing embryo needs 4.617 liters of oxygen and will produce 3.864 liters of carbon dioxide. Thus, there is a need for adequate air flow (ventilation) in the incubator and in the room where the incubator is located. Reducing the oxygen levels in the incubator below 17% can reduce hatchability (normal oxygen levels in air are about 20%). For carbon dioxide, levels above 1% in the incubator air reduce hatchability and levels above 2% are lethal to embryos. This is most important when a large number of eggs are being incubated and all the eggs are using oxygen and producing carbon dioxide. There is a slight difference in urban air versus country air, with urban air running around 0.08% carbon dioxide versus 0.03% in country air, although this difference is probably negligible to a developing egg. A GQF incubator is shown (**157a**). The ventilation fans are located on the back of the top shelf (**157b**). A Lyon table top incubator with the ventilation fan located in the lid is shown (**157c**). A close-up of the ventilation fan is also shown (**157d**).

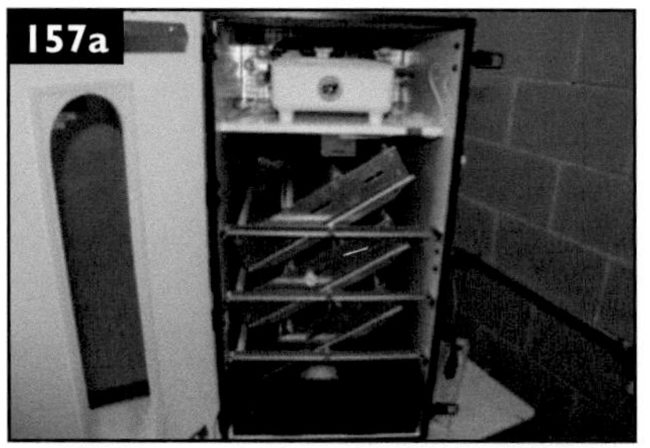
157a

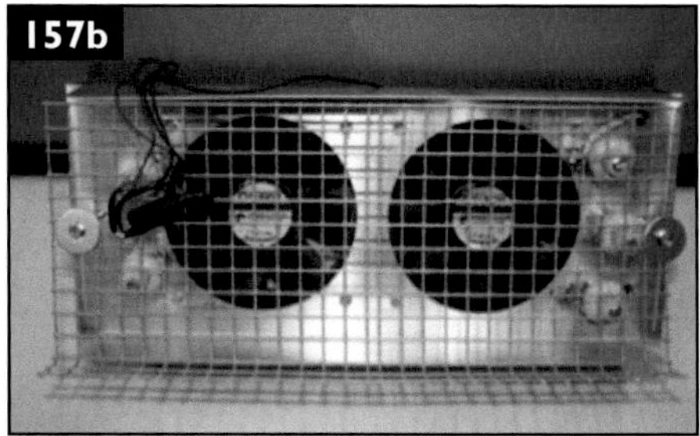
157b

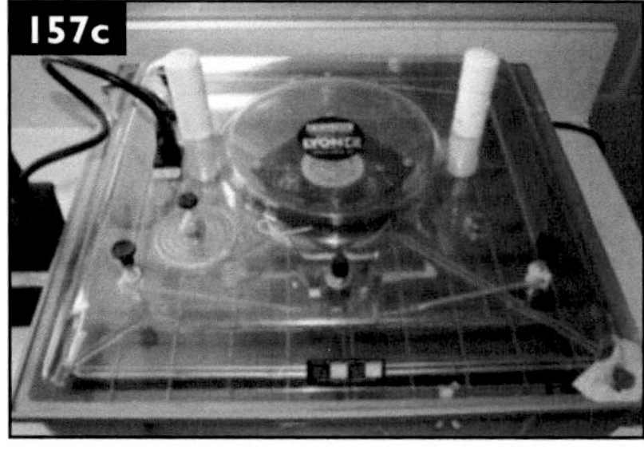
157c

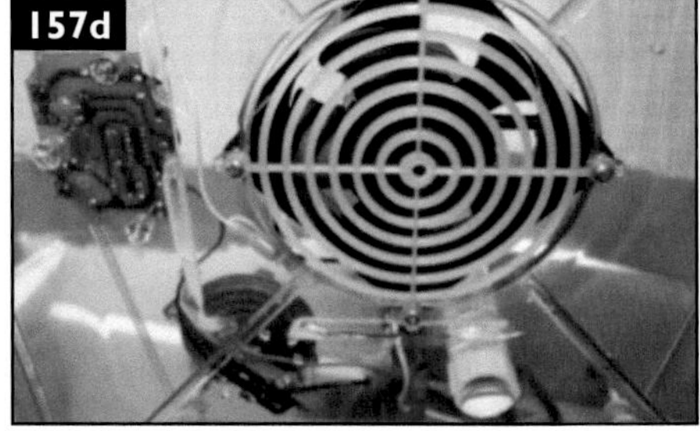
157d

Further reading

Anderson Brown AF, Robbins GES (2002) The physical conditions needed for successful hatching. In: *The New Incubation Book*. Hancock House Publishers, Surrey, pp. 96–134.

CASE 158

1 What is the main differential diagnosis? Psittacine beak and feather disease, caused by psittacine circovirus, results in feather loss and abnormal feather coloration, as seen in this bird.

2 What is your advice to the owner in respect of these birds? Do not move any birds in or out. Have the three young birds tested and, if negative, move them into accommodation that cannot be contaminated with circovirus. If positive, keep and retest in 30 days; if still positive after this, clinical disease will ensue, typically within months.

3 What treatment can be provided to these young birds? There is one peer reviewed published report of the clearance of circovirus from young infected but not clinically affected young parrots, using repeated doses of avian interferon. Antibiotics and antifungals might be indicated if the birds are immunosuppressed.

Further reading

Stanford M (2004) Interferon treatment of circovirus infection in grey parrots (*Psittacus e erithacus*). *Vet Rec* **154**:435–436.

CASE 159

1 What is the lesion shown? The image shows a typical cross-section through the crop wall, including the various layers (mucosa, submucosa, muscularis, and adventitia). The arrow points towards a myenteric ganglion on the adventitial surface. The ganglion is heavily infiltrated by small, dark-staining, mononuclear cells. The image shows lymphoplasmacytic myenteric ganglioneuritis.

2 In what disease is this lesion characteristic? This lesion is considered pathognomonic for proventricular dilatation disease. Note that proventricular dilatation disease and avian bornavirus infection are not synonymous, as some birds may be subclinical carriers of these viruses.

3 What are the key points for collection and preparation of a crop biopsy? Obtaining a biopsy of sufficient size (e.g. 12 × 8 mm). The biopsy should include a prominent blood vessel along its long axis, as this will increase the probability of including sufficient nervous tissue in the sample, and thus the sensitivity of the test. Following fixation in 10% buffered formalin for at least 24 hours, the biopsy should be carefully sliced perpendicular to its long axis to produce as many thin slices (approximately 1 mm thick) as possible. Preparing 6–10 such sections is recommended. A small tissue sample should be kept without fixation for bornavirus real-time PCR testing.

Further reading

Gancz AY, Clubb S, Shivaprasad HL (2010) Advanced diagnostic approaches and current management of proventricular dilatation disease. *Vet Clin North Am Exot Anim Pract* **13(3)**:471–494.

CASE 160

1 What dermatologic physical examination findings are present? The image shows a budgerigar with proliferative lesions of the rhinotheca and cere. The lesions are characteristically 'honeycombed' in appearance.

2 What organism is associated with this physical examination finding, and what diagnostic tests would aid in identification? *Knemidocoptes* (*Cnemidicoptes*) *pilae* is a burrowing mite in the order Sarcoptiformes that is classically associated with this presentation. A skin scraping, as traditionally performed in mammals, and microscopic examination would aid in identification of the mite. As a sarcoptiform mite, the organism would be round to oval in shape; adults have four legs with five segments on each leg.

3 How would you treat this bird? Treatment for the primary cause of the lesions is focused on antiparasitic agents; however, some birds with severe lesions may require antibiotics to treat secondary bacterial infection or general supportive care (analgesics, rehydration, assisted feeding). Antiparasitic agents that have been reported include ivermectin and other avermectins (moxidectin, selamectin) and topical paraffin oil. It is vital that all in-contact birds are treated, as subclinical carriers may subsequently reinfect this bird. Treatment involves weekly application for 4–6 weeks. Ivermectin is dosed at 200 μg/kg and in itself has a very wide safety margin; however, ivermectin is typically diluted in propylene glycol, which can cause toxic effects. It is safest to use a diluted aqueous formulation (e.g. aqueous oral sheep drench) and administer by mouth, rather than the propylene glycol formulation topically.

Further reading

Schmidt RE, Lightfoot TL (2006) Integument. In: *Clinical Avian Medicine*, Vol. 1. (eds. GJ Harrison, TL Lightfoot) Spix Publishing, Palm Beach, pp. 395–410.

CASE 161

1 What abnormalities of the droppings are present? Lipid droplets, voluminous feces, and polyuria.

2 What is the most likely underlying cause? Exocrine pancreatic insufficiency (EPI). EPI in parrots is not a common presentation. It can arise after any inflammatory insult caused by an infectious agent or immune-mediated condition, or, alternatively, by toxins, leading to pancreatic atrophy. Viral diseases that also affect the pancreas are paramyxovirus 3, avian polyomavirus, adenoviruses, and psittacine herpesvirus 1; these are all known to have affinity for the pancreas in parrots. Bacteria, such as *Chlamydia psittaci* and many others, can affect the pancreas as an extension of systemic disease. Zinc, a common toxin of caged birds, can cause pancreatic acinar degranulation. Cyclopiazonic acid, a toxin produced by fungi, such as *Penicillium* spp., *Aspergillus versicolor*, *A. oryzae*, *A. flavus*, and *A. tamari*, causes degeneration and necrosis of the exocrine pancreas.

3 What simple fecal test can be performed to confirm the diagnosis? Lugol's iodine test (**161b**). In EPI cases, undigested starch will be present in the feces; adding Lugol's solution (iodine disinfectant solutions can be used instead) will result in a dark-blue-to-black color change (A). A healthy bird's feces should be used as control (B).

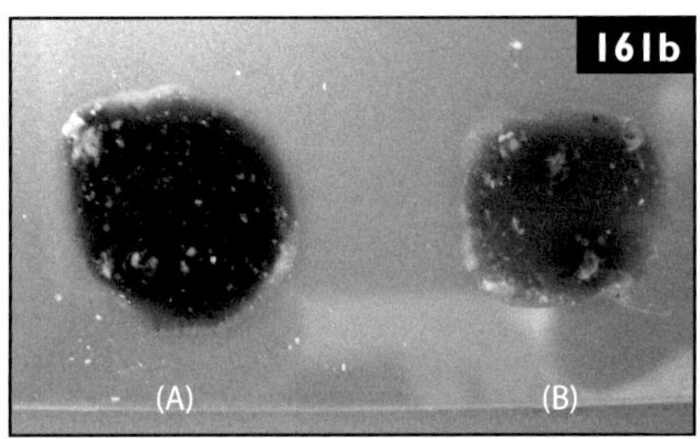

161b

Further reading

Lumeij JT (1994) Gastroenterology. In: *Avian Medicine: Principles and Application.* (eds. BW Ritchie, GJ Harrison, LR Harrison) Wingers Publishing, Lake Worth, p. 513.

CASE 162

1 What are some of the clinical indications for esophagostomy tube placement in avian patients (162a)? Esophagostomy tube placement is indicated in cases of severe trauma or disease involving the beak, as well as diseases of the oropharynx, proximal esophagus, or crop, such as abscesses and neoplasms. They are not recommended for regurgitating or vomiting individuals or for patients with respiratory disease. Esophagostomy tubes may also be used to bypass the crop in cases of severe crop trauma such as burn injury, crop laceration, or refractory crop dysfunction. They can also prove useful postoperatively in proventriculotomy patients. The technique is also useful in patients who are well trained and will tolerate tube use without restraint; where tube use for medication, feeding, or fluids is required four or more times a day; or where the patient would otherwise be extremely stressed by physical restraint for gavage tube administration.

2 Are esophagostomy tubes generally well tolerated in birds? Yes. In a case series of 18 birds of prey, esophagostomy tubes were well tolerated in all but two patients. A cloth cover may be fitted over the bird's back, with ties joining from right shoulder to left caudal and left shoulder to right caudal, to prevent the bird interfering with the tube end when not in use (**162b**).

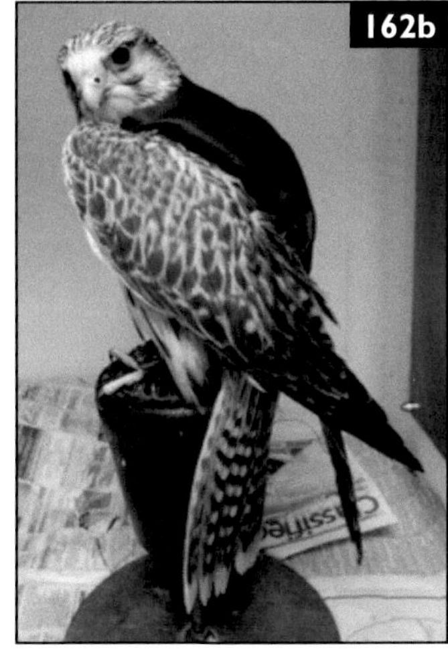
162b

3 When preparing to place an esophagostomy tube in raptorial species, at what level do you aim to place the distal tube end, and why? The distal tube end should be positioned at the cranial proventricular level. If it is further distal, the sensation of the tube within the proventriculus may trigger the bird to attempt to 'cast up' the tube, as it naturally would a 'casting' (i.e. the indigestible part of its diet).

Further reading

Huynh M, Sabater M, Brandao J *et al.* (2014) Use of an esophagostomy tube as a method of nutritional management in raptors: a case series. *J Avian Med Surg* **28(1)**:24–30.

CASE 163

1 What abnormalities can be seen in the histologic section? The histologic features show distension at the base of the glands, with pink proteinaceous fluid and sloughing of glandular epithelial cells with karyomegaly and basophilic intranuclear inclusions consistent with an acute DNA virus infection.
2 What etiologic agents should be considered? Avian polyomavirus is the most likely cause of the inclusions but adenovirus, herpesvirus, and finch circovirus should also be considered as possibilities.
3 What other diagnostic tests should be performed to confirm a specific etiologic diagnosis? Similar intranuclear inclusions were also seen in the liver and this case was confirmed positive for avian polyomavirus infection by PCR testing.

Further reading

Raidal SR (2012) Avian circovirus and polyomavirus diseases. In: *Fowler's Zoo and Wild Animal Medicine, Current Therapy*, Vol. 7. (eds. RE Miller, ME Fowler) Elsevier Saunders, St. Louis, pp. 297–303.

CASE 164

1 What are the main differential diagnoses? Hepatic granulomas and abscesses can be found in several avian diseases caused by viruses (avian reovirus), bacteria (*Mycobacterium, Yersinia, E. coli, Salmonella* spp., *Staphylococcus* spp., *Streptococcus* spp.), fungi (*Aspergillus* spp.), or parasites (coccidia, ascaridia).
2 What complementary examination would you perform? Liver impression smears were prepared for cytology and Gram stain. While cytology confirmed a large number of unidentified bacteria, Gram stain showed a large number of small, gram-negative, and bipolar stained bacteria, suggestive of *Yersinia pseudotuberculosis* (**164b**). The diagnosis was confirmed by PCR testing.

3 How would you prevent this disease? Access by wild birds or vermin, such as cockroaches, rodents, and flies, into the aviaries of susceptible birds must be controlled as much as possible. Soil should be changed periodically and water should always be kept clean. Potential sources of stress, such as overcrowding and any other environmental or social stressors, should be investigated and addressed.

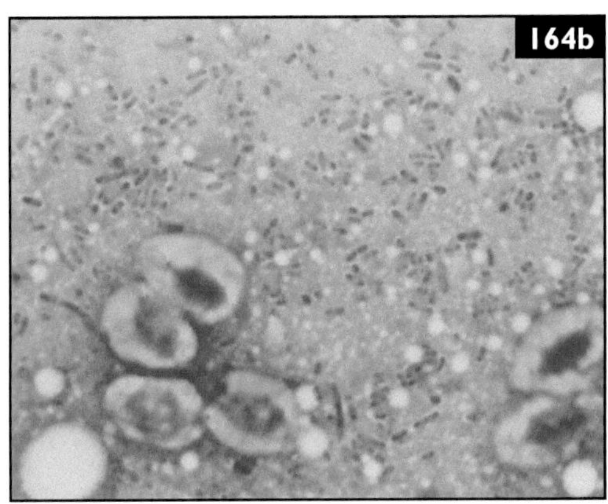

Further reading

Allchurch AF (2003) Yersiniosis. In: *Zoo and Wild Animal Medicine*, 5th edn. (eds. RE Miller, MR Fowler) Elsevier, St. Louis, pp. 724–727.

CASE 165

1 Describe the anatomic entry points for a triple-entry salpingohysterectomy. The first entry point is made just cranial to the pubis bone and ventral to the flexor cruris medialis muscle (**165b**, 2). Following insertion of a telescope through this incision, a second port is created under endoscopic guidance, caudal to the pubis bone and ventral to the flexor cruris medialis muscle (**165b**, 3; white arrow). The third entry point is made immediately caudal to the last rib (**165b**, 1; black arrow) and ventral to the flexor cruris medialis muscle (**165b**, m).

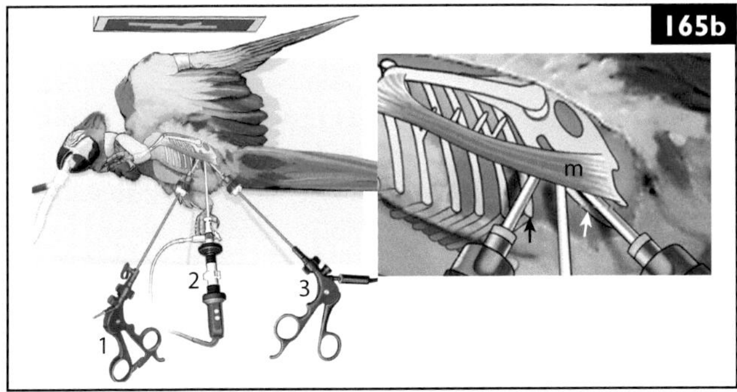

Courtesy of Educational Resources, UGA

2 What structures, labeled (1), (2), and (3) in image 165a, is the uterus (4) closely associated with and that need to be avoided during salpingohysterectomy? The immature uterus is closely associated with the kidney (1), the ureter (2), and the renal vein (3). Therefore, it is important to provide traction and keep the reproductive tract elevated away from these structures during dissection. In larger, mature females the reproductive tract may be so large that intracorporeal manipulation becomes difficult.

3 What are the limitations and contraindications of salpingohysterectomy in birds? Apart from the size limitations of avian patients and surgical and anesthetic complications, salpingohysterectomy does not involve removal of the ovary. In contrast to salpingohysterectomy, ovariectomy still remains a high-risk procedure in birds, and is reserved for cases where severe disease is present and/or euthanasia is being considered. Ovariectomy is rarely, if ever, considered an elective procedure in companion birds. Salpingohysterectomy does not appear to prevent ovulation and therefore carries a risk of future egg yolk coelomitis, particularly in high fecundity species like chickens. Salpingohysterectomy should therefore not be a recommended treatment option for chronic egg laying birds or high fecundity species, unless additional steps are taken to prevent ovulation. The procedure should be reserved for cases of nonovarian reproductive tract pathology and, if performed, may need to be coupled with long-term GnRH agonist administration.

Further reading

Hernandez-Divers SJ, Stahl S, Wilson GH *et al.* (2007) Endoscopic orchidectomy and salpingohysterectomy of pigeons (*Columba livia*): an avian model for minimally invasive endosurgery. *J Avian Med Surg* **21**(**1**):22–37.

CASE 166

1 What is the normal position for the embryo when hatching? In the normal position the head moves from between the legs in the narrow end of the egg to under the right wing in the wide end of the egg. The egg tooth on the bill is pointed at the air cell membrane (**166c**).

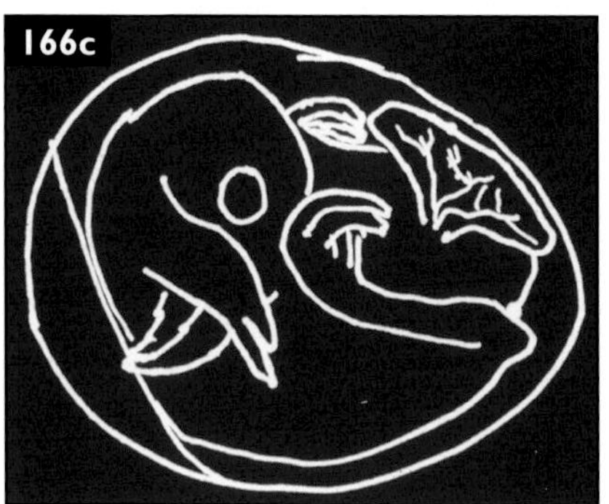
166c

2 Identify the number of this malposition and the prognosis for the embryo. Malposition 2 (**166a**). In this position, characterized by the head being located in the small end of the egg, the entire embryo is upside down in the egg as compared to normal orientation. The feet and yolk sac are located up near the air cell. If the embryo succeeds in pipping (breaking through the shell), a normal hatch can happen. About 50% of embryos in this position will die.

In malposition 6 (**166b**), the head is over rather than under the right wing. This position is likely to result in a live hatch with few complications.

3 Describe the effect each of the other types of malpositioning can have on hatching death. The other types of malposition are as follows:

- Malposition 1: the embryo's head is found between the thighs; this is a normal position early in incubation. However, during the last third of incubation, the embryo should move its head up and under the right wing. Malposition 1 is always fatal; it can be associated with above normal incubation temperatures.
- Malposition 3: this occurs when the chick rotates its head under the left wing instead of the right wing. This malposition is nearly always lethal and is associated with malnutrition in laying females, high incubation temperatures, or improper positioning of the egg during incubation.
- Malposition 4: the body is rotated in the long axis of the egg. The head is, therefore, away from the air cell and along the side of the egg. Without assistance, this malposition is often fatal as the embryo never breaks through to breathe.
- Malposition 5: this occurs when the feet are located over the head. Because of this malposition, the legs are not located properly to kick and cause the body to rotate as the chick is cutting out. Unless hatching is assisted, the results will often prove fatal.
- Malposition 7: this occurs when the embryo is small or the egg is spherical. The embryo is found lying crosswise in the egg instead of in the normal orientation with the head up near the air cell. This malposition is often fatal.

Further reading

Clubb S, Phillips A (1992) Psittacine embryonic mortality. In: *Psittacine Aviculture, Perspectives, Techniques and Research*. (eds. R Schubot, KJ Clubb, SL Clubb) Aviculture Breeding and Research Center, Laxahatchee, pp. 10-1 to 10-9.

Olsen GH (2000) Embryological considerations. In: *Manual of Avian Medicine*. (eds. GH Olsen, SE Orosz) Mosby, St. Louis, pp. 189–212.

CASE 167

1 What are the contraindications for tube feeding in the avian patient? The most important contraindication for tube feeding is lack of experience, since improper tube feeding can result in aspiration and potentially patient death. In general terms, the largest feeding tube (with the biggest roundest end) should be used, as the chances of esophageal damage or gavage into the trachea are reduced. Additional contraindications for tube feeding include birds that are regurgitating or unable to keep their heads elevated. Tube feeding should also not be performed until the patient has been rehydrated.

2 What is the estimated crop volume? Estimated crop volume is 20–50 mL/kg (2–5%) of body weight, varying between species and with respect to age. Generally, administration commences with a small volume (1–1.5% of body weight) and once tolerated increased to 3–5%. Juveniles tend to have a proportionately larger crop capacity than adults. Owls, toucans, gulls, and penguins have no crop and hence food should be administered more slowly. Irrespective of frequency and volume of feeding, the patient should be weighed first thing each morning (prior to feeding or medicating) to ensure that weight is being maintained or increased. If the latter is not being achieved, volume fed or frequency of feeding must be increased.
3 List the potential complications of tube feeding. Aspiration and possible death are potential complications of tube feeding. If the tube is passed forcefully, it may lacerate the oropharynx or perforate the crop. If continued, food may be injected through the laceration and into the surrounding tissue, potentially causing life-threatening cellulitis, or into the clavicular air sac resulting in airsacculitis and possible aspiration pneumonia.

Further reading

Roset K (2013) Clinical technique: tube feeding the avian patient. *J Exot Pet Med* **21(2):** 149–157.

CASE 168

1 What will you tell your client? You should tell your client that the egg is fertile. The blood vessels indicate fertility. This egg is viable. Lack of blood vessels would indicate a nonfertile or an infected or diseased egg.
2 By what day should you see blood vessels in a candled psittacine egg? By day 3 to 4 you should see blood vessels in a healthy fertilized psittacine egg. While blood vessel development can occur later, it is rarely apparent before day 3 to 4.
3 What do you see in this egg besides blood vessels? Besides blood vessels there is a tiny embryo visible in this egg. If the embryo dies, candling will reveal a blood ring. A blood ring indicates a dead and probably genetically abnormal or diseased embryo from a fertilized egg. It can also indicate early embryonic loss due to questionable incubation parameters, including improper temperature, humidity, rotation, rough handling and excessive vibrations, or poor ventilation.

Further reading

Romagnano A (2005) Reproduction and paediatrics. In: *BSAVA Manual of Psittacine Birds*, 2nd edn. (eds. N Harcourt-Brown, JR Chitty). British Small Animal Veterinary Association, Gloucester, pp. 222–233.

CASE 169

1 What disease condition is affecting this young rhea? The changes seen in the ribcage of this rhea are consistent with rickets. The ribs are deformed and there are rounded, white cartilaginous nodules present at the junctions of the vertebral and sternal ribs (costochondral junctions), as well as at sites of pathologic fractures.

2 Describe the pathogenesis of the lesions shown. Rickets is a nutritional disease of young growing birds and can be caused by absolute deficiencies of vitamin D, calcium, or phosphorus, or by imbalances in the ratio of calcium to phosphorus in the diet. Vitamin D deficiency results in reduced gastrointestinal calcium absorption, increased secretion of parathyroid hormone from hyperplastic parathyroid glands, and failure of mineralization of developing bone, particularly in the hypertrophic zone of the epiphyseal plate. Calcium and phosphorus deficiencies result in similar lesions; histopathology of bone may help differentiate among the three main causes of rickets.

3 What management actions should be taken to reduce disease associated with the condition shown? Evaluation and correction of dietary imbalances are required to address the cause of rickets and other metabolic bone diseases. This may require a nutritional evaluation of the diet or testing of feeds to ensure that the listed nutritional composition is correct. In rare cases, malabsorption from gastrointestinal disease may mimic nutritional deficiency. Injection with vitamin D_3 and calcium supplementation may be used therapeutically in addition to correction of the diet.

Further reading

Klasing KC (2013) Nutritional disease. In: *Diseases of Poultry*, 13th edn. (eds. DA Swayne, JR Glisson, LR McDougald *et al.*) Wiley-Blackwell, Ames, pp. 1205–1232.

CASE 170

1 What is the main concern in this bird? A bird's crop is not a stomach, being more akin to a shopping basket. The crop will normally start to empty soon after feeding, being empty within 6–8 hours. There is no acid or enzyme to prevent putrefaction and any meat is being held close to 41°C (105.8°F). The meat will rapidly go off, producing toxins that enter the blood stream rapidly, creating a potentially critical situation. This condition is termed 'sour crop'.

2 When is this clinical presentation most likely to occur? The situation is most likely to arise when a bird that is in very thin (low) condition is given an over full crop. Most commonly this is when a bird first enters (kills for the first time). The falconer may well have had to reduce the bird's weight further and further to make the bird keener to catch and kill quarry, and the bird may have had to fly particularly hard to make that kill. The falconer may be tempted to reward the bird well for making its first kill, allowing it to consume a large crop of food. The same scenario can arise if a bird is recovered in very low condition having been 'absent without leave' for a few days; the falconer gives a large meal in an attempt to increase the bird's weight quickly.

3 What treatment is recommended? Such patients are far sicker than they appear. They are emergencies and must be provided with critical care irrespective of the time of day. The crop must be emptied and flushed out, and fluid therapy and antibiotics should be provided. There are a number of ways of emptying the crop. Manual retrieval from the crop to the mouth is long-winded and stressful. The quickest, most efficient, and stress free method is indicated (i.e. a brief gaseous anesthetic for ingluviotomy to empty and then saline flush the crop). If by this point the patient is not sufficiently stable for prolonged anesthesia (to facilitate surgical closure), then repair is delayed until the following day when the patient is likely to be more stable.

Further reading

Forbes NA (2015) Raptor nutrition masterclass. In: *Proceedings International Conference on Avian, Herpetological and Exotic Mammal Medicine*, Paris, pp. 33–36.

CASE 171

1 List the main differential diagnoses for this lesion. The top differential diagnoses are squamous cell carcinoma (SCC), papillomatosis, and poxvirus. Other less likely differentials include mycobacteriosis, trichomoniasis, severe hypovitaminosis A with secondary infection, fungal disease, other neoplasia, or primary bacterial infection.

2 List diagnostic tests that would be appropriate to aid in the diagnosis of this lesion. Removal of the superficial plaque with a biopsy of deeper tissues is the best approach to reaching a diagnosis. Acid-fast staining could be helpful to rule out mycobacterial organisms. Cytologic examination (particularly saline wet mount or Gram stain) of underlying exudate may also provide additional information. Fungal or bacterial culture and sensitivity could be considered to determine further information about potential secondary infections. CT could be considered to better assess the nasal passages and extent of disease.

3 Discuss likely progression timeline, treatment options, and prognosis. These lesions are generally slow/chronic in progression, although poxvirus can progress more rapidly. This bird was determined to have a SCC on deep tissue biopsy. The ideal treatment for this lesion is complete surgical excision. Due to the location and extent of disease, complete excision is unlikely and adjunct therapy should be considered. Adjunct therapies to treat oral SCC in avian patients include intralesional chemotherapy, cryotherapy, radiation therapy, NSAIDs, and phototherapy. The prognosis is good in the case of complete surgical excision (unlikely). Recurrence is likely in the case of incomplete surgical resection, but adjunct therapy may slow progression of the lesion.

Further reading

Zehnder A, Graham J, Reavill D *et al.* (2016) Neoplastic diseases in avian species. In: *Current Therapy in Avian Medicine and Practice.* (ed. BL Speer) Elsevier, St. Louis, pp. 107–141.

CASE 172

1 Describe the surgical approach for proventriculotomy and ventriculotomy. The left lateral tranverse coeliotomy approach preferably or the ventral midline with flap coeliotomy approach is used to access the proventriculus and ventriculus. The suspensory structures must be dissected bluntly to retract the proventriculus caudally. Stay sutures are placed in the wall of the ventriculus to exteriorize both organs. The proventriculotomy is initiated at the dorsal isthmus (junction between the ventriculus and the proventriculus) and extended cranially as needed. The ventriculus may be accessed through a proventriculotomy preferably or through a ventriculotomy through the caudoventral thin muscle. This part of the ventriculus is located just caudal to the caudal border of the sternum and is easily accessed for ventriculotomy.

2 What precautions are needed during these procedures? When this incision is made, gastrointestinal fluid might escape the incision and contaminate the coelom. To prevent this happening, exteriorize the ventriculus as much as possible, using stay sutures placed in the lateral tendinous fascia, and then pack off as much as possible around the incision site with laparotomy pads or gauze. The proventriculus is fragile and might tear if manipulated with toothed forceps or if stay sutures are placed. At the moment of incision, suction should be available and positioned adjacent to the incision. As soon as an incision is created, suction is used to remove all fluid from the gut lumen.

3 Describe how would you close the surgical incisions in these organs. The proventriculotomy or isthmus incision in most common companion avian species is closed with a fine 4-0 to 6-0 monofilament absorbable material on a small atraumatic taper needle using a simple continuous pattern with a second inverting continuous pattern. The normal isthmus incision site can be covered by caudal apices of the right liver lobe. Following proventricular closure this lobe of the liver is sutured down over the repaired incision, to adhese over the incision and reduce the risk of breakdown. The ventriculus is closed with a simple interrupted pattern using a 3-0 to 5-0 absorbable suture. The placement of collagen patches to cover the site of the proventriculotomy, or a coelomic fat patch over the ventriculotomy site, does not reduce the risk of wound dehiscence and is not recommended.

Further reading
Guzman DS (2016) Avian soft tissue surgery. *Vet Clin North Am Exot Anim Pract* **19(1)**: 133–157.

CASE 173

1 What is the currently preferred anesthetic gas for avian species, and why? Isoflurane is currently the preferred choice for avian anesthesia due to its low relative cost, comparatively rapid induction and recovery, low blood solubility, and minimal metabolism.

2 When using isoflurane for raptor anesthesia, what undesirable side-effects may be observed? In addition to causing dose-dependent cardiopulmonary depression, isoflurane may cause cardiac arrhythmias. Cardiac arrhythmias, with second-degree heart block being most prevalent, have been noted in 35–75% of bald eagles anesthetized with isoflurane. In one study, they occurred during induction and recovery in 80% of the cases. Catecholamine release was suspected to be the cause. Cardiac arrhythmias are also commonly detected in other avian species such as Pekin ducks and pigeons, but many authors feel they are more common in raptor species.

3 What are the pros and cons of using sevoflurane? Sevoflurane has better solubility than isoflurane and this allows for faster induction and recovery, as well as more rapid changes in anesthetic depth. In pigeons and bald eagles, induction and recovery times were more rapid with sevoflurane (pigeons: 95 ± 9 sec; bald eagles: 166.1 ± 16.5 sec) than with isoflurane (pigeons: 154 ± 12 sec; bald eagles: 200.3 ± 16.5 sec). In bald eagles, temperature, heart rate, and blood pressure were significantly higher with isoflurane. In red-tailed hawks, only the time to visual tracking was faster with sevoflurane compared with isoflurane. Sevoflurane has a less irritating smell than isoflurane, which may reduce stress and help prevent struggling during mask induction.

Further reading
Aguilar RF, Smith VE, Ogburn P *et al.* (1995) Arrhythmias associated with isoflurane anesthesia in bald eagles (*Haliaeetus leucocephalus*). *J Zoo Wildlife Med* **26(4)**:508–516.
Hawkins MG, Zehnder AM, Pascoe PJ (2014) Cagebirds. In: *Zoo Animal and Wildlife Immobilization and Anesthesia*, 2nd edn. (eds. G West, D Heard, N Caulkett) Wiley-Blackwell, Ames, pp. 299–434.
Joyner PH, Jones MP, Ward D *et al.* (2008) Induction and recovery characteristics and cardiopulmonary effects of sevoflurane and isoflurane in bald eagles. *Am J Vet Res* **69(1)**:13–22.
Quandt JE, Greenacre CB (1999) Sevoflurane anesthesia in psittacines. *J Zoo Wildlife Med* **30(2)**:308–309.

CASE 174

1 When is the air cell formed? The air cell is the light colored area of the inside of the egg, which forms shortly after laying. Eggs are at the body temperature of the laying female bird and cool down to environmental or ambient temperature after laying. As the egg cools, the contents shrink and air is drawn into the egg through the porous shell.

2 Where is it located in most eggs, and why is it located there? The air cell usually forms in the wide or blunt end of the egg because this is the end of the egg normally orientated upwards when the egg is resting in a cup-shaped nest.

3 What function does the air cell perform during the hatching process? The air cell functions in hatching during the first part of the hatching process, termed the internal pip. This is when the bill of the embryo breaks through the air cell membrane into the air cell itself, and the respiratory system of the embryo begins functioning for the first time by breathing the air in the air cell. Often the embryo will vocalize for the first time when this occurs.

Further reading

Olsen GH (2000) Embryological considerations. In: *Manual of Avian Medicine.* (eds. GH Olsen, SE Orosz) Mosby, St. Louis, pp. 189–212.

CASE 175

1 What is inappropriate about this initial pin placement? The IM pin was retrograded into the humero-ulnar joint space. This joint does not tolerate insult and damage by an IM pin retrograded into it through either an ulna or humerus is very likely to cause complications (i.e. postoperative joint ankyloses and loss of flight). It is not possible to retrograde an IM pin through the ulna without damaging either joint.

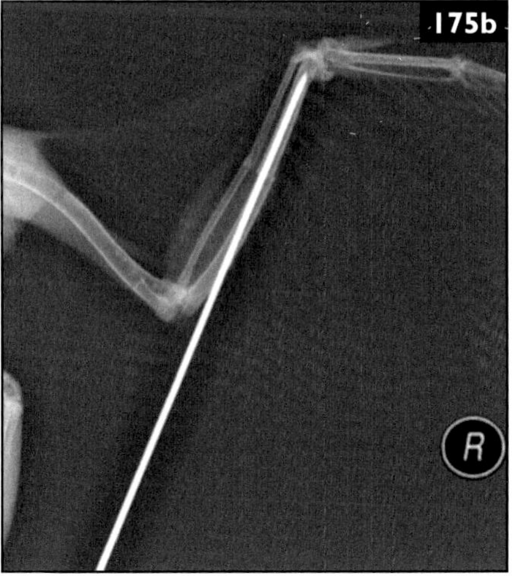

2 What is the recommended technique for pin placement? The IM pin should be driven normograde, entering the caudal ulna between the insertions of the 3rd and 4th secondary feathers from medial (i.e. count from the elbow laterally) so as to avoid the elbow joint (see intraoperative image, **175b**). This technique is made possible by the natural curvature of the proximal ulna, as present in most species.

3 What final construct would you use to repair this type of fracture? A tie-in ESF–IM pin in the ulna and an IM pin in the radius driven normograde through the distal fragment. In this fracture, an alternative repair would be to pin the radius first, passing a pin from the fracture site, normograde through the distal radius (which does not interfere with the carpal joint), then after reducing the fracture, retrograde back into the proximal radius. Once this is done the ulna is pulled back into good alignment. So long as there are no longitudinal fissures running down the ulna fragments, the ulna may be stabilized with two ESF pins in each of the proximal and distal segments, on the dorsal aspect. All four pins are then joined with a connecting bar.

Further reading

Redig PT, Cruz L (2008) Fractures. In: *Avian Medicine*, 2nd edn. (ed. J Samour) Mosby, St. Louis, pp. 215–248.

CASE 176

1 Which parasite would you consider as the etiologic agent based on the information provided? *Syngamus* spp., also known as gape worm.

2 If you decide to perform a tracheoscopy, what anatomic considerations should you consider in this species? In many crane species, the trachea is not straight and has multiple loops extending into the sternum to enhance their vocalization. This makes tracheoscopy in these species very difficult.

3 What treatment and control method would you recommend to the owner to reduce the prevalence in his collection of cranes? Benzimidazole anthelmintics such as fenbendazole (50–100 mg/kg PO daily for 5 days, repeated after 14 days) have been demonstrated to be effective. Ivermectin (0.2 mg/kg IM, SC, PO, two dosages 10–14 days apart) has also shown variable success. Avoid overcrowding; rear young birds on clean pasture (netted to prevent feral bird access). Avoid heavily contaminated paddocks. *Syngamus* spp. have direct and indirect life cycles. Earthworms act as intermediate hosts in the indirect life cycle, and play a role in the persistence of the environmental infection, as the third-stage larvae can survive in the earthworms, disappearing underground to reappear sometimes months later and, once ingested, causing disease again. Pasture rotation using a nonavian grazing species may lessen the impact of earthworms in their reservoir role. Alternatively, having an impervious substrate (concrete or plastic sheeting), covered with shallow soil or turf, could prevent earthworms burrowing and coming back up later. In the event of infection, the turf and soil are removed and replaced with clean material.

Further reading

Fernando MA, Barta JR (2014) Tracheal worms. In: *Parasitic Diseases of Wild Birds*. (eds. CT Atkinson, NJ Thomas, DB Hunter) Wiley-Blackwell, Ames, pp. 343–354.

CASE 177

1 Name three avian Orders that may be considered intermediate or definitive hosts for this parasite. Columbiformes and Psittaciformes have been reported as intermediate hosts while Falconiformes are considered the definitive hosts and may serve as source of infection for the intermediate hosts.

2 What clinical signs have been observed in intermediate hosts? Neurologic signs including torticollis, nystagmus, ataxia, inability to stand, and decreased proprioception.

3 What lesions would you expect during postmortem examination? Gross lesions may not be present. Encephalitis and meningitis are the most common histologic findings. Additionally, myositis has been described in some cases.

Further reading

Rimoldi G, Speer B, Wellehan Jr JF *et al.* (2013) An outbreak of *Sarcocystis calchasi* encephalitis in multiple psittacine species within an enclosed zoological aviary. *J Vet Diagn Invest* **25**(**6**):775–781.

CASE 178

1 What diagnostic tests should be performed? Uropygial secretion cytology and culture (bacterial and fungal) should be performed. Cytology revealed an inflammatory response with cocci bacteria present. Fungal culture did not reveal any growth. Bacterial culture yielded a methicillin-resistant *Staphylococcus aureus* (MRSA) growth. Further testing allowed the identification of staphylococcal cassette chromosome mec type IV (community-acquired).

2 Preliminary results from the laboratory are consistent with a *Staphylococcus* spp. infection. What is the significance of this finding? Staphylococcal cutaneous colonization in captive psittacines is reported to be less common than in other species; nevertheless, cutaneous staphylococci were identified in 89/180 captive psittacines in one study. The most common *Staphylococcus* spp. were *S. intermedius*, *S. epidermidis*, and *S. hominis* subsp. *hominis*, while *S. aureus* was isolated in 4/113 isolates. In another study assessing the normal cutaneous flora of apparently healthy captive African grey parrots (*Psittacus erithacus*), budgerigars (*Melopsittacus undulates*), and cockatiels (*Nymphicus hollandicus*), positive skin cultures were identified in 52/75 birds, which allowed the identification of 89 bacterial colonies. *Staphylococcus* and *Corynebacterium* spp. were the most common genera. In the current case, it is unclear if the MRSA was commensal or acquired from either the environment or humans to which the bird was exposed. Based on the cytologic evidence of inflammation and infection, it appears that bacterial involvement is expected. MRSA (community-acquired) associated dermatitis has been reported in a Congo African grey parrot. Ulcerative dermatitis and valvular endocarditis associated with *S. aureus* in a Hyacinth macaw (*Anodorhynchus hyacinthinus*) has also been reported. It was suggested that endocarditis associated with *S. aureus* septicemia was a potential complication of feather damaging behavior.

3 What are the zoonotic concerns? Not much is known about the zoonotic transmission of MRSA in companion animals. While *S. aureus* is considered to be mainly a human pathogen, it can be found in many animal species. Transmission of MRSA from birds to humans appears to be underreported; nevertheless, zoonotic capability should be considered and care should be taken to prevent transmission of such disease to owners and medical staff.

Further reading

Briscoe JA, Morris DO, Rankin SC *et al.* (2008) Methicillin-resistant *Staphylococcus aureus*-associated dermatitis in a Congo African grey parrot (*Psittacus erithacus erithacus*). *J Avian Med Surg* **22**:336–343.

Briscoe JA, Morris DO, Rosenthal KL *et al.* (2009) Evaluation of mucosal and seborrheic sites for staphylococci in two populations of captive psittacines. *J Am Vet Med Assoc* **234**:901–905.

Huynh M, Carnaccini S, Driggers T *et al.* (2014) Ulcerative dermatitis and valvular endocarditis associated with *Staphylococcus aureus* in a hyacinth macaw (*Anadorhynchus hyacinthinus*). *Avian Dis* **58**:223–227.

Lamb S, Sobczynski A, Starks D *et al.* (2014) Bacteria isolated from the skin of Congo African grey parrots (*Psittacus erithacus*), budgerigars (*Melopsittacus undulatus*), and cockatiels (*Nymphicus hollandicus*). *J Avian Med Surg* **28**:275–279.

CASE 179

1 What is the structure labeled 1, and what is its function? The propatagium, a triangular fold of skin. It increases the surface area of the wing and forms the aerofoil shape.

2 Name the structure labeled 2. It is the leading edge of the propatagium and is supported by the *ligament propatagialis pars longus*. This ligament has a small, fleshy belly mainly attaching to the clavicle. The distal fifth of the tendon is fibrous and unyielding, but the majority of the tendon is elastic and will maintain the tension of the leading edge of the wing even when it is not fully extended, thereby keeping the aerofoil shape while flying.

3 What effect does damage to this structure have on the function of the wing, and how should it be repaired? Any injury to this area will prevent the bird from flying.

When the propatagium is repaired, the elastic tendon must be found and, if damaged, must be repaired by suturing the ends together. Birds can fly well even when they have lost a significant part of the ligament provided it is repaired correctly.

CASE 180

1 What factors may lead to the development of hunger traces? Hunger traces can be identified as dark lines located transversely across one, several, or many pairs of feathers. An adrenocortical surge occurring while the flight feathers are developing will result in these lesions. Glucocorticoids strongly suppress growth and increase protein catabolism. These lesions probably reflect a short period of decreased amino acid availability during the development of the feather.

2 Taking into consideration the time at which these hunger lines were caused, what event took place in these pigeons that may explain the same signs in every one of the 10 pigeons? Leg bands are placed around the legs of pigeons at approximately 7 days of age.

3 Provide a possible explanation that could be the reason for these stress lines. To allow easier placement of the leg bands in these pigeons the fancier used a hand cream. On inspection of the cream, it turned out that it contained triamcinolone, a potent glucocorticoid. Triamcinolone is readily absorbed through the skin, resulting in high concentrations of circulating glucocorticoids, just as seen after any stressful event. The stress lines were likely caused by the triamcinolone used to place the leg bands. Fenbendazole treatment, administered to pigeons while feathers are growing, can also result in hunger traces.

Further reading

Westerhof I, Van den Brom WE, Mol JA *et al.* (1994) Sensitivity of the hypothalamic-pituitary-adrenal system of pigeons (*Columba livia domestica*) to suppression by dexamethasone, cortisol, and prednisolone. *Avian Dis* **38**:435–445.

CASE 181

1 Which type of photoreceptor (cone or rod) is more numerous in the nervous layer of a nocturnal bird's retina? Nocturnal birds, including owls, have some cones (responsible for visual acuity and color vision) but mostly rods (sensitive to the intensity of light), whereas diurnal birds have more cones than rods.

2 What is your diagnosis in this owl? Chorioretinitis: acute punctuate lesions (black dots) and chronic postinflammatory lesions (atrophic retinal changes) (white area).

3 List some potential etiologies. Chorioretinal lesions including chorioretinitis, choroiditis varying from focal pigmented areas, and generalized retinal degeneration with hyperreflectivity and synchysis scintillans are common in owls. Multiple etiologies for these lesions have been considered: trauma, toxoplasmosis, nutritional, and effects of sun on the retina. Results from a retrospective study of ocular findings in tawny owls (*Strix aluco*) demonstrated that cicatricial retinal lesions were not associated with high titers of antibodies to *Toxoplasma* spp., but correlated with those observed in humans with ocular injuries secondary to high-speed blunt trauma. In canaries, tachyzoites of *T. gondii* were confirmed in the choroid, vitreous, lens, and nerve layer of the retina of birds showing severe choroiditis, focal necrosis, and retinal detachment.

Further reading

Williams DL, González Villavincencio CM, Wilson S (2006) Chronic ocular lesions in tawny owls (*Strix aluco*) injured by road traffic. *Vet Rec* **159**:148–153.

CASE 182

1 Based on the history and clinical presentation, what are the differential diagnoses? Fungal pneumonia and/or airsacculitis (e.g. *Aspergillus* spp.); bacterial pneumonia and/or airsacculitis; bacterial or fungal tracheitis; aspiration pneumonia; parasitic airsacculitis.
2 What diagnostic tests would you perform to confirm the diagnosis? Survey radiography (ventrodorsal and laterolateral projections); hematology and plasma chemistry panel; coelomic endoscopic examination; fecal parasite examination.
3 On direct fecal examination using 0.9% NaCl, numerous thick-shelled embryonated ova could be observed (182, ×400). Can you identify the ova in the fecal preparation? The ova are from *Serratospiculum seurati*, a nematode commonly (65%) found in falcons in the Middle East. Several arthropods (e.g. beetles) have been identified as intermediate hosts of *S. seurati*. The adult worms are commonly found in the air sacs, resulting in the clinical signs observed in this bird.

Further reading

Zucca P (2008) Infectious diseases, parasites, nematodes. In: *Avian Medicine*, 2nd edn. (ed. J Samour). Elsevier, St. Louis, p. 330–336.

CASE 183

1 What are the most commonly used methods for semen collection in birds? Which method applied in Falconiformes uses males imprinted onto the handlers to

collect viable semen samples? Voluntary donation, massage method, and electro-ejaculation methods. The voluntary donation method is used in Falconiformes to collect viable semen samples.

2 What prompted falconers, primarily in the USA, to develop methods for semen collection and artificial insemination in raptors? Which organization was at the forefront in the development of artificial breeding techniques in falcons? The decline in the population of certain North American raptors such as the peregrine falcon (*Falco peregrinus*) prompted falconers in the USA to develop artificial breeding techniques in order to maximize the number of captive bred falcons suitable for release into strategic locations throughout the USA. The organization at the forefront was the The Peregrine Fund under the umbrella of Cornell University, Ithaca, New York, USA.

3 What is the preferred method of semen collection in most Passeriformes, as shown in this house sparrow (*Passer domesticus*) (183) and similar to that used in budgerigars (*Melopsittacus undulatus*)? What anatomic structure facilitates semen collection in the house sparrow? The massage method. The seminal glomus facilitates semen collection in the house sparrow. These are paired structures located on both sides of the cloaca. The seminal glomus is formed by multiple convolutions of the terminal sections of the vas deferens located on either side of the proctodeum.

Further reading

Samour J (2004) Semen collection, spermatozoa cryopreservation and artificial insemination in non-domesticated birds. *J Avian Med Surg* 18(4):219–223.

CASE 184

1 Which drugs are commonly administered by intracameral injections, and what are the potential complications of this route of administration? Different drugs commonly administered into the anterior chamber of the eye are viscoelastic substances to maintain the anterior chamber pressure, adrenalin to control iris hemorrhage or induce mydriasis, tissue plasminogen activator to manage anterior and/or posterior chamber fibrin formation or carbachol to achieve myosis, and mydriatics such as D-tubocurarine. D-tubocurarine provokes a consistent moderate to maximal mydriasis in pigeons and several raptor species. Potential complications of intracameral injections are: structural damage, hyphema, intraocular pressure increase, infectious uveitis, and systemic effects. Few complications have been reported with anterior chamber paracentesis in humans and complications in birds have not been studied.

2 When does a clinician induce mydriasis in birds? Mydriasis allows posterior segment visual examination and surgery. A high percentage of raptors admitted

into rehabilitation centers because of flight trauma present with abnormalities involving the posterior segment of the eye, which may preclude their successful release.
3 What alternatives may be used to induce mydriasis in birds? Variable mydriasis can be fairly consistently achieved under general anesthesia. In raptors, short-acting anesthesia (ketamine hydrochloride and xylazine) provokes mydriasis. Air sac perfusion anesthesia has been reported to be successful in inducing mydriasis in pigeons, but appears not to achieve this in cockatoos. Topical parasympatholytic agents are ineffective due to the predominance of striated muscular fibers in the avian iris. The iris muscles may be partially paralyzed by neuromuscular paralyzing agents. Topical rocuronium bromide provokes mydriasis in European kestrels (*Falco tinnunculus*), common buzzards (*Buteo buteo*), little owls (*Athene noctua*), tawny owls (*Strix aluco*), and Hispaniolan Amazon parrots (*Amazona ventralis*). Topical vecuronium bromide was effective in kestrels (*Falco tinnunculus*), citron-crested and sulphur-crested cockatoos (*Cacatua sulphurea citrinocristata* and *Cacatua galerita)*, African grey parrots (*Psittacus erithacus*), and blue-fronted Amazon parrots (*Amazona aestiva*), although Amazon parrots showed mild transitory systemic side-effects. However, topical vecuronium bromide was not effective at tested doses in South African black-footed penguins (*Spheniscus demersus*). A topical combination of atropine, phenilephrine, and vecuronium bromide was effective in double-crested cormorants (*Phalacrocorax auritus*). Topical D-tubocurarine induced mydriasis in some avian species (e.g. pigeons [*Columba livia domestica*]) but not in others. Topical alcuronium chloride resulted in mydriasis in kestrels (*Falco tinnunculus*) but eyelid paralysis was observed in most of the birds and one developed neck paralysis. Topical pancuronium bromide showed inconsistent mydriasis in kestrels (*Falco tinnunculus*) and mild to severe systemic effects in some cockatoos (*Cacatua sulphurea*).

CASE 185

1 Based on the gross image, what type of testicular tumor do you suspect? Seminoma. Seminomas generally retain the shape of the testicle and are creamy white soft masses supported on a fine fibrovascular stroma. The exfoliative cytology will generally be of a dense population of round cells.
2 What is the likely cause of the clinical signs? The mass effect of the tumor displacing and compressing coelomic organs can account for the respiratory changes and contribute to the lethargy and anorexia. Nerve compression (ischiadic [sciatic] and/or pudendal) from the enlarging mass can result in a peripheral neuropathy presenting as lameness.
3 Can you determine malignancy by cytology or even by a small biopsy section? It is usually difficult to determine the malignant potential of this tumor based solely on histologic or cytologic evaluation of the primary neoplasm.

Examination of the entire testis for infiltration into the tunica albuginea, epididymis, or spermatic cord, as well as other organs, is required. Complete work up including hematology, plasma biochemistry, radiographs, and even ultrasound would be needed to stage this neoplasm.

Further reading

Mutinelli F, Vascellari M, Bozzato E (2006) Unilateral seminoma with multiple visceral metastases in a duck (*Anas platyrhynchos*). *Avian Pathol* **35(4)**:327–329.

CASE 186

1 Why is a lateral coelioscopy contraindicated in this patient for evaluation of the liver? Coelioscopic evaluation of the liver via a left or right lateral approach would create a communication between the air sac system and the hepatoperitoneal cavity, which in the presence of ascites would flood the respiratory system and potentially drown the patient or result in aspiration pneumonia.

2 What is the preferred coelioscopic approach in this patient? Ventral coelioscopy is the preferred approach in this case as the hepatoperitoneal cavity is distended with fluid, forcing the air sacs laterally (**186a**). Therefore, a ventral midline approach permits entry into the hepatoperitoneal cavity without entering the air sacs.

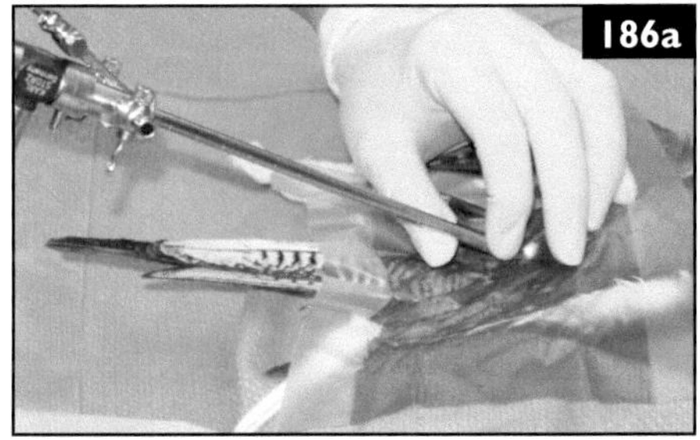

186a

3 Describe the technique for obtaining a liver biopsy in this patient. How does this differ from obtaining a biopsy via a lateral approach? A liver biopsy can be obtained from the caudal edge of the liver (**186b**) using 5-Fr biopsy forceps. With a lateral approach, the hepatoperitoneal membrane needs to be incised with scissors prior to biopsy, as biopsy through the membrane results in greater crush artifact.

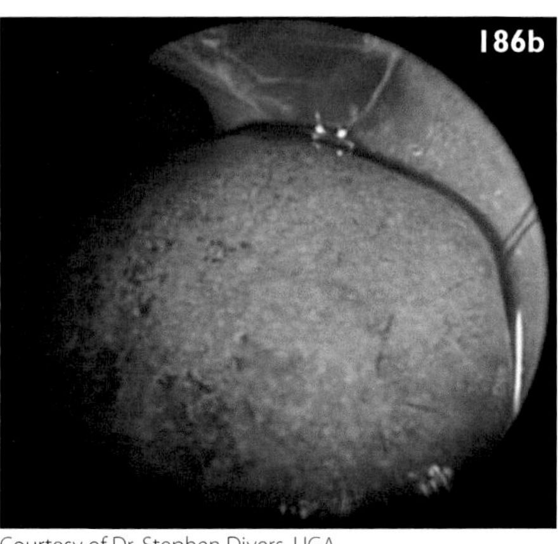

186b

Courtesy of Dr. Stephen Divers, UGA

Further reading

Divers SJ (2010) Avian diagnostic endoscopy. *Vet Clin North Am Exot Anim Pract* **13(2)**:187–202.

CASE 187

1 How can a bird be losing body condition and yet not be losing weight? A space occupying lesion in the coelom would expand at the expense of the air sacs, as such air is replaced by soft tissue, fluid, or even gastrointestinal contents, which are heavier than air. This would result in an increase in body weight offsetting the body condition and muscle loss from the pectoral muscles.

2 What condition is this bird suffering from, and what are the three main etiologies? This bird is suffering from ascites (the diagonal fluid density line from the heart to the kidneys is characteristic). The most likely causes of ascites are heart disease causing portal hypertension, liver disease causing hypoproteinemia, or portal hypertension. Reproductive disease, gastrointestinal or renal disease (e.g. protein-losing enteropathy or nephropathy), or neoplasia in other organs of the coelomic cavitiy (e.g. spleen, pancreas) can all cause increased coelomic fluid, presenting with similar signs.

3 What steps would you take to further investigate this condition? CBC and plasma biochemistry panel; plain radiography and contrast radiography, achieved by passing a silicone feeding tube via the oropharyngeal cavity and crop directly into the proventriculus to deliver barium; coelomic ultrasound; and coelomocentesis with fluid analysis. Coelomocentesis is better performed in the ventral midline, just caudal to the point of historic yolk sac connection. Further cranially is best avoided as the liver may be enlarged, while laterally might result in penetration of the air sac, resulting ultimately in fluid being able to flow into the air sac, and may cause drowning.

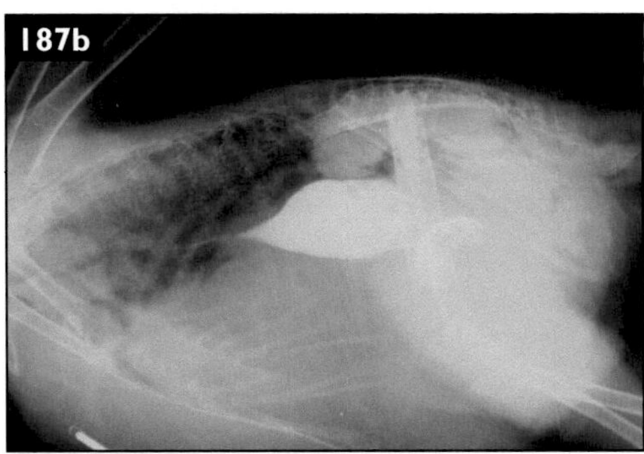

The barium contrast radiograph shown (**187b**) is of the same patient as in the question, and it confirms hepatomegaly. Ultrasound would do likewise.

Further reading

Krautwald-Junghanns ME, Schmidt V (2011) Special diagnostic, pathological findings. In: *Diagnostic Imaging of Exotic Pets*. (eds. ME Krautwald-Jinghanns, M Pees, S Reese, T Tully) Schlutersche, Hannover, pp. 89–91.

CASE 188

1 In what diseases is this lesion characteristic? It can be seen in birds with proventricular dilatation disease, as well as with other viral diseases causing encephalitis including West Nile virus disease, paramyxovirus disease, and other similar viral diseases.

2 Is this lesion always associated with neurologic signs in psittacines? No. This lesion is commonly seen in birds with the gastrointestinal form of proventricular dilatation disease that show no obvious neurologic signs.

3 What other histologic lesions would you expect to find in this bird? Lymphoplasmacytic myenteric ganglioneuritis; lymphoplasmacytic infiltration of medullary areas within the adrenal gland; lymphoplasmacytic myositis of the ventriculus; lymphoplasmacytic infiltration of epicedial ganglia; lymphoplasmacytic cardiomyositis; lymphoplasmacytic cuffing of peripheral nerves; perivascular cuffing in the optic nerves, choroid, ciliary body, and occasionally in the iris and pectin; retinal lymphoplasmacytic infiltration; and retinal degeneration.

Further reading

Gancz AY, Clubb S, Shivaprasad HL (2010) Advanced diagnostic approaches and current management of proventricular dilatation disease. *Vet Clin North Am Exot Anim Pract* 13(3):471–494.

CASE 189

1 How do you approach and handle an adult ostrich? Ostriches can be dangerous due to their size and their powerful legs and feet. A minimum of two people are required to handle an ostrich (**189**). Ostriches kick forwards, therefore a handler should not stand in front of a bird unless they already have hold of the head or neck.

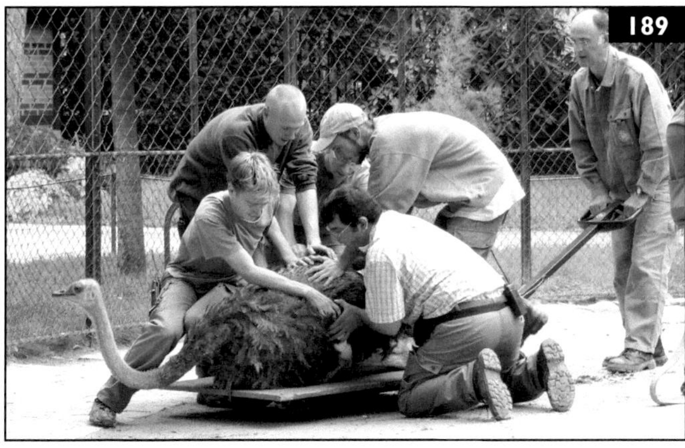
189

One handler should approach the bird from the side or behind (keeping out of the way of the legs) and grasp the neck; at this point the second handler grasp the bird's tail or wing to prevent it from swiveling round. The neck is pulled down, the head grasped, and a head cover pulled over it. Once the head is in the dark, the bird will become calmed and can be restrained safely.

2 Where are the microchip implantation sites in adults and chicks in this species? The recommended electronic microchip implantation site in birds is the left pectoral muscle. However, ratites do not possess a keel and have reduced pectoral muscle, which prevents microchip implantation in that site. The recommendation is that ostrich chicks are implanted at one day of age by placing the chip into the pipping muscle, just below the ear, on the left side (this muscle shrinks away within a few days of hatching). In adults, the microchip is implanted subcutaneously in the left side of the neck.

3 How do you differentiate between male and female ostriches? In adult (3–4 years) ostriches the male is black and the female brown. These feather color changes commence from 14 months onwards. When in breeding condition the male bird's beak is red, as opposed to pale silvery yellow in the female. Male ostriches, like waterfowl but unlike other avian species have a phallus. Ostrich chicks may be vent sexed at 1 day of age; in experienced hands accuracy is stated to be 95%. PCR sexing can be carried out on feather samples at any age.

Further reading

Kummrow M (2015) Ratites: Tinamiformes and Struthioniformes, Rheiiformes, Cassuariformes. In: *Fowler's Zoo and Wild Animal Medicine*, Vol. 8, 1st edn. (eds. RE Miller, ME Fowler) Elsevier/Saunders, St. Louis, pp. 75–82.

CASE 190

1 What is the most likely cause of the mass in this canary? What is another differential diagnosis for a crusty mass on the skin of a canary? The most likely cause of the mass on the wing is a feather follicle cyst (folliculoma). Avian pox lesions can look similar and cause crusty lesions, as classically described in canaries; however, they are typically on the unfeathered regions of the skin. Xanthoma may also occur on the wing tip, but is unlikely in this location.

2 The client would like to know the cause of this abnormality. What information can you share with them? Feather follicle cysts are genetically predisposed in certain lines of canaries including Norwich, Gloucester, and crested type varieties and some new color varieties. In addition, a feather follicle cyst may occur in any bird secondary to trauma to the feather follicle.

3 How would you treat this bird? Surgical resection of the abnormal feather follicle, including the dermal papilla (which the feather grows from), is required to prevent recurrence. The dermal papilla is soft (jelly-like) and located immediately in front of the inferior umbilicus (at the tip of the calamus or quill).

Further reading

Bowles HL, Odberg E, Harrison GJ *et al.* (2006) Surgical resolution of soft tissue disorders. In: *Clinical Avian Medicine*, Vol. 2. (eds. GJ Harrison, TL Lightfoot) Spix Publishing, Palm Beach, pp. 775–830.

CASE 191

1 Many veterinarians include sedation prior to IV injection of euthanasia solution. Provide examples of parenteral sedation that can be used when the owner requests to be present for the procedure. Intranasal administration or IM administration of midazolam with additional sedative agents such as dexmedetomidine or ketamine.

2 Pentobarbital may need to be administered by a route other than IV if the bird is under general anesthesia. What other routes are acceptable for the unconscious bird? Intraosseous: euthanasia drugs should not be administered via the IO route into the humerus or femur because drowning or irritation to the respiratory system may occur. IO catheters can, however, be safely placed in birds, preferably in the distal ulna or proximal tibiotarsus. Intracardiac or hepatic injection can also be used.

3 IM, SC, intrathoracic, intrapulmonary, intrathecal, and other nonvascular injections are not acceptable routes of administration for injectable euthanasia agents in awake animals. Why? Barbiturate salts and other euthanasia solutions are alkaline and considered painful at the site of injection. There is limited information available regarding the effectiveness of these nonvascular sites. Injection into an air sac or pneumatic bone may be poorly absorbed and could cause distress and drowning rather than unconsciousness.

Further reading

Hess L (2005) Euthanasia techniques in birds – roundtable discussion. *J Avian Med Surg* **19**:242–245.

Latimer KS, Rakich PM (1994) Necropsy examination. In: *Avian Medicine: Principles and Application*. (eds. BW Ritchie, GJ Harrison, LR Harrison) Wingers Publishing, Lake Worth, pp. 355–379.

Miller EA (2000) Euthanasia of nonconventional species: zoo, wild, aquatic, and ectothermic animals. In: *Minimum Standards for Wildlife Rehabilitation*, 3rd edn. (ed. EA Miller) National Wildlife Rehabilitators Association, St Cloud, p. 77.

Orosz S (2006) Birds. In: *Guidelines for Euthanasia of Nondomestic Animals*. American Association of Zoo Veterinarians, pp. 46–49.

Rae M (2006) Necropsy. In: *Clinical Avian Medicine*, Vol. 2. (eds. GJ Harrison, TL Lightfoot) Spix Publishing, Palm Beach, pp. 661–678.

CASE 192

1 What is the most likely diagnosis? *Serratospiculum* spp. infection.

2 Describe the life cycle of this parasite. The cycle is indirect. Ova containing fully developed larvae are passed in the feces and swallowed by the intermediate hosts (beetles and other insects) in which the parasites reach the third larval stage and become infective. Once the intermediate host is eaten by a bird, larvae penetrate the proventricular and ventricular walls and migrate to the respiratory system. Female nematodes lay eggs within the air sacs, which are coughed into the mouth, swallowed, and passed in the feces.

3 What treatment options would you consider? Historically a combination of ivermectin and mechanical removal of the parasites from the air sacs using endoscopy was recommended. Research has shown that an elevated dose of ivermectin or moxidectin (1 mg/kg SC or PO, repeated in 7–14 days) is effective in killing the worms, which do not then require removal. NSAIDs and antibiotics for secondary bacterial infection are recommended.

Further reading

Lloyd C (2003) Control of nematodes in captive birds. *In Pract* **25**:198, 201–206.

Samour J, Naldo J (2001) Serratospiculiasis in captive falcons in the Middle East: a review. *J Avian Med Surg* **15**(**1**):2–9.

CASE 193

1 What additional diagnostic test would you perform? A direct ophthalmoscope or a slit-lamp biomicroscope facilitates the assessment of more subtle changes in the lens and lens-induced uveitis. Tonometry could be valuable to check for cataract-related uveitis or glaucoma. Ocular ultrasonography is useful to detect retinal detachment. An electroretinogram is useful to evaluate the electrical function of the retina.

2 Which causes have been reported to provoke this condition in birds? Senile and traumatic cataracts are the most common cataracts observed in birds. Other reported causes in birds include: genetic (Yorkshire and Norwich canaries), nutritional (e.g. vitamin E deficiency in turkey embryos), electric, infectious (Marek's disease), toxic, post uveitis, and secondary to retinal degeneration.

3 How would you treat this condition? Surgery is the only therapeutic option for cataracts. Cataract removal requires specialized microsurgery and magnification equipment as well as advanced ophthalmologic skills. Two surgical techniques have been reported in large eyes: phacoemulsification and extracapsular extraction of the lens. Aspiration with an irrigation/aspiration hand-piece or even with a cannula could be an option for species with smaller eyes. Lens-induced post-traumatic uveitis should be managed with topical and systemic anti-inflammatories (e.g. diclofenac or meloxicam) and mydriatics.

Further reading

Wilson D, Pettifer GR (2004) Anesthesia case of the month. Mallard undergoing phacoemulsification of a cataract. *J Am Vet Med Assoc* **225**(5):685–688.

CASE 194

1 The energy cost of maintaining an egg's temperature, whether by natural or artificial incubation, depends on three factors. What are these factors? The three factors important in maintaining incubation temperature in an egg are: (1) ambient temperature; (2) heat produced by the embryo at different stages of incubation – as the embryo develops in the egg, it begins to thermoregulate or begins to produce its own body heat by utilizing some of the nutrients in the egg; and (3) thermal conductivity of the egg itself; not all eggs are equal.

2 There are two types of incubation strategies used by different species of birds. Describe each strategy. The two types of incubation strategies used by birds are: (1) steady state incubation where the parent bird(s) incubate the egg almost constantly from laying the last egg (clutch completion) to hatching; and (2) intermittent incubation where the parent bird(s) will leave the nest unattended for varying lengths of time, more than required for a parental shift in incubation duties or to turn (rotate) the eggs. The parent birds may use their time away from incubation to feed, ward off intruders (nest protection), groom, or just loaf. Parental absence from the nest results in a degree of egg cooling; the quantum is affected by the duration of absence and the ambient temperature. The embryos of different species have adapted to tolerate varying degrees of cooling. Tolerance to intervals in incubation is generally greater in the last trimester.

3 When using an artificial incubation process, what type of incubation behavior (from the question above) is being duplicated with different types of incubators? Steady state incubation is usually being duplicated when eggs are placed in a forced-air incubator or a still-air incubator. These are the two most common types of incubators. The newer contact incubators have more capability to duplicate the brood patch incubation of birds and the intermittent type of natural incubation. Measuring egg temperatures in the nest or in an incubator can be done with data-logger eggs. A sandhill crane (*Grus canadensis*) plastic egg dummy, with a small data-logger in the egg to record temperature throughout incubation, is shown (**194a, b**).

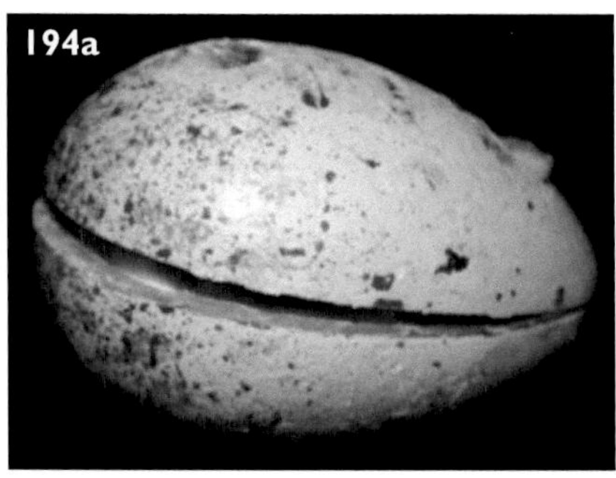

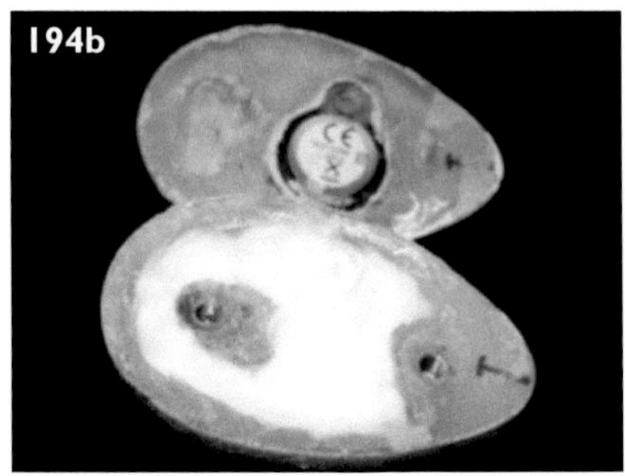

Further reading

Turner JS (2002) Maintenance of egg temperatures. In: *Avian Incubation, Behavior, Environment, and Evolution*. (ed. DC Deeming) Oxford University Press, Oxford, pp. 119–142.

CASE 195

1 What is the most likely cause of the distended proventriculus seen in the image? How could you confirm your presumptive diagnosis? *Macrorhabdus ornithogaster* (gastric yeast, formerly termed megabacteria) infection. Identification of the organism can be confirmed on a nonstained or Gram-stained fecal sample in live birds or an impression smear of the proventricular mucosa at postmortem examination.

2 List other differential diagnoses. Bacterial or mycotic proventriculitis, parasitic infections such as *Atoxoplasma, Isospora* and *Cochlosoma*, avian bornavirus, toxins such as lead or other heavy metals, neoplasia, foreign body.

3 What would be the treatment plan for a canary breeder confronted with this problem? Acidify the drinking water using, for example, cider vinegar at 10 mL/L drinking water. Screen fecal samples for *Macrorhabdus ornithogaster*, being mindful that not all affected canaries will shed *Macrorhabdus* at all times. Treat affected birds with amphotericin B (1,000 mg/L in drinking water for 10 days).

Further reading

Rubbenstroth D, Rinder M, Stein M *et al.* (2013) Avian bornaviruses are widely distributed in canary birds (*Serinus canaria f. domestica*). *Vet Microbiol* **165(3-4)**:287–295.

Sandmeier P, Coutteel P (2006) Management of canaries, finches and mynahs. In: *Clinical Avian Medicine*, Vol. 2. (eds. GJ Harrison, TL Lightfoot) Spix Publishing, Palm Beach, p. 899.

CASE 196

1 What virus would most likely cause these problems in nestling Passeriformes? Avian polyomavirus (APV).

2 What findings would you expect on histopathology? How would you confirm your diagnosis? Large basophilic intranuclear inclusion bodies in many organs and often a membranous glomerulopathy. The diagnosis would be confirmed with PCR techniques.

3 What steps would be necessary to clear the virus from this collection? Stop all breeding for a complete season to minimize virus shedding. Using choanal and cloacal swabs, test all breeding birds for APV by PCR, but be aware that not all APV carriers will shed virus at all times. Eliminate all birds that test positive. Test all new birds that are introduced into the collection. Instigate a hygiene system including a closed aviary (not open to visitors) and use of foot disinfection at the entrance to the aviary, as well as disinfection of hands, food and water bowls, and tools within the aviary.

Further reading

Sandmeier P, Coutteel P (2006) Management of canaries, finches and mynahs. In: *Clinical Avian Medicine*, Vol. 2. (eds. GJ Harrison, TL Lightfoot) Spix Publishing, Palm Beach, pp. 892–893.

CASE 197

1 What would be your differential diagnosis for this condition? Which would be your primary differential based on the dietary history? Differential diagnoses that should be considered in this case include infectious diseases (such as West Nile virus and Newcastle disease virus), intoxication (such as heavy metal toxicity, organophosphates), and nutritional deficiencies, primarily thiamine deficiency but also calcium or vitamin D deficiency and hyperglycemia, which lead to similar signs. The primary differential in this case would be thiamine deficiency as it is a vitamin that may be low in frozen food due to limited stability. In addition, raw fish may contain thiaminase, which breaks down thiamine.

2 What specific tests would you run to rule out your primary differential? What additional body system could be affected in addition to the central nervous system if your primary suspicion is confirmed? Thiamine deficiency can be established by measuring blood thiamine levels by high performance liquid chromatography. Alternatively, erythrocyte transketolase activity may also be measured to provide a surrogate marker for thiamine status. Diet analysis to establish thiamine values may also provide evidence of this deficiency. In addition to neurologic signs, thiamine deficiency has been documented to cause cardiac arrhythmias and cardiac failure in several species including pigeons.

3 What would be your treatment plan to rectify the nutritional status of these birds? Thiamine supplementation may be provided by either enteral or parenteral routes. Doses of 2–4 mg/kg thiamine hydrochloride PO or IM twice daily have been documented to improve the clinical signs of thiamine deficiency in juvenile goshawks. While supplementation of B vitamins is generally considered safe as excess may be excreted in the urine, clinical signs and mortality following oversupplementation of certain B vitamins are documented. Therefore monitoring thiamine levels following treatment may help determine treatment efficacy and duration. Diet correction by including adult whole prey and limited storage duration prior to feeding is required to address potential additional nutritional deficiencies (such as deficiencies in calcium, phosphorus, and vitamin D).

Further reading

Carnarius M, Hafez HM, Henning A *et al.* (2008) Clinical signs and diagnosis of thiamine deficiency in juvenile goshawks (*Accipiter gentilis*). *Vet Rec* **163**:215–217.

CASE 198

1 What is the tentative diagnosis? Based on the clinical signs, including lack of feather regrowth, lethargy, and obesity, hypothyroidism is highly suspected.

2 What diagnostic tests may be used to confirm the tentative diagnosis? Diagnostic tests that may be used to confirm hypothyroidism include:

- Measurement of plasma or serum T_4 concentration. However, a definite diagnosis of hypothyroidism cannot be based on a single low T_4 result, as plasma levels may fluctuate.
- A thyroid-stimulating hormone (TSH) stimulation test whereby serum or plasma T_4 concentrations are measured prior to and 6 hours following IM injection of 1 IU/kg of human recombinant TSH. Hypothyroidism may be suspected based on lack of response to the administration of TSH, with T_4 concentrations increasing less than 2.5 fold compared with baseline.
- Thyroid scintigraphy using sodium pertechnetate Tc99m was found useful in detecting thyroid hypofunction in radiothyroidectomized cockatiels. This technique is not readily available, thus limiting its use in avian practice.
- Thyroid biopsies may be collected to histologically confirm a nonfunctional thyroid gland as well as potential causes for the underlying dysfunction (e.g. thyroiditis). Such biopsies are, however, rarely performed in practice.

3 If the tentative diagnosis is confirmed, what would be the recommended treatment for this bird? In cases of confirmed hypothyroidism, treatment consists of oral L-thyroxine supplementation (20 µg/kg PO q12h).

Further reading

Oglesbee BL (1992) Hypothyroidism in a scarlet macaw. *J Am Vet Med Assoc* **201(10):** 1599–1601.

Schmidt RE, Reavill DR (2008) The avian thyroid gland. *Vet Clin North Am Exot Anim Pract* **11(1):**15–23.

CASE 199

1 Describe how this procedure should be performed. Cloacoscopy is performed with the bird in dorsal recumbency. Warm saline irrigation is provided via the ingress port of the operating sheath for visualization. Endotracheal intubation is important to protect the airway, as oral regurgitation can occur from excessive fluid administration. During irrigation, digital pressure is applied externally to the edge of the vent to prevent the infused saline leaking out, ensuring dilation of the cloacal lumen. Only a minimal amount of saline irrigation is required to provide visualization.

2 Name the labeled structures in the image shown (199), obtained during a cloacoscopy in a pigeon. 1 = coprodeum; 2 = oviductal opening; 3 = ureteral papilla on the dorsal uroproctadeal fold.

3 What difference in cloacal anatomy can be observed during cloacoscopy between a pigeon and a psittacine? Within the coprodeum, the opening to the rectum in a pigeon is on the bird's right side and in a psittacine it is on the bird's left side.

Further reading

Divers SJ (2010) Avian diagnostic endoscopy. *Vet Clin North Am Exot Anim Pract* **13(2):**187–202.

CASE 200

1 Which one of these vitamins has been reported to cause lethal toxicity in gyrfalcons? Vitamin B_6, or pyridoxine, at doses of 15 mg/kg and higher. The recommended dosage depends on protein ingestion. LD50 has not yet been documented.

2 What are the associated clinical signs? Emesis, pistachio green-colored urates, anorexia, lethargy, and death 24–36 hours post injection.

3 List three food items that naturally contain vitamin B_6. Meat, liver, and kidney of prey species, and also within the digestive tract of prey items, cereal seeds, pistachio nuts, and chickpeas.

Further reading

Samour J (2013) Acute toxicity after administration of high doses of vitamin B6 in falcons. *Proceedings of the International Conference on Avian Herpetological and Exotic Mammal Medicine, April 2013*, Wiesbaden, pp. 100–102.

Scherer CS, Baker DH (2000) Excess dietary methionine markedly increases the vitamin B6 requirement of young chicks. *J Nutr* **130(12)**:3055–3058.

CASE 201

1 What are the toxic effects of avocados in birds? Effects of avocado poisoning are mainly cardiac with the presence of pericardial effusion, cardiac tamponade, and myocardial toxicity. Subcutaneous edema has also been reported in birds, in particular ostriches.

2 What is the toxin contained within avocados? The toxin contained in the avocado plant is persin.

3 What parts of the avocado are toxic? All parts of the fruit and plant (leaves, bark, seeds, fruit) are toxic, but toxicity varies between avocado varieties.

Further reading

Burger WP, Naudé TW, Van Rensburg IB *et al.* (1994) Cardiomyopathy in ostriches (*Struthio camelus*) due to avocado (*Persea americana* var. *guatemalensis*) intoxication. *J South Afr Vet Assoc* **65(3)**:113–118.

Dumonceaux G, Harrison GJ (1994) Toxins. In: *Avian Medicine: Principles and Applications*. (eds. BW Ritchie, GJ Harrison, LR Harrison) Wingers Publishing, Lake Worth, pp. 1030–1052.

Hargis AM, Stauber E, Casteel S *et al.* (1989) Avocado (*Persea americana*) intoxication in caged birds. *J Am Vet Med Assoc* **194(1)**:64–66.

CASE 202

1 What diseases can cause a firm coelomic distension in an adult hen? Diseases that can cause a firm coelomic distension in an egg laying hen include egg-related peritonitis (ERP), lymphoid leukosis +/– involving the reproductive tract, ovarian adenocarcinoma, cystic right oviduct, egg impaction, an ectopic egg loose within the coelomic cavity, hernia, and coelomic effusion of any cause. This particular hen had ERP. The reluctance to ambulate was due to associated pain. This is a very common presentation for a hen with ERP.

2 What would be the possible treatment for each of the diseases listed above? ERP can be septic or not. If septic it is usually secondary to an *E. coli* diarrhea, so antibiotic treatment is indicated. While (in the USA) no antibiotics are labeled for use in egg laying hens where the eggs are to be eaten, trimethoprim sulfamethoxazole is often used and eggs discarded for at least 2 weeks after the last dose. Ideally, antibiotic use should be based on culture and after consulting with www.farad.org for withdrawal information. **Note:** Fluorquinolones and cephalosporins are prohibited drugs in poultry in the USA (i.e. they cannot be given to poultry in any circumstance, irrespective of life role (e.g. pet/egg or meat production). Even owner consent does not circumvent this legal restriction. The use of antibiotics in poultry aids the development of antibiotic resistant *Campylobacter* organisms, which would in turn make the treatment of infected humans more difficult. There are other drugs that fall under the rules of extra-label drug use (ELDU), such as sulfamethoxazole, and www.farad.org should be contacted for specific information and instructions on ELDU in poultry. Drugs used in poultry in Europe must be listed in Table 1(EU) No 37/2010. Drugs approved for use in poultry in the UK can be verified at veterinaryformulary.com. ERP can also arise concurrent with an egg or eggs loose in the coelomic cavity or a hernia, or egg impaction, necessitating surgical intervention. Radiographs or ultrasound will provide information on presence, number, and position of shelled and unshelled eggs. An attempt should be made to remove as much of the egg material as possible at the time of surgery, while appreciating that usually it cannot all be removed and surgical time must be kept to a minimum. A salpingohysterectomy is recommended for ERP or right cystic oviduct. Unfortunately, there is no treatment for lymphoid leukosis or ovarian adenocarcinoma. If coelomic effusion is present, this can be determined radiographically or by ultrasound and can be due to a variety of causes including heart disease.

Further reading

Greenacre CB (2015) Reproductive diseases of the backyard hen. *J Exot Pet Med* **24(2)**: 164–171.

CASE 203

1 What is the methodology for placement of an air sac tube? While an inhalation agent is delivered via the trachea, the patient is placed in right lateral recumbency with the wings extended dorsally and the legs stretched caudally. Feathers covering a triangle formed by the cranial thigh muscles, the musculature covering the synsacrum, and the last rib are plucked. Standard aseptic preparation is performed and a clear, sterile adhesive drape is placed over the entry site. A small skin incision is performed using a scalpel blade behind the last rib or between the last two ribs, and the underlying muscle and subcutaneous tissues are bluntly dissected. The air sac is perforated using a hemostat and an air sac tube is inserted. The diameter of the air sac tube should be similar to the bird's tracheal diameter and the length of tube inserted within the skin should not exceed one-third of the width of the coelom at the entry point. The tube must have multiple holes along its length within the air sac, such that airflow is maintained. The tube is fixed in place to ensure that it cannot come out of the air sac using nonabsorbable suture and a Chinese finger trap knot, taking care not obstruct the tube's lumen.

2 What are the indications to maintain anesthesia using an air sac tube? Air sac anesthesia is indicated to maintain anesthesia in patients requiring surgery or diagnostic tests involving the head, oropharyngeal cavity, eyes, or upper airway, where the presence of an endotracheal tube within the glottis will interfere with the procedure. It is also indicated where there is a partial or complete obstruction of the trachea.

3 How does air sac tube delivery of isoflurane compare with endotracheal administration of isoflurane? A study performed in sulphur-crested cockatoos (*Cacatua galerita*) showed both endotracheal and caudal thoracic air sac administration provided a reliable method of maintaining anesthesia and resulted in minimal alteration in respiratory function. However, transient apnea while applying caudal thoracic air sac anesthesia has been noted in a number of publications, and it is recommended that oxygen flow rates are reduced to 250 mL/kg/min and birds are ventilated with positive pressure. In chickens (*Gallus gallus domesticus*), measured partial pressure of carbon dioxide in expired gas ($PeCO_2$) could not be used in a simple linear fashion to predict partial pressure of carbon dioxide in arterial blood ($PaCO_2$) during air sac insufflation anesthesia. In that study in chickens, it was found that the $PeCO_2$ at which apnea occurs during air sac insufflation anesthesia was not predictable. Anesthetic gas introduced via the air sac tube into the caudal thoracic air sac should naturally pass over the gas exchange surface in the paleopulmonic parabronchi.

Further reading

Hawkins MG, Zehnder AM, Pascoe PJ (2014) Caged birds. In: *Zoo Animal and Wildlife Immobilization and Anaesthesia*. (eds. G West, D Heard, N Caulkett) Wiley-Blackwell, Ames, pp. 399–405.

Jaensch SM, Cullen L, Raidal SR (2001) Comparison of endotracheal, caudal thoracic air sac and clavicular air sac administration of isoflurane in sulphur-crested cockatoos (*Cacatua galerita*). *J Avian Med Surg* **15(3)**:170–177.

CASE 204

1 What possible differentials should be considered? There is marked thickening and scale encasing the rachis, with distortion of the inner groove. Differential diagnoses that should be considered include ectoparasites and bacterial and viral infections such as avian circoviruses.

2 What diagnostic tests should be performed to investigate the cause? A dissecting microscopic should be used to rule out ectoparasites and histopathologic examination of developing feather follicles can be performed. Laboratory investigation for avian circoviruses is also recommended and this case was positive for avian circovirus by

PCR using degenerate avian circovirus PCR primers. A wide range of bird species, including corvids, are susceptible to avian circovirus infection with increasing evidence indicating that broader host susceptibility should be considered for beak and feather disease virus (BFDV), since this infection has been detected in nonpsittacine birds including raptors.

3 What is the likely prognosis for birds with such lesions? Recent evidence suggests that BFDV, which is mainly a pathogen of psittacine birds, can also infect and cause transient disease in nonpsittacine birds with some recovering normal plumage. At least one molt should be permitted to assess the degree of damage to pterylae.

Further reading

Stewart ME, Perry R, Raidal SR (2006) Identification of a novel circovirus in Australian ravens (*Corvus coronoides*) with feather disease. *Avian Pathol* **35:(2):**86–92.

CASE 205

1 What are your differential diagnoses for a distended coelomic cavity in a canary? Intestinal disease (coccidiosis, flagellates such as *Cochlosoma* spp., bacterial enteritis, sudden nutritional change); reproductive tract disease (egg binding, salpingitis/impacted oviduct, egg-related peritonitis, ovarian cysts); liver disease (atoxoplasmosis, yersiniosis, mycobacteriosis, chlamydiosis, neoplasia, noninfectious hepatitis or hepatic lipidosis); cardiac disease (congestive heart failure); neoplasia of any coelomic organs.

2 At what age are canaries most likely to be affected by intestinal coccidiosis, and why? Juvenile birds, because of their poorly developed immune system (no vertical transfer of coccidial immunity) and regular contact with the excretions of their subclinically (and hence oocyst shedding) infected parents.

3 What is the life cycle of intestinal coccidiosis (*Ispora canaria*) in canaries? Orally ingested oocysts excyst to form sporozoites within the intestinal tract. These sporozoites undergo several generations of asexual schizogony and produce merozoites. The sexual gametogony of these merozoites then produces oocysts, which are excreted in the feces. In intestinal coccidiosis all stages develop within the intestinal wall.

Further reading

Sandmeier P, Coutteel P (2006) Management of canaries, finches and mynahs. In: *Clinical Avian Medicine*, Vol. 2. (eds. GJ Harrison, TL Lightfoot) Spix Publishing, Palm Beach, pp. 901–903.

CASE 206

1 What are the differential diagnoses? What is the most likely diagnosis? Stress-induced hyperglycemia, hypoglycemia induced by weight reduction and re-entering flights at quarry, lead poisoning (due to risk of having been fed shot quarry), hypocalcemia (due to failure to feed or consume a whole carcase diet), West Nile virus infection, organophosphate poisoning (due to mobilization of organophosphates from fat stores during weight loss), hepatopathy, septicemia. For an accipiter with this presentation, specifically during training or retraining, the most likely cause is 'stress-induced hyperglycemia' (otherwise known as stress-induced diabetes).

2 What is your diagnostic plan? How would you treat this bird if you confirm your suspicion? A CBC and plasma biochemistry panel would be a first step. Normal blood glucose levels in a resting, trained, and unstressed northern goshawk are 18–22 mmol/L (324–396 mg/dL). If the blood level exceeds 23 mmol/L (414 mg/dL), then a subtle and abnormal startle response may be seen, with a high risk of a generalized tonic–clonic seizures when the blood glucose level is >27 mmol/L (>486 mg/dL). With blood levels between 23 and 27 mmol/L (414 and 486 mg/dL), administration of midazolam or diazepam, together with a darkened, quiet, and calm environment, will typically allow clinical signs to resolve and normalize within 2–3 days. If blood glucose levels exceed 27 mmol/L (>486 mg/dL), once daily administration of 1–2 units of 24-hour insulin for 1–2 days is likely to be required in order to control seizures.

3 What action can be taken to avoid this situation? Accipiters are prone to stress, especially during initial training or retraining. In part this is caused by the enforced proximity to humans at that time, to whom they are unhabituated. Traditionally, these birds would have been placed on perches at ground level during this training. Such birds would naturally perch in the branches of trees, waiting to fly down into quarry. It is unnatural and stressful for them to be held at ground level. By placing the accipiter on a high perch (2–3 meters above ground level) so they can look down on their handlers and immediate environment during initial training, they can become habituated to close proximity to handlers from a safe position. When handling by the austringer (a goshawk falconer) is increased, it is not as stressful as it would otherwise have been, and hyperglycemia does not occur.

Further reading

Forbes NA (1995) Stress hyperglycaemia in Northern goshawks (*Accipiter gentilis*). In: *Proceedings of European Association of Avian Veterinarians Conference*, Jerusalem, pp. 127–131.

CASE 207

1 Describe the abnormal radiographic findings. This laterolateral radiographic projection shows a large caudoventral coelomic homogeneous soft tissue mass in the region of the liver, displacing caudodorsally the contrast filled proventriculus and ventriculus and compressing the thoracic air sacs.

2 List the differential diagnoses for this radiographic finding. Hepatopathy including neoplastic, infectious (bacterial, viral, parasitic, fungal), or inflammatory etiologies. There is also the possibility of cardiomegaly. As no ventrodorsal view is provided, it is difficult to assess for air sac disease, but severe granulomatous disease cannot be excluded.

3 Based on the suspected concurrent papillomatous lesion, what is your top differential diagnosis? Cholangiocarcinoma of the liver. Gastrointestinal adenocarcinoma and intrahepatic cholangiocarcinoma can occur concurrently with internal papillomatosis in New World psittacine parrots, as the latter is now known to be caused by oncogenic herpesviruses.

Further reading

Gibbons PM, Busch MD, Tell LA *et al.* (2002) Internal papillomatosis with intrahepatic cholangiocarcinoma and gastrointestinal adenocarcinoma in a peach-fronted conure (*Aratinga aurea*). *Avian Dis* **46(4)**:1062–1066.

CASE 208

1 What are the goals of traumatic brain injury treatment? Traumatic brain injury medical treatment is aimed at preventing or reducing the effects of secondary brain injury through maintaining adequate cerebral perfusion pressure, preventing or decreasing cerebral edema, and controlling intracranial pressure.

2 How would you treat traumatic brain injury in this bird? The bird should be placed in a dark, quiet area with an environmental temperature of 73°F (23°C), not warmer as hyperthermia may contribute to greater post-traumatic brain damage. Elevation of the head (up to 30°) may decrease intracranial pressure by facilitating venous and cerebrospinal fluid drainage. Administration of oxygen in an oxygen cage is recommended for moderate to severe cases. Intravenous hypertonic saline (7–7.8% NaCl; 3 mL/kg over 15 minutes) followed by crystalloid fluids at 50% of the normal rate, can be used instead of mannitol in hypovolemic or euvolemic patients to decrease intracranial pressure. Hypertonic saline is contraindicated in hyponatremic patients. Slow administration over 15 minutes of mannitol (0.25–1 mg/kg IV q4–6h as needed for up to three boluses) should be considered, together with crystalloid fluids at 50% of the normal rate. Mannitol is contraindicated in hypovolemic patients. If there is an insufficient response to the first dose of mannitol, an additional bolus can be given 40–60 minutes later. Corticosteroids are not recommended to treat traumatic brain injury.

3 How would you manage pain? Slow administration of opioid drugs (e.g. buprenorphine in raptors) is recommended to treat pain and avoid intracranial pressure elevation secondary to the sympathetic response pain, but caution is warranted for patients unable to adequately ventilate. The use of NSAIDs in cases of traumatic brain injury in birds is only recommended once the patient is stabilized.

Further reading

Sanchez-Migallon Guzman D (2016) Systemic diseases: disorders of the neurological system. In: *Avian Medicine*, 3rd edn. (ed. J Samour) Elsevier, St. Louis, pp. 421–433.

CASE 209

1 Which blood vessels are suitable for venipuncture? The three major blood vessels that can used for venipuncture are: (1) The right jugular vein, located under the right lateral cervical apteria. The left jugular vein can be used, but is smaller than the right. (2) Either of the basilic veins, located on the ventral aspect of the elbow joint. (3) Either of the medial metatarsal veins, located on the medial aspect of the podotheca (the scaled part of the leg, below the tibiotarsal–tarsometatarsal joint). This vein is aligned with the second digit, the medial forward directed toe. It is very shallow, but can often not be visualized because of the keratinized skin overlying it.

2 How much blood can be safely collected from this bird? 9.45 ml of blood. The circulating blood volume of parrots is approximately 10% of their body weight. The amount of blood that can be collected from a healthy bird is 10% of the circulating blood volume (i.e. 1% of the bird's body weight).

3 How would you handle the blood sample after collection to maximize the quality of the laboratory results? Immediately after collection the blood sample should be processed as follows: (1) Fresh blood smears should be made. Erythrocytes, after prolonged mixing with an anticoagulant such as K_2EDTA, will often be distorted and have other artifactual changes that can affect assessment of their morphology. For this reason, fresh blood smears are preferred to smears made in the laboratory. (2) Blood intended for biochemical analysis is usually placed in lithium heparin, unless requested otherwise by an external laboratory. The sample should be gently mixed to prevent hemolysis associated with rough handling. If testing is likely to be delayed by more than 2 hours, the sample should be centrifuged and the plasma decanted into another container without anticoagulant and submitted to the laboratory. This prevents artifactual errors associated with prolonged contact between erythrocytes and plasma. (3) Blood intended for hematologic analysis should be placed in K_2EDTA. Although white cell counts are often inaccurate using automated cell counters (due to the nucleated erythrocytes in avian blood), other parameters such as hematocrit and some secondary indices (e.g. MCV) can be measured accurately.

Further reading

Doneley R (2011) Clinical techniques. In: *Avian Medicine and Surgery in Practice*. CRC Press, Boca Raton, pp. 55–68.

CASE 210

1 **What is your primary differential?** Xanthoma or xanthomatous inflammation.
2 **What is a unique characteristic of this lesion?** Xanthomas are masses consisting of multinucleated giant cells, macrophages, and cholesterol clefts, occurring most commonly at sites of previous trauma or hemorrhage.
3 **What is the recommendation for treatment?** Surgical excision (with care as this tissues tends to be highly vascular and tends not to heal well); the surgical site may also be prone to trauma. Dietary improvement is recommended.

Further reading

Souza MJ, Johnstone-Mclean NS, Ward D *et al.* (2009) Conjunctival xanthoma in a blue and gold macaw (*Ara ararauna*). *Vet Ophthalmol* **12(1)**:53–55.

CASE 211

1 **What anatomic features must be considered for intubation (211)?** The trachea bifurcates typically closer to the glottis in most penguin species, because they possess a septum, variable in length depending on the species, which divides the trachea into right and left channels. Use of a large size endotracheal tube may result in mucosal trauma. Penguins also possess a horn-like projection arising from the ventral wall of the glottal opening (i.e. in the proximal trachea [*crista ventralis*]), which may also interfere with intubation. Therefore, a smaller number 1 or 2 endotracheal tube should be used.
2 **What methods should be considered to maintain body temperature?** Cold climate species require the use of ice, ice packs, or other ways to control/prevent hyperthermia, especially during the initial phase of anesthesia. However, with prolonged procedures, penguins (like other bird species) need to be warmed to maintain body temperature.
3 **Which body position is best suited for penguins under general anesthesia?** Recent studies performed in Humboldt penguins (*Spheniscus humboldti*)

indicated that significant changes in lung density and air sac volume occur in penguins with respect to recumbent orientation while anesthetized. These changes may have significant physiologic consequences, especially for birds in dorsal recumbency. Therefore, positioning in dorsal recumbency during anesthesia may not be appropriate for penguins because of their unique body shape and anatomy. Ventral recumbency should be prioritized for this species, particularly for long procedures.

Further reading

Nevitt BN, Langan JN, Adkesson MJ (2014) Comparison of air sac volume, lung volume, and lung densities determined by use of computed tomography in conscious and anesthetized Humboldt penguins (*Spheniscus humboldti*) positioned in ventral, dorsal, and right lateral recumbency. *Am J Vet Res* 75(8):739–745.

CASE 212

1 **How does the healing rate of avian bone differ from mammalian bone?** In general, bird bones heal at a much faster rate than mammalian bones. A repaired simple, uncomplicated closed humeral fracture will heal in 3 weeks in an adult healthy bird compared with an average of 8 weeks in a mammal.

2 **What is the relative healing rate of various long bones in birds?** The average healing time for avian long bones varies by location. For simple, repaired, uncomplicated closed fractures the following times are common:

- Humerus: 3 weeks.
- Radius/ulna: 4 weeks.
- Metacarpus: 5–6 weeks.
- Femur: 3 weeks.
- Tibiotarsus: 4 weeks
- Metatarsus: 6+ weeks.

3 **Do bird bones heal by periosteal or endosteal callus formation?** While avian bones produce both periosteal and endosteal callus, the fixation methods most commonly used in birds, such as IM–ESF tie-in and ESF, result in periosteal callus formation that creates a bridging osteosynthesis. In contrast, plate fixation results in less callus formation and more endosteal healing.

Further reading

Redig PT, Ponder J (2016) Management of orthopedic issues in birds. In: *Avian Medicine*, 3rd edn. (ed. J Samour) Mosby, St. Louis, pp. 312–350.

CASE 213

1 What is the most likely diagnosis of these lesions, and how could this diagnosis be confirmed? The most likely diagnosis is an Avipoxvirus infection. Confirmation of the diagnosis can be achieved by histologic evaluation of the nodules, which are characterized by a palisade-like arrangement of epithelial cords with large granular intracytoplasmic inclusion bodies (also known as Bollinger bodies).

2 What is the mode of transmission for this disease? Mosquitoes are the most common vectors for transmission of Avipoxvirus. Mosquitoes obtain the virus by feeding on an infected bird with the virus circulating in the bloodstream, after which they feed on a susceptible host, transferring virus infection to the new host. On occasions, if there are abrasions of the mucous membranes or skin, the virus may also be transmitted indirectly from contaminated surfaces (e.g. food or drinking bowls) or airborne particles. Following infection, a bird remains viremic for a long time (up to 1 year), thereby acting as a reservoir of infection.

3 What therapeutic and preventive measures can be taken? Include the prognosis in your answer. No specific treatment is available. The skin lesions are often self-limiting, although severe infections may result in immunosuppression. Systemic antibiotic treatment may then be indicated. When the lesions on the beak prevent eating, force feeding (by gavage or ingluviotomy tube) is necessary. If the pigeons are not force fed, it is likely they will die due to inanition. In pigeons, commercial vaccines are available to prevent infection. Action can be taken to reduce mosquito numbers in the vicinity of pigeons (e.g. treating surfaces or shade netting with safe insecticidal surface spray). Once an outbreak has commenced, great care must be taken in handling and medicating patients to avoid transferring infection from bird to bird on your hands or clothing. With supportive care (and potentially the use of antibiotics) the prognosis is fair.

Further reading

Cooper JE, Harrison GJ (1994) Dermatology. In: *Avian Medicine, Principles and Application.* (eds. BW Ritchie, GJ Harrison, LR Harrison) Wingers Publishing, Lake Worth, pp. 607–639.

CASE 214

1 What is the most important role of the ceca? The precise role of ceca in digestion remains unclear but it appears that bacteria in the ceca further digest and partially ferment digested foods into usable biochemical compounds that are absorbed through the cecal walls. Ceca may also function to separate the nutrient-rich fluid in partially digested food from the fibrous portion, which is eventually eliminated.

2 Not all birds have functional ceca. Which group of birds lack a functional cecum? Ceca are poorly developed or nonexistent in most arboreal birds (e.g. psittacines and pigeons), perhaps because of the unacceptable weight of the watery, partially digested food in the intestine and the large structures required to handle it. Indeed, well-developed cecal fermentation is restricted to ground-dwelling as well as flightless birds (e.g. ratites) and is much more common in mammals than in birds.

CASE 215

1 What is the most probable diagnosis? What other clinical signs are often seen? Spiral bacterial infection (organisms are suspected to belong to the genus *Helicobacter*). Common clinical signs reported in cases of spiral bacterial infection include red clogged nares, sneezing, reddened and blunted choanal papillae, oropharyngeal hyperemia, conjunctivitis, sinusitis, and periorbital swelling. Infected birds may also show general signs of illness, including lethargy, anorexia, and weight loss.

2 What is the method of choice for antemortem diagnosis? The method of choice for antemortem diagnosis is cytologic examination of swabs from the choana and the oropharynx, as efforts to culture spiral bacteria from cockatiels have been unsuccessful. Bacteria can be identified on smears stained with Gram stain or Romanowsky stain.

3 What is the recommended treatment regimen? Spiral bacterial infections have been treated successfully using doxycycline orally (25 mg/kg q12h for 3 weeks) or via the drinking water using doxycycline hyclate (400 mg/L for 30 days). As oral medication requires twice daily capture over several weeks and as intake of medication via the drinking water may not be guaranteed in severely ill birds, injectable doxycycline is preferred. As vitamin A deficiency contributes to respiratory disease in birds, a diet change to a more balanced, commercially available pelleted diet after treatment may also be beneficial.

Further reading

Evans EE, Wade LL, Flammer K (2008) Administration of doxycycline in drinking water for treatment of spiral bacterial infection in cockatiels. *J Am Vet Med Assoc* **232(3)**:389–393.

CASE 216

1 Name at least four criteria that can be used to determine the gender of a pigeon. The gender of pigeons cannot always be morphologically distinguished with complete certainty, but body size (larger in male), shape of the head (plumper in male), cere and eye cere (larger in male), and differences in specific behavior (males 'coo' more, walk more upright, have more fluffed up feathers) can be used as indications of gender determination.

2 The genes for the color of hair in mammals and feathers in birds are in part localized on the sex chromosomes. What is the major difference between sex chromosomes in birds compared with mammals? In mammals the X chromosome is the sex chromosome that carries the genes, while the Y chromosome does not. Female mammals carry two X chromosomes, while males carry the XY chromosomes. In birds, females (hens) have a Z and a W chromosome, while the cocks have two Z chromosomes. The Z chromosomes carry the genes (similar to the X chromosomes in mammals).

3 What is the gender of this pigeon? Based on what criteria can 100% accuracy be given that this is actually the gender? This is a male pigeon (cock). This can be determined with 100% accuracy as this bird has the color characteristics of a heterozygote. The genes for the (ash) red and blue (wild type) color of pigeons are located on the sex chromosomes. Red is the dominant color over the wild type color in pigeons. In this red pigeon, in many of the covert feathers and in particular on the tail feathers. The fact that blue streaks are seen in this ash-red pigeon, indicates that it must be a heterozygote for the color and therefore has to be a male pigeon.

Further reading

Arif Mümtaz. Pigeon genetics. Web page: http://mumtazticloft.com/m_ash-red.asp

CASE 217

1 What is the most likely etiology of this abnormality? Lead toxicosis. Proventricular impactions are commonly reported in lead poisoned waterfowl, consisting of grass or other vegetation fibers, corn or other grains, sand, or a combination of these items. Occasionally, impactions can include portions of the caudal esophagus, and even the entire length of the esophagus in severe cases. Other gross lesions in lead poisoned waterfowl may include emaciation, green discolored liver, bile-stained ventricular lining, pale streaked myocardium, and often the presence of lead shot or sinkers (fishing weights) in the ventriculus.

2 What is the most appropriate tissue to submit to confirm your presumptive diagnosis? Liver is the best tissue to submit to confirm a diagnosis. Liver lead levels >6 ppm (wet weight) are diagnostic for acute toxic exposure. If antemortem sampling is possible, whole, EDTA or heparinized blood (check with the laboratory what their requirement is) may be used for lead analysis. Blood lead levels >0.97 µmol/L (>20 µg/dL) indicate exposure, and clinical signs are generally present with levels >2.41 µmol/L (>50 µg/dL).

3 What are the most common environmental sources for this etiology in waterfowl? Spent lead shot from hunting activities over, or near, bodies of water, and discarded or lost lead fishing sinkers (weights) or fishing tackle, are the most common sources of lead poisoning globally. It has been proposed that waterfowl inadvertently ingest lead shot or sinkers when they are foraging for food or ingesting grit (ingested to assist with ventricular grinding function). In the USA, lead shot was banned for use during waterfowl hunting in 1991. However, residual lead shot persists in lakes and wetlands for many years after the cessation of use and lead toxicosis continues to cause problems in waterfowl (and scavenging carnivorous birds) in many areas. In situations where a lake water level is reduced due to weather factors or extraction, high incidence of lead toxicity can occur in a flock previously unaffected, due to access to lead on the substrate that was previously beyond reach.

Further reading

Wobeser GA (1997) Lead and other metals. In: *Diseases of Wild Waterfowl*, 2nd edn. Plenum Press, New York, pp. 163–178.

CASE 218

1 What is the most likely diagnosis? How would you confirm the diagnosis? This is the classical appearance of a cloacal papillomatous lesion, most often found in New World psittacines such as Amazon parrots, macaws, and conures. Most lesions are confined to the oropharyngeal and cloacal mucosa, although lesions might, more rarely, be found along the gastrointestinal tract. Initial confirmation can be obtained by applying 5% acetic acid topically and assessing for blanching of the surface. Histopathology and PCR techniques should also be performed on a biopsy sample. These papillomatous lesions have been associated with infections with psittacid herpesvirus (genotypes 1, 2, and 3). Psittacid herpesviruses are a heterogeneous group of viruses, currently divided into four genotypes and four serotypes, which have also been associated with an acute fatal infection in parrots (Pacheco's disease). However, some birds survive the acute manifestations of the disease and may become latently infected, while others appear to become latently infected following an inapparent infection.

2 What surgical treatment would you perform? Several techniques for surgical removal of these masses have been described including blade excision, application of caustic substances, radiosurgical excision, cryosurgical removal, and laser surgery. Some of these methods might result in ablation or excision of the mass, but recurrence is common. These surgical procedures are very painful and require appropriate administration of analgesics and systemic antibiotics during the postoperative period and until the wounds heal.

3 What are your recommendations to the owner? What is the long-term prognosis for this bird? The owner should not keep this bird as a breeder. Depending on the genotype of the viruses and the species involved, these viruses can disseminate through a collection. The prognosis for curing the problem is guarded to poor. While surgery could relieve some of the discomfort for some time, recurrence is common as is development of internal papillomatous lesions (e.g. oropharyngeal) or neoplasia (e.g. biliary and pancreatic adenocarcinoma), which is often fatal.

Further reading

Styles DK, Tomaszewski EK, Jaeger LA *et al.* (2004) Psittacid herpesviruses associated with mucosal papillomas in neotropical parrots. *Virology* **325(1)**:24–35.

CASE 219

1 What is the most likely underlying cause? Frounce caused by *Trichomonas gallinae*. Other differential diagnoses are: candidiasis, trauma, *Capillaria* spp. infestation with secondary bacterial infection, bacterial stomatitis (e.g. *Pseudomonas* spp.), oral neoplasia with secondary bacterial infection, and poxvirus infection with secondary bacterial infection. A diagnosis in this bird cannot be made without cytology and microbiology. To confirm the diagnosis the flagellate can be collected from the oropharynx or esophagus by advancing a slightly moistened (in warm saline) cotton tipped applicator into the esophagus and moving this up and down a couple of times. After removing the swab, it can be compressed so that some fluid is expelled onto a slide. The fluid on the slide should then be examined immediately so that the flagellate can be seen swimming (circling) in the wet sample. A magnification of 10 × 20 is usually sufficient to see the typical movement of the flagellates. Thirty minutes to 1 hour after collection of the sample, the parasites will be difficult to recognize, as by then they will have stopped moving. A wet mount sample stained with Giemsa will allow identification of trichomonads, even when movement has ceased.

2 What is the most likely source of infection? Pigeon or dove prey ingestion.

3 What is the recommended treatment? Nitroimidazole class drug. The preferred drug is carnidazole (20–50 mg/kg one-off dose) or ronidazole (6–10 mg/kg PO q24h for 7 days). Metronidazole (50 mg/kg PO q24h for 5 days) may be used as well, but is considered less effective for the treatment of trichomoniasis. In any bird with severe oropharyngeal, esophageal, or crop (owls do not have one) disease, especially when they are already thin, supplementary feeding by gavage is essential. If gavage is challenging or stressful for the patient, an indwelling proventriculotomy tube, placed via the upper esophagus, is a good option.

Further reading

Greiner EC, Ritchie BW (1994) Parasites. In: *Avian Medicine: Principles and Application.* (eds. BW Ritchie, GJ Harrison, LR Harrison) Wingers Publishing, Lake Worth, p. 1013.

CASE 220

1 What pectoral limb fractures can be adequately stabilized with a wing wrap, and when should a body wrap be incorporated into the wrap? A figure-of-eight wrap provides adequate support for fractures involving the antebrachium, carpometacarpus, and digits. Wing wraps can be effective for some fractures of the pectoral girdle and humerus when used in conjunction with a body wrap or 'belly band'.

2 Depending on patient size, what bandaging options can be considered for fractures of the tibiotarsus? A tape splint can be used to stabilize tibiotarsal fractures in small patients weighing <300 grams. For larger birds, a foam-backed aluminum splint may be placed from mid femur to mid tarsometatarsus. The splint is effective so long as the joint above and the joint below the fracture are immobilized. Alternatively, a modified Thomas-Schroeder splint or a modified Robert Jones bandage may be used.

3 Cage rest is recommended for most birds fitted with a bandage. List three items involved in cage resting the avian patient. (1) Confinement of the bird to a small, smooth-sided enclosure such as an aquarium, cardboard box, or acrylic pet cage to prevent climbing and falling. (2) Provision of low or no perches. (3) If the bird is agitated, reduction of light levels to reduce activity. Adequate ventilation and light levels must be provided.

Further reading

Chavez W, Scott Echols M (2007) Bandaging, endoscopy, and surgery in the avian patient. *Vet Clin North Am Exot Anim Pract* **10(2)**:423–425.

CASE 221

1 What is the main radiographic abnormal finding? There is a simple (likely closed), mid-shaft transverse fracture of the left coracoid.

2 Provide a treatment plan for this patient. Treatment of pectoral girdle fractures consists of providing support to the affected shoulder with a body wrap, performing physical therapy to maintain range of motion and evaluate extension, and managing the bird with cage rest and pain medications such as meloxicam. Physical therapy consists of removing coaptation and conducting passive range of motion exercises, using anesthesia as appropriate for management of pain and stress. This should be done 2–3 times weekly. The body wrap may be removed once there is a stable fibrous callus felt on palpation or seen on a digital radiograph – a bony callus is not typically present within the first few weeks of treatment.

3 What is the prognosis for release? Pectoral girdle fractures treated in this way have a good prognosis, and even birds with radically displaced fractures often (82%) heal well enough for release to the wild. Complications are rare and large calluses rarely cause any reduced function. The shoulder joint should be monitored for development of osteoarthritis secondary to traumatic impact. Conservative treatment has been shown to have a much greater success rate than surgery (45% release rate); for this reason surgical repair is not recommended. While there are few long-term studies, band return data have shown good survival post release in many cases treated conservatively.

Further reading

Scheelings TF (2014) Coracoid fractures in wild birds: a comparison of surgical repair versus conservative treatment. *J Avian Med Surg* **28(4)**:304–308.

CASE 222

1 Which protozoal parasite would you consider as the most likely etiologic agent? *Cryptosporidium baileyi* has been reported to cause upper respiratory signs, conjunctivitis, and otitis in falcons and owls.

2 What additional diagnostic procedures would you perform? Cytology performed from swabs collected from conjunctiva, oropharyngeal cavity, and trachea, stained with Giemsa stain, may reveal the presence of pale blue circular structures 4 μm diameter, consistent with the parasite. Molecular diagnostics should be carried out to confirm the diagnosis.

3 What therapeutic options would you consider? What prognosis would you offer? Paromomycin (100 mg/kg PO q12h) and azithromycin (40 mg/kg PO q24h) have shown variable responses in the cases reported in the literature. Supportive treatment may have an important role in the patient's recovery, but prognosis is considered guarded to poor.

Further reading

Rodriguez Barbon A, Forbes NA (2007) Use of paromomycin in the treatment of *Cryptosporidium* in two falcons. *Falco* **30**:22–24.

CASE 223

1 What is the black structure observed in the upper left side of the image? The pecten, a choroidal structure protruding into the vitreous, which hides the optic nerve papilla.

2 List the different types of pecten in birds and the species they belong to. According to the type of pecten, avian species could be classified as:

- Species with a plicated pecten: most of the species.
- Species with a veined pecten: ostrich, rhea, and tinamou.
- Species with a conical pecten: kiwi.

3 List potential functions of the pecten. Nutritional, thermal, intraocular pressure regulation, secretory, light absorption, and vision.

Further reading

King AS, McLelland J (1984) Special sense organs. In: *Birds: Their Structure and Function*, 2nd edn. (eds. AS King, J McLelland) Ballière Tindall, Philadelphia, pp. 284–314.

CASE 224

1 What is the problem with its legs? Developmental deformities of the bones of the leg are common in young, rapidly growing ratite chicks. Outward rotation along the length of the tibiotarsus is one of the most common deformities. Changes can occur rapidly and are generally progressive, with malformation of the joints occurring primarily or secondarily.

2 How can this problem be managed? Developmental leg deformities are difficult to prevent and manage as their causation is complex and incompletely understood. Genetic factors may be important. Ensuring appropriate nutrition, encouraging exercise on nonslip surfaces, and avoiding too rapid growth are all recommended. Applying tape splints in the early stages may prevent worsening and on occasion correct developing abnormalities. Once the bones are well formed, orthopedic surgical intervention, which carries a poor prognosis and is impractical in production animals, is the only possible treatment.

3 Incidental to the bird's primary issue, what management procedure has been carried out on its feet? Emus have three forward-facing toes that have at their tips a strong toenail. This emu has been 'declawed'; the distal phalanx has been amputated. This procedure is sometimes carried out by the producer on recently hatched chicks to reduce the damage birds can do to themselves and each other. Integumentary scarring will result in downgrading of the hides and economic loss.

Further reading

Speer BL (1996) Development problems in young ratites. In: *Ratite Management, Medicine and Surgery*. (eds. TN Tully, SM Shane) Krieger Publishing Company, Malabar, pp. 147–154.

CASE 225

1 How can the two diseases be differentiated from each other based on clinical signs? The clinical signs of paratyphoid infection caused by *Salmonella typhimurium* var. Copenhagen infection may include loose stool and a torticollis. Loose stool may be the result of polyuria and/or diarrhea. Loose stool as a result of a paratyphoid infection is caused by diarrhea, while loose stool as a result of a paramyxovirus infection is caused by polyuria.

2 What paramyxovirus serotype is most likely to be responsible? What other serotypes of this virus have been associated with disease in birds? Avian paramyxovirus (APMV) serotype 1 (pigeon strain). Twelve different avian paramyxovirus serotypes have currently been identified that may cause infection in birds. APMV serotype 1 is the most common serotype, and is the causative agent of Newcastle disease. Although the paramyxovirus infection in pigeons also belongs to serotype 1, this disease is not referred to as Newcastle disease, as this term is reserved for highly pathogenic strains of APMV-1. Bird species in which the different serotypes have been isolated are: APMV-2: chicken and turkey; APMV-3: turkey and parakeet; APMV-4: wild- and mallard duck, goose, and chicken; APMV-5: budgerigar; APMV-6: domestic and mallard duck, goose, and turkey; APMV-7: wild dove, turkey, and ostrich; APMV-8: wild Canada goose and pintail; APMV-9: domestic and feral duck: APMV-10: rockhopper penguin: APMV-11: common snipe: APMV-12: wigeon.

3 What therapeutic and preventive measures can be taken for the viral disease responsible for the clinical signs observed in these pigeons? No specific treatment is available. The condition is self-limiting, although infections may last for months and remnants of renal disease may persist. In pigeons, commercial vaccines are available to prevent infection. These vaccinations are mandatory in some European countries due to the close relationship between paramyxovirus-1 infections in pigeons and Newcastle disease.

Further reading

Gerlach H (1994) Viruses. In: *Avian Medicine: Principles and Application*. (eds. BW Ritchie, GJ Harrison, LR Harrison) Wingers Publishing, Inc., Lake Worth, pp. 920–929.

Gogoi P, Ganar K, Kumar S (2015) Avian paramyxovirus: a brief review. *Transbound Emerg Dis* doi:10.1111/tbed.12355.

CASE 226

1 What is the name of the parasite shown in the image (226) responsible for these clinical signs? Tracheal mites (*Sternostoma tracheacolum*).

2 What are your differential diagnoses for these clinical signs in finches and canaries? *Enterococcus faecalis, Chlamydia psittaci* and other bacterial causes of upper respiratory disease; *Syngamus trachea*; *Aspergillus fumigatus*; avian poxvirus; *Atoxoplasma* spp.; *Trichomonas gallinae*; inhalant toxins; abdominal distension.

3 How can you evaluate for the presence of this parasite antemortem? What treatment regimens would you recommend? Tracheal transillumination after wetting the feathers may show mites in the lumen of the trachea, recognized as small black spots. Lack of visualization does not rule out their presence. Individual birds can be treated with ivermectin or doramectin. The commercial formulation of ivermectin or doramectin is diluted to 10% (i.e. 1:10) with medical grade propylene glycol or sesame oil, respectively. Apply as 'spot on' to the bare skin dorsolaterally over the neck at the site of jugular blood collection at a dosage of 0.4 mg/kg (approximately one drop). Repeat after 10 days.

Further reading

Sandmeier P, Coutteel P (2006) Management of canaries, finches and mynahs. In: *Clinical Avian Medicine*, Vol. 2. (eds. GJ Harrison, TL Lightfoot) Spix Publishing, Palm Beach, p. 906.

CASE 227

1 What toxins may cause inhalation toxicity in birds? Nicotine from tobacco smoke; undiluted sodium hypochlorite solution (inhalation of produced gases); Teflon toxicity (PFTE, nonstick cookware, waterproofing on outdoor clothing, working parts in hair dryers, hardening agents in gloss paint, heat lamps, ironing board covers, etc.); nonirritant gases: carbon monoxide, carbon dioxide, hydrogen cyanide; irritant gases: aldehydes, hydrogen chloride, sulfur dioxide; miscellaneous airborne toxins: air fresheners, hair products, nail polish, scented candles and plugs, aerosols, gasoline fumes, paints, mothballs, fumigants, solvents, aerosol propellants, cleaning products, plastic overheated in the microwave.

2 List the common clinical signs reported in birds suffering from inhalation toxicity. Include depression, somnolence, anorexia, coughing, sneezing, wheezing, tachypnea, dyspnea, rhinitis, sinusitis, and conjunctivitis, but also dermatitis and feather-destructive behavior (e.g. nicotine toxicity). Severe toxicity may lead to sudden death due to pulmonary edema, congestion, necrosis, or hemorrhage (e.g. sodium hypochlorite inhalation toxicity). In some cases, incoordination and convulsions may be seen (e.g. Telfon toxicity). Sometimes, clinical signs will develop several hours or even days after initial exposure to the toxin.

3 What is the advised treatment regimen in case of inhalation toxicity in birds? If inhalation toxicity is suspected, affected birds should immediately be transferred to well-ventilated areas (e.g. oxygen cages). Supportive care with fluid therapy, antibiotics, analgesics, anti-inflammatory drugs, and bronchodilators may prevent secondary infections (e.g. leading to pneumonia). Diuretics might be indicated in some cases of suspected pulmonary edema. Although still often mentioned in the literature, corticosteroids are no longer recommended in the treatment of gaseous toxicities, as no beneficial effects have been proven and immunosuppression may increase the risk of secondary infections. Prognosis of birds with inhalation toxicity is generally poor, especially in birds suffering from PTFE intoxication. Sudden death typically occurs, before supportive treatments can be initiated.

Further reading

Arca-Ruibal B (2016) Systemic diseases. In: *Avian Medicine*, 3rd edn. (ed. J Samour) Elsevier, St. Louis, pp. 385–395.

CASE 228

1 What anatomic parts of the beak seem to be affected? In this case, clearly, bone, dermis, and keratin have been lost, with exposure of the nasal diverticulum of the frontal sinus. The upper beak or bill (rostrum maxillare) is composed of keratin, soft tissues (dermis), and bone. The term used to describe the upper beak keratin layer is the rhinotheca, and often these injuries are incorrectly described as rhinothecal amputations.

2 How can this injury be treated? Wound management, supportive and nursing care, antimicrobial therapy, and appropriate pain management should be applied in concert in the ultimate treatment strategy for this patient. For a fresh wound, topical analgesia with lidocaine gel may help, prior to cleaning of the wound itself. Bimodal parenteral analgesia should be considered, including popular drugs such as butorphanol (1–4 mg/kg IM) and meloxicam (1 mg/kg IM). The wound can be cleaned topically with chlorhexidine or dilute povidone iodine, taking care not to flood the exposed sinus space where appropriate. Systemic antibacterial treatments may be prudent for this injury. Supportive and nursing care treatments may include parenteral fluids (~30–50 mL/kg SC q12–24h) and gavage feeding as needed to maintain body weight and gastrointestinal transit. The attachment of acrylic caps over this wound may be fair to consider in time, but most are treated as open wounds. Prosthetic reconstruction of an artificial beak is not a viable option for most of these injuries.

3 What is the prognosis for a traumatic amputation of the bill? When bone is lost (as contrasted to keratin only), the prognosis for regrowth is minimal. Regardless of a lack of potential for regrowth of the beak, many of these patients heal their wounds over, and can learn to eat and maintain themselves with time. Some birds will need to learn to eat an altered diet that is softer and more readily prehended and swallowed with tongue and lower bill action.

Further reading

King AS, McLelland J (1984) Integument. In: *Birds: Their Structure and Function*, 2nd edn. (eds. AS King, J McLelland) Baillière-Tindall, Philadelphia, pp. 24–26.

CASE 229

1 What will you tell your client? You should tell your client that the egg is a nonfertile clear egg. Clear eggs are nonfertile or infected or diseased eggs that do not develop.

2 Should you remove the egg from the incubator? If so, by what day? You should remove clear eggs from the incubator by day 7. By this time you should know if an egg is viable or not. Viable incubated eggs, especially those of endangered psittacines, are valuable and should not be exposed to potentially infectious clear eggs. Clear eggs containing infectious agents such as bacteria or fungi can contaminate viable eggs and even explode in the incubator.

3 What is missing from this egg? Blood vessels and an embryo are missing from this egg, hence the term clear egg. By day 3 to 4 you should be able to see blood vessels in a healthy fertilized psittacine egg.

Further reading

Romagnano A (2005) Reproduction and paediatrics. In: *BSAVA Manual of Psittacine Birds*, 2nd edn. (eds. N Harcourt-Brown, JR Chitty). British Small Animal Veterinary Association, Gloucester, pp. 222–233.

CASE 230

1 What procedure may be considered to stabilize this patient prior to anesthesia? Coelomocentesis should be performed prior to general anesthesia in order to reduce the volume of fluid in the coelom and improve the patient's ability to breathe.

2 When performing coelomic surgery in patients with coelomic effusion, what measures should be implemented to avert possible respiratory complications? These patients should be maintained in an upright position to prevent coelomic fluid and debris from entering the lungs through perforation of the air sacs. The surgery table must be tilted to a minimum of 30° so that the patient's head is elevated. Proper intubation is mandatory to ensure airway patency. Gentle intermittent positive pressure ventilation will help maintain adequate oxygenation. Pressure placed on the breathing bag should not exceed 15 cmH_2O.

3 If an air sac is inadvertently perforated during surgery, how will this affect the anesthesia? If the air sacs are penetrated, anesthetic gas may escape making it difficult to maintain the patient under anesthesia. If the puncture in the air sac is identified, a moistened cotton-tip applicator may be used to decrease loss of anesthetic gas, thus limiting personnel exposure. If the leaking cannot be controlled, the required pressure placed on the breathing bag will need to be increased to reach 15 cmH_2O. The vaporizer setting and the rate of intermittent positive pressure ventilation may need to be increased when there is severe gas leakage, which might result in respiratory alkalosis and hypotension. Use caution when using any ventilator during surgical procedures in the coelomic cavity, especially if there is an opening in the air sac system. Because volume-limited ventilators (e.g. Hallowell) deliver only a preset volume of anesthetic gas, it is almost impossible to control ventilation and anesthesia because most of the anesthetic gas leaks from the opening in the air sac. Although difficult, it is possible to control ventilation under the same circumstances with a pressure-limited ventilator (e.g. Vetronics, Bird) because this type of system will continue to supply anesthetic gas until the preset pressure is achieved.

Further reading

Edling TM (2005) Updates in anesthesia and monitoring. In: *Clinical Avian Medicine*, Vol. 2. (eds. GJ Harrison, TL Lightfoot) Spix Publishing, Palm Beach, pp. 747–760.

Guzman DS (2016) Avian soft tissue surgery. *Vet Clin North Am Exot Anim Pract* **19(1)**: 133–157.

Sinn LC (1994) Anesthesiology. In: *Avian Medicine: Principles and Application.* (eds. BW Ritchie, GJ Harrison, LR Harrison) Wingers Publishing, Lake Worth, pp. 1066–1080.

CASE 231

1 How would you stabilize this bird prior to performing additional diagnostic tests? Preoxygenation may be indicated prior to handling, in a small, clean and warm (85–95°F [29.5–35°C]) hospital cage. Perform a physical examination, being certain to protect the prolapsed oviduct to prevent iatrogenic and self-trauma. Parenteral fluid therapy (SC, IV, or IO) should be started as soon as possible. Opioid analgesia (butorphanol, 1–4 mg/kg SC or IM) is indicated to manage pain and provide sedation. NSAIDs are contraindicated in cases of severe dehydration and shock. The tissue could be covered with K-Y gel to prevent further contamination.

2 What diagnostic tests would you perform? CBC and plasma chemistry panel (including ionized calcium) to evaluate for any evidence of systemic disease; whole body radiography and coelomic ultrasound to evaluate possible underlying reproductive pathology, including eggs. An oviductal swab for bacterial culture and sensitivity of the oviduct might be collected.

3 How would you surgically manage this condition? What are the possible complications? After anesthesia is induced, the bird is placed in dorsal recumbency. The oviduct is lavaged copiously with warm saline. If there is severe inflammation, hypertonic solutions (e.g. dextrose 50%) can be used as well to decrease the edema. Since the tissue appears viable, the prolapsed tissue is gently replaced within the cloaca using moistened cotton tip applicators. Simple interrupted or mattress sutures should be placed on both sides of the vent to prevent re-prolapse while the underlying cause is investigated or treated (**231b**). Systemic antibiotics and NSAIDs are administered as needed following recovery from anesthesia. The use of GnRH agonists (e.g. deslorelin acetate implant) would be recommended to downregulate

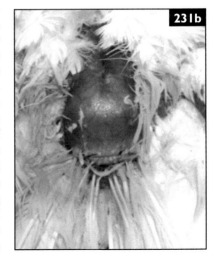
231b

the reproductive system. The sutures are removed carefully a few days later, while monitoring for recurrence of the prolapse.

Further reading

Rosen LB (2012) Avian reproductive disorders. *J Exotic Pet Med* **21**(**2**):124–131

CASE 232

1 What is your diagnosis? Capillariasis. The characteristic eggs, with bipolar opercula, can be seen in the stools.

2 How would you treat this condition? *Capillaria* worms can be treated with fenbendazole, albendazole, levamisole, or ivermectin. This parasite is difficult to get rid of and may become resistant to different drugs, so an aggressive protocol should be used. Fenbendazole (50 mg/kg PO q24h for 5 days) has been used anecdotally in toucans without apparent adverse effects. Levamisole (15 mg/kg SC once weekly for 3 weeks) can also be used, but adverse side-effects (vomiting and hypersalivation) can occur.

3 What sanitary measures should be undertaken to prevent this condition? *Capillaria* life cycle is direct (bird feces, ground, bird) or indirect via earthworms. Worms will be picked up from the ground, so any measure to reduce or prevent worm infection, entry into the enclosure, or worm ability to burrow (e.g. an impervious substrate in the aviary) should be applied to limit capillariasis. Feeders and water bowls should be put in a high position; many perches and high roosting sites should be available to encourage the toucans to live in the upper levels of the aviary. Although *Capillaria* eggs are very resistant, they can be destroyed with hot steam. Boiling water has been used anecdotally on surfaces. Ground, gravel, and sand should be replaced whenever possible. Finally, the use of suspended cages is recommended in breeding facilities.

Further reading

Dislich M (2014) Piciformes. In: *Tratado de Animais Selvagens*, 2nd edn. (eds. ZS Cubas, JCR Silva, JL Catão-Dias) Roca, Brasil, pp. 598–625.

CASE 233

1 What clinical signs do you anticipate after ingestion of this product? Trichlorphon is an organophosphate cholinesterase inhibitor. Hyperstimulation of muscarinic cholinergic synapses causes bradycardia progressing to asystole, bronchoconstriction, increased respiratory and salivary secretions, digestive stasis, regurgitation, ataxia, seizures, lethargy, and protrusion of the nictitans, as illustrated in the image. This is followed by hyperstimulation of nicotinic synapses resulting in skeletal muscle paralysis including the voluntary respiratory muscles. Death results from cardiopulmonary failure.

2 How can you confirm ingestion? Intoxication can be confirmed by measuring the concentration of plasma butyrylcholinesterases, which would typically be decreased in case of ingestion. In Amazon parrots of various species, plasma butyrylcholinesterases levels have been reported to range between 0.24 and 6.94 kU/L.

3 How would you treat this bird? Depending on the timing of ingestion, crop and proventricular lavage and/or activated charcoal (1–3 g/kg PO q12h) may be indicated. Care should be taken to avoid gavage feeding to prevent aspiration if regurgitation is already present. In addition, activated charcoal without sorbitol should be chosen to avoid secondary diarrhea. To antagonize the cholinergic effects, pralidoxime iodide (2-PAM) has been recommended at doses ranging from 10 to 100 mg/kg q6–48h. Note that 2-PAM would be contraindicated in cases of carbamate intoxication. Atropine (0.01–0.5 mg/kg) has also been described, although it only antagonizes muscarinic effects and not nicotinic effects responsible for muscular paralysis, and dosing needs to be frequently repeated. Symptomatic treatment of seizures is administered as needed and parenteral fluid therapy may enhance trichlorphon clearance and prevent dehydration from digestive signs.

Further reading

Carpenter JW (2005) *Exotic Animal Formulary*, 3rd edn. Saunders, Philadelphia, pp. 293–296.

Grosset C, Bougerol C, Sanchez-Migallon Guzman D (2014) Plasma butyrylcholinesterase concentrations in psittacine birds: reference values, factors of variation, and association with feather-damaging behavior. *J Avian Med Surg* **28(1)**:6–15.

Lightfoot TL, Yeager JM (2008) Pet bird toxicity and related environmental concerns. *Vet Clin North Am Exot Anim Pract* **11(2)**:229–259.

Redig PT, Arent LR (2008) Raptor toxicology. *Vet Clin North Am Exot Anim Pract* **11(2)**:261–282.

CASE 234

1 Would you consider fasting such a patient prior to general anesthesia? The pediatric patient should be fasted prior to general anesthesia, since the proventriculus, ventriculus, and intestines are normally enlarged in unweaned birds. The fasting period should be as short as possible. Typically, a 2–3-hour fast is adequate.

2 How do you minimize hypoglycemia? Feeding should occur soon after recovery to prevent hypoglycemia. If concerned, fluid therapy with added dextrose can be used during the procedure, although this is not normally indicated unless the procedure is prolonged.

3 How do you prevent hypothermia in this patient? Some studies suggest the use of forced-air warming system (convective) is superior to traditional heating methods (conductive with heating pad, radiation with infrared lamp) in restricting heat loss. However, in other studies the use of the conductive device is recommended in preference to convective devices when performing anesthetic procedures in birds. Nevertheless, both convective and conductive modalities are effective for the reduction of hypothermia during inhalation anesthesia of birds. Monitoring body temperature is essential and may be performed using an esophageal or cloacal thermometer. The normal body temperature of pet birds usually ranges from 101 to 107°F (38.3 to 41.7°C).

Further reading

Rembert MS, Smith JA, Hosgood G *et al.* (2001) Comparison of traditional thermal support devices with the forced-air warmer system in anesthetized Hispaniolan Amazon parrots (*Amazona ventralis*). *J Avian Med Surg* **15(3)**:187–193.

Romagnano A (2012) Psittacine incubation and pediatrics. *Vet Clin North Am Exot Anim Pract* **15**:163–182.

van Zeeland YRA, Cardona T, Schoemaker NJ (2012) Maintenance of core body temperature in anaesthetised pigeons (*Columba livia domestica*): a comparison of two thermal devices. *Vet J* **194**:429–432.

CASE 235

1 Which nematodes would you consider as etiologic agents? *Echinuria* spp. and *Streptocara* spp. are two nematodes reported to cause lesions in the upper gastrointestinal tract in waterfowl.

2 What additional diagnostic test would you perform? Fecal examination may reveal 35–37 × 18–20 µm ova, although fecal examination alone is not a reliable diagnostic method, as ova are not present at all stages of pathogenesis.

3 What treatment and control methods would you implement in the collection? Ivermectin (0.2 mg/kg IM) has been proven a successful therapeutic option but surgical débridement and fluid and nutritional support may be required in severely affected specimens. Minimizing exposure to wild birds and eliminating the intermediate host (species of crustaceans from the *Daphnia* spp.) from aquatic areas in the enclosures are advisable. Copper sulfate added to the water has been used to eradicate this intermediate host. The median lethal dose has been reported at 0.38 mg/L in some *Daphnia* spp. Targeted anthelmintic treatment during the rearing period is advisable. An alternative management strategy is to rear all young waterfowl away from the source of infection, so that young are born in an environment where infection is unlikely. If birds hatch in an environment where infection is likely, then targeted routine anthelmintic therapy (e.g. from 2 weeks of age, every 2 weeks, on four occasions) can be provided.

Further reading

Carreno RA (2014) *Dispharynx*, *Echinuria*, and *Streptocara*. In: *Parasitic Diseases of Wild Birds*. (eds. CT Atkinson, NJ Thomas, DB Hunter) Wiley-Blackwell, Ames, pp. 326–342.

CASE 236

1 Based on the history and clinical findings, what are your differential diagnoses? Coccidiosis; salmonellosis; pseudomoniasis.
2 What diagnostic tests would you perform to confirm the diagnosis? Fecal direct and flotation parasite examination; Giemsa staining of fecal smears; bacterial culture.
3 Which parasitic genera could be implicated? Which one is most likely? What treatment would be recommended? *Caryospora* spp., *Isospora* spp., and *Eimeria* spp. Most likely *Caryospora neofalconis*, and the recommended pharmaceutical therapy is toltrazuril (15–25 mg/kg PO daily for 2 consecutive days, repeated 1 week later). There are at least six species of *Caryospora* spp. pathogenic to falcons. There is no cross-antigen protection conferred by one *Caryospora* species to another. Sixty-five percent of first year falcons are infected with *Caryospora* spp. Parent birds are infected; they demonstrate an increased level of fecal oocyst shedding prior to the breeding season, resulting in oocyst contamination of the nest environment. Young falcons have no maternal protection against the parasite. Young birds are exposed, infected, and gradually develop their own immunity. If stressed during this period, prior to developing an immunity, they will suffer clinical disease. Birds commonly show weight loss, poor performance, and diarrhea (on occasions with hemorrhage). Merlins (*Falco columbarius*) are particularly prone to severe disease, and may simply be found dead subsequent to minor stress in this period. Depending on the age of exposure and level of challenge, young birds may be target treated (e.g. toltrazuril at 30, 50, 75 days), the aim being to treat the eyass (a young first year raptor) after infection has occurred (during the prepatent period) but before clinical disease occurs. In this way the parasite is killed and an immunity generated prior to the bird suffering clinical disease. The ideal timing of target treatments may vary year on year, as the level of infection within the collection is gradually reduced. The duration of immunity is host and *Caryospora* spp. dependent, typically ranging from 12 to 24 weeks. Once a collection is infected it is not desirable to exclude the parasite from the environment, as it is the repeated challenge of the bird by environmental oocysts that maintains the bird's protective immunity.

Further reading

Forbes NA, Simpson GN (1997) *Caryospora neofalconis*: an emerging threat to captive-bred raptors in the United Kingdom. *J Avian Med Surg* **11**:110–114.
Samour J (2008) Infectious diseases, parasites, protozoa. In: *Avian Medicine*, 2nd edn. (ed. J Samour) Elsevier, St. Louis, pp. 318–325.

CASE 237

1 What are your differential diagnoses for these liver lesions seen at postmortem examination (220)? Yersiniosis, salmonellosis, mycobacteriosis, other bacterial infections.

2 What clinical signs would you expect to see in canaries with this disease, from this breeder? Sudden death, fluffed bird, distended coelomic cavity, pasted vent, diarrhea, biliverdinuria.

3 What diagnostic test would you perform to confirm the diagnosis, and what treatment regimens would you recommend? Gram stain and Ziehl–Neelsen stain of an impression smear. Aerobic culture of liver. Mycobacteria can be differentiated in specialized laboratories by culture and PCR. There is no suitable flock treatment for mycobacteriosis. Yersiniosis and salmonellosis can be treated by separating diseased birds and treating clinically healthy in-contact birds with a gram-negative spectrum antibiotic such as enrofloxacin in drinking water (200 mg/L for 10 days). Diseased birds need supportive treatment and direct oral application of a suitable antibiotic. Zoonotic implications of salmonellosis need to be considered. In all cases, the source of infection needs to be considered and tested to prevent reoccurrence.

Further reading

Sandmeier P, Coutteel P (2006) Management of canaries, finches and mynahs. In: *Clinical Avian Medicine*, Vol. 2. (eds. GJ Harrison, TL Lightfoot) Spix Publishing, Palm Beach, pp. 896–897.

CASE 238

1 What is the most likely diagnosis? Tick bite. Soft ticks (Argasidae) and hard ticks (Ixodidae) have been reported as a cause of disease in raptors from tropical and temperate areas, respectively. Ticks may act as vectors for viruses, bacteria, and parasites. *Ixodes frontalis* has been associated with an avian tick-related syndrome of unknown etiology in the UK. With respect to *I. frontalis* attachment, a regional and seasonal (typically lasting only 2 weeks) disease outbreak can affect all areas of the country simultaneously. In the UK, 70% of outbreaks occur in August and September and cause significant mortality and morbidity in cage and aviary birds (50% of affected birds being raptors). Wild birds with ticks attached perch on branches above aviaries, dropping the ticks onto the ground close to the aviary. When weather and seasonal changes stimulate the tick, it seeks to find a natural host (potentially the raptor in the aviary) and attaches to that bird. Birds will remove attached ticks during preening in all the parts of the body that they can reach with their beak. If ticks are attached around the head and neck, they are unable to remove them, these being the ticks that then engorge with blood, at the same time injecting pathogens subcutaneously into the bird. The bird is found dead, or presented lethargic for treatment, with an area of surrounding subcutaneous hemorrhage. In any bird presenting with cranial or cervical subcutaneous hemorrhage, a tick bite should be included in the differential diagnoses list.

2 What treatment should be provided to the bird? According to results from two different studies, 48–75% of treated birds recovered after receiving prompt veterinary care, the remaining birds dying. However, survival rates increased to 100% when the antibiotic administered was changed to doxycycline or oxytetracycline.

3 What additional actions should be taken? As the disease is strictly seasonal, when one bird is affected, all other birds on site are at risk at that time. All in-contact birds should be treated with a single dose of fipronil spray (7.5 mg/kg applied directly to the skin). The aviary should be treated with a bird-safe environmental parasiticide. This may be repeated prophylactically prior to the anticipated tick season in subsequent years. An ecologically friendly alternative could be the use of suspended flights or the periodic removal of a raptor from its aviary for 7–10 days, during which time poultry are kept in the aviary. The poultry will scratch about and consume any insects or arthropods they find on the aviary floor (ticks included), thereby reducing or eliminating the tick risk to the raptor when it is returned to its aviary.

Further reading

Monks DI, Fisher M, Forbes NA (2006) *Ixodes frontalis* and avian tick-related syndrome in the United Kingdom. *J Small Anim Pract* **47(8)**:451–455.

CASE 239

1 How do you perform an ECG in a bird? The avian ECG is typically obtained in the frontal plane by placing two front electrodes on the propatagia and one (left) or two (earth on right) back electrodes on the knee webs using needle electrodes or flat clips. Each lead evaluates the cardiac electrical activity on a different plane and a standard examination classically includes three bipolar leads (I, II, and III) and three augmented unipolar leads (aVR, aVL, aVF). A proper ECG recording is easier to obtain on anesthetized birds, as few will tolerate the procedure and movement or muscle tremors may impair the recordings. However, ECG tracings on conscious birds can still be obtained on pigeons, some raptors, and lethargic birds. Recordings need to be performed at 50–100 mm/s with 100 mm/s being optimal to better assess the morphology of the QRS complexes. Electrocardiographic measurements are typically performed on lead II tracings.

2 What is your diagnosis with regard to the bradycardia present in this bird? Similar to the mammalian ECG, a normal avian ECG is usually composed of

P waves, QRS complexes, and T waves. In certain birds a Ta wave is present. The QRS complexes are mainly of the rS type on lead II, meaning the S wave is the most prominent and the Q wave is absent.

In this case the P waves are not consistently followed by an rS complex. This is indicative of a second-degree atrioventricular (AV) block whereby AV conductance is interrupted intermittently. The second-degree AV block may be further subdivided into two types: the Mobitz type I (Wenkebach phenomenon), which is characterized by a progressive lengthening of the PR interval until a P wave is blocked; and type II, which is characterized by a constant PR interval with a fixed relationship between the atrial and ventricular rate. In this bird, the PR interval is constant, thus indicating a type II second-degree AV block with a ratio of 3:1, meaning three P waves to every rS complex.

3 What test can be performed to diagnose an underlying increase in vagal tone? To determine whether bradycardia is the result of an increased vagal tone, an atropine response test is warranted. For this purpose, an atropine injection (0.01–0.02 mg/kg IM) may be given, following which the ECG may be repeated 15–30 minutes post injection. A subsequent increase in heart rate indicates an increased vagal tone. In birds with atropine-responsive bradycardia, therapy may be initiated with long-acting parasympathicolytic (e.g. propantheline, 0.03 mg/kg PO q8h) or sympathicomimetic drugs.

Further reading

Lumeij JT, Ritchie BW (1994) Cardiology. In: *Avian Medicine: Principles and Application.* (eds. BW Ritchie, GJ Harrison, LR Harrison) Wingers Publishing, Inc., Lake Worth, pp. 695–722.

van Zeeland YRA, Schoemaker NJ, Lumeij JT (2010) Syncopes associated with second-degree atrioventricular block in a cockatoo. In: *Proc 31st Ann Conf Assoc Avian Vet*, San Diego, pp. 345–346.

Zandvliet MMJM (2005). Electrocardiography in psittacine birds and ferrets. *Sem Avian Exot Pet Med* **14(1)**:34–51.

CASE 240

1 Where is it located? It is located on the dorsal surface of the rump, cranial to the point of attachment of the major tail feathers or rectrices.

2 What does it produce? It secretes a rich oil of waxes, fatty acids, fat, and water.

3 What are the main functions of its product? When applied externally with the bill it cleans feathers and preserves feather moisture and flexibility, which assists in the durability and longevity of the feathers. Regular applications of the secretion to the plumage sustain its functions as an insulating and waterproofing layer. Water birds typically have large preen glands, but whether the secretions of this organ are essential for keeping feathers dry and maintaining buoyancy remains to be verified.

The waxy secretion of the preen gland also helps to regulate the bacterial and fungal flora of feathers and skin. Finally, it has been suggested that components of the oil, when exposed to sunlight, become converted to activated vitamin D_3.

4 Name some birds that totally lack a preen gland. Ostrich, emu, cassowary, and some doves, parrots, and woodpeckers.

5 What clinical abnormalities may affect the preen gland, and how would each be treated? Obstruction of the preen gland duct (manual expression), neoplasia (surgery if possible), abscessation (débridement, culture, and antibiosis), periuropygial dermatitis (control of self-trauma, antibiosis, anti-inflammatory agents, and topical cleansing agents).

CASE 241

1 How would you manage pain in this patient (1) during the preoperative period, (2) during the intraoperative period, and (3) during the postoperative period?

- **Preoperative period.** Combinations of an opioid and a NSAID are often administered to birds when initially presenting for orthopedic trauma. General anesthesia can cause hypotension and reduce renal perfusion, therefore it is still recommended to avoid NSAID administration in the immediate pre- and perioperative period. Opioids (e.g. hydromorphone, 0.3–0.6 mg/kg) coupled with benzodiazepines (e.g. midazolam, 0.5–1 mg/kg) administered IM are frequently recommended for the immediate preanesthetic period and may assist in reducing the amount of inhalation anesthetic needed for induction and maintenance of anesthesia.
- **Intraoperative period.** CRI using opioids (e.g. fentanyl, 30–60 µg/kg/h IV) has been used as an adjunct to inhalation anesthesia for orthopedic pain. An effective local anesthetic block (e.g. lidocaine, 2 mg/kg) at the surgical site and splash blocks on nerves in the surgical area of the fracture can decrease sensitization and wind-up that might otherwise occur during tissue handling. Brachial plexus block techniques with local anesthetics could be attempted as well, blindly or with the aid of a nerve stimulator, but this has proved to be an unreliable technique in birds, with inconsistent results.
- **Postoperative period:**
    - Immediate postoperative period (24–48 hours). Assuming the patient is well hydrated, a combination of a NSAID (e.g. meloxicam, 1 mg/kg SC) drug and continued opioid CRI or parenteral opioid (e.g. buprenorphine, 0.3–0.6 mg/kg q8–12h) administration with gradual reduction in doses during the 24–48-hour postoperative period are recommended. Adjunctive protocols, including physical therapy and cold or warm thermal therapy, may be added as needed. Cold therapy will help reduce swelling, whereas warm therapy may stimulate blood flow to specific areas.

- Later postoperative period. Opioid administration with titration to effect and gradual discontinuation. NSAIDS (e.g. meloxicam, 1.6 mg/kg PO q12h) or tramadol (5 mg/kg PO q8–12h) may be utilized when the patient returns to home care. Cold therapy of the affected regions should be continued for a minimum of 3 days if tolerated, at which point it can be alternated with heat therapy prior to stretching (with icing following these therapies).

Further reading

Hawkins H, Paul-Murphy J, Sanchez-Migallon Guzman D (2015) Recognition, assessment and management of pain in birds. In: *Current Therapy in Avian Medicine and Surgery*. (ed. BL Speer) Elsevier, St. Louis, pp. 616–630.

CASE 242

1 What are your main concerns with a predator bite? Birds that have been exposed to a dog, cat or other carnivore mouth will often die within 24–48 hours from bacterial sepsis without antibiotic treatment. Other concerns in cat and dog encounters include crush and tear trauma, leading to air sac rupture, internal organ damage, fractures, and significant hemorrhage. A common mistake is to assume that antibiotics are not needed if the bird has no physical evidence of a puncture or scratch. Birds have extremely thin skin and often the injury cannot be detected with the naked eye.

2 What is the normal flora of the oral cavity of the dog and cat? Most bite wounds from both species contain a mixed aerobic and anaerobic population. In a study in humans, 50% of dog bites contained *Pasteurella* spp., while 75% of cats contained the same organism. Other aerobic organisms seen in both species were *Streptococcus* spp., *Staphylococcus* spp., *Neisseria* spp., *Corynebacterium* spp., *Moraxella* spp., and *Enterococcus* spp. Anaerobic organisms seen in both species included *Fusobacterium* spp., *Bacteroides* spp., and *Prevotella* spp.

3 How would you treat birds bitten by dogs or cats? Fluid therapy, pain management, thermal support, and oxygen when needed. Superficial wounds can be flushed with warm sterile saline or 0.05% chlorhexidine. Any large lacerations should be cleaned, débrided, and sutured once the bird is stable, but in most cases can be left to heal by secondary intention. Fractures can be temporally immobilized with a splint. For infected bites, combination antibiotic therapy is recommended. Antimicrobial suggestions for dog or cat bite wounds include combinations of: (1) amoxicillin–clavulanate or azithromycin; (2) enrofloxacin and clindamycin; and (3) enrofloxacin and amoxicillin–clavulanate.

Further reading

Wade L (2002) Dog and cat bites in birds: why Baytril is NOT enough. *AAV Newsletter and Clinical Forum* September-November: 9–11, 121.

CASE 243

1 What is your most important differential diagnosis for this case? List other differential diagnoses. Diabetes mellitus (DM). Diabetes insipidus with stress hyperglycemia, pancreatitis, or steroid-induced (exogenous or endogenous) hyperglycemia would also be possible but unlikely.

2 What other diagnostic tests should be considered for this bird? Since DM in birds appears to be secondary to other diseases, a complete diagnostic work up should be considered, including CBC, biochemistry panel, survey radiographs, infectious disease testing (*Chlamydia psittaci*, polyomavirus, PMV-3, PsHV, adenovirus), and blood levels of zinc. Pancreatic biopsy and possibly liver and/or kidney biopsy may be needed in some cases for a definitive diagnosis of the primary cause. Blood levels of insulin, glucagon, fructosamine, and beta-hydroxybutyric acid (a ketone) have been used in several case reports to aid diagnosis and management of DM in birds, with variable results.

3 What treatment options have been used in birds with this condition? Recommended treatment protocols for DM in birds include the use of insulin or oral hypoglycemic agents (such as glipizide). Dietary changes, weight management, and discontinuing the use of diabetogenic drugs are also recommended, as for mammalian species with DM.

Further reading

Hudelson KS, Hudelson PM (2006) Endocrine considerations. In: *Clinical Avian Medicine.* (eds. GJ Harrison, TL Lightfoot) Spix Publishing, Palm Beach, pp. 541–557.

Schmidt RE, Reavill DR (2014) Lesions of the avian pancreas. *Vet Clin North Am Exot Anim Pract* **17**:1–11.

CASE 244

1 What is the most likely diagnosis? How often is this seen in waterfowl collections? Avian mycobacteriosis caused by *Mycobacterium avium*. It is common in captive waterfowl collections, typically being the single most common cause of mortality and responsible for a large percentage of losses.

2 How can this disease be prevented from entering a collection? New stock should be introduced as eggs or first season birds from clean collections reared on clean pasture. Most importantly, free flying waterfowl should be kept physically separated from resident stock by the use of netted enclosures for captive stock. The water supply to the stock should be clean and free of infection. Reed bed technology may be used to clean inflow and outflow water of *M. avium*.

3 What can you do to decrease the risk of spreading the disease in a collection? The course of *M. avium* infection is typically long (e.g. 12–18 months), often involving the intestine and liver. This commonly results in fecal excretion of *M. avium* bacilli for a prolonged period prior to apparent ill health or death, resulting in massive environmental contamination. Once *M. avium* is in a collection, actions should be designed to minimize the risk of excessive environmental contamination, as well as reducing the risk of ingestion of bacilli. In addition, the following measures are recommended: individually identify all birds and postmortem any losses; keep species that are inherently more resistant to tuberculosis; always rear juvenile birds on clean pasture that is only used for young birds; determine at what age species die of tuberculosis and cull others of the same species (if appropriate) prior to the age of likely bacilli shedding; manage water–land interfaces (dabbling areas) – these are the commonest environments to become infected and result in fresh infection; cut back vegetation to maximize UV light on and around the pond in order to reduce the likelihood of survival of *M. avium* in the environment.

Further reading

Drewe JA, Mwangi D, Donoghue HD *et al.* (2009) PCR analysis of the presence and location of *Mycobacterium avium* in a constructed reed bed, with implications for avian tuberculosis control. *FEMS Microbiol Ecol* 67(2):320–328.

CASE 245

1 What is this presentation called? Constricted toe syndrome, which is seen most commonly in Eclectus, macaws, and African grey parrots, but others may also be affected. An annular constricting band of fibrous tissue forms at a joint on one or more digits. Other chicks in a clutch could be affected. The band prevents venous drainage from the distal toe, which swells.

2 What is the etiology? The full etiology remains unproven, but it is considered to be related to rearing in an environment with low humidity.

3 What treatment and preventive actions should be taken? Firstly, careful examination of the constriction using magnification is required to ensure that there are no filaments of fibrous material causing the constriction. Under general anesthesia, the digit should be surgically prepared. Using a fine scalpel blade or edge of a hypodermic needle, four incisions (longitudinal in respect to the digit alignment) should be made at 90, 180, 270, and 360 degrees, being careful to avoid the lateral veins and arteries. The digit should then be carefully covered with a supportive, hydrocolloidal, nonconstrictive dressing. Antibiotics and NSAID medication should be maintained for 5 days. The rearing environment humidity should be increased in an attempt to prevent reoccurrence or problems with subsequent chicks.

Further reading

Romagnano A (2005) Psittacine paediatrics and neonatology. In: *Manual of Psittacine Birds*, 2nd edn. (eds. N Harcourt-Brown, J Chitty) British Small Animal Veterinary Association, Gloucester, pp. 222–233.

CASE 246

1 What is the structure indicated by the white arrow? The syringeal bulla.

2 In what avian family is this structure found? This structure is unique to members of the family Anatidae (ducks, geese, and swans) but is most commonly found in males of the subfamily Anatinae, including the domestic duck. It is not found in geese or swans. The syringeal bulla is an asymmetrical dilatation of the left side of the syrinx. The coalesced final rings of the trachea form the cranial portion of the bulla, whereas the first rings of the left bronchus form the caudal portion. The bulla is most often partly or completely ossified, although it may be membranous in some species. Interestingly, the bulla is on the right side of the syrinx in the shelduck (*Tadorna* spp.) and may be symmetrical in ducks of the subfamily Dendrocygnini, genus *Dendrocygna* (the whistling ducks).

3 Which cranial nerve innervates this structure? The syringeal bulla is innervated by cranial nerve XII (hypoglossal nerve), which arises from a collection of rootlets emerging from ventral medulla oblongata. These rootlets combine to form two nerves that exit the skull via two hypoglossal canals or foramina. Once the nerves exit the skull they combine with the first and second cervical nerves to form the hypoglossocervical nerve. This nerve passes over and anastomoses with cranial nerves X and IX. Shortly after anastomosing with cranial nerve X the hypoglossocervical nerve gives off the descending cervical nerve, which innervates the tracheal muscles. At the level of the larynx the hypoglossocervical nerve further bifurcates into the laryngolingual branch, which innervates the tongue, and the tracheal branch, which innervates the tracheal muscles and the intrinsic muscles of the syrinx.

Further reading

King AS, McLelland J (1984) *Birds: Their Structure and Function*. Baillière Tindall, London, pp. 119–120, 264–265.

Orosz SE, Bradshaw GA (2007) Avian neuroanatomy revisited: from clinical principles to avian cognition. *Vet Clin North Am Exot Anim Pract* **10(3)**:775–802.

Pierko M (2007) Morphological comparison of the upper respiratory tract in mallard *Anas platyrhynchos* and scaup *Aythya marila*. *Electr J Pol Agric Univ* **10(4)**: http://www.ejpau.media.pl/volume10/issue4/art-08.html.

CASE 247

1 Give a possible differential for these lesions. Ingestion of perennial ryegrass (also called English ryegrass) (*Lolium perenne*), which is shown in the image.
2 What is the name of this dermatologic disorder? Photosensitization-induced dermatitis (primary photosensitization due to ingestion of a photodynamic agent).
3 What is the name of the toxin? Perloline, which is the photodynamic agent in perennial ryegrass.

Further reading

Rostami A, Madani SA, Vajhi A (2011) Necrotic dermatitis in waterfowl associated with consumption of perennial rye-grass (*Lolium perenne*). *J Avian Med Surg* **25(1)**:44–49.

CASE 248

1 What abnormalities can be seen in the impression smear? The cytologic features show marked karyomegaly consistent with an acute DNA virus infection. In the large cell on the left the nucleus is massively expanded, with cellular DNA forming a darker staining margin of chromatin encircling a viral intranuclear inclusion.
2 What etiologic agents should be considered? Avian polyomavirus and psittacine adenovirus are the two most likely causes of karyomegaly.
3 What other diagnostic tests should be performed to confirm an etiologic diagnosis? This case was confirmed positive for adenovirus infection by PCR testing and was negative for avian polyomavirus. Histopathology was also used to confirm the presence of necrosis in the liver and spleen, again associated with basophilic intranuclear inclusions and karyomegaly, which can occur with acute adenovirus and polyomavirus infection.

Further reading

Raidal SR (2012) Avian circovirus and polyomavirus diseases. In: *Fowler's Zoo and Wild Animal Medicine, Current Therapy*, Vol. 7. (eds. RE Miller, ME Fowler) Elsevier Saunders, St. Louis, pp. 297–303.

CASE 249

1 What abnormality is evident in the excrement? The picture shows voluminous excrement that contains whole, undigested seeds.
2 What diseases could result in similar clinical signs? This finding is not pathognomonic as it may be seen with proventricular dilatation disease, *Macrorhabdus ornithogaster* infection, and potentially other conditions that impair the grinding function of the ventriculus.

3 What diagnostic tests would you use to investigate the cause of the clinical signs? (1) Fecal cytology could demonstrate the presence of *Macrorhabdus ornithogaster*. (2) Fecal parasitology to exclude endoparasites and microbiology to investigate for bacterial or fungal gastrointestinal disease. (3) Plain radiographs and endoscopy for evidence of proventricular or ventricular neoplasia or foreign body. (4) Fluoroscopy with contrast to assess proventricular and ventricular function and assess luminal dilation.

Crop biopsy could demonstrate the pathognomonic changes of proventricular dilatation disease (76% sensitive in one study), and bornavirus real-time (RT) PCR testing may also be useful. Urofecal RT-PCR testing could identify bornavirus RNA, but the shedding is intermittent in some birds and some birds may shed the virus without developing the disease. There is no apparent difference in results between collecting fresh droppings or swabbing the cloaca. Avian bornavirus serology may also be conducted but a positive result does not prove bornavirus is the etiology of the disease. Blood PCR testing, while performed by some veterinarians routinely, may yield false-negative results given that viremia does not seem to be a common feature of avian bornavirus-related pathology.

Further reading

Gancz AY, Clubb S, Shivaprasad HL (2010) Advanced diagnostic approaches and current management of proventricular dilatation disease. *Vet Clin North Am Exot Anim Pract* 13(3):471–494.

CASE 250

1 What is the most likely diagnosis? Neoplasia (e.g. proventricular adenoma, adenocarcinoma, or squamous cell carcinoma). The junction of the proventriculus and ventriculus is the most common site for these neoplasms. Other differential diagnoses are perforating foreign body or gastric nematode infection, either of which may be complicated by secondary bacterial or fungal infections.

2 What further diagnostics are recommended? Biopsy for histopathology and microbiology.

3 What is the prognosis? Poor to grave. If a neoplasm is confirmed (as is likely), it does not lend itself to surgery. Chemotherapy or radiation therapy have been used with mixed to poor results.

Further reading

Yonemaru K, Sakai H, Asaoka Y *et al.* (2004) Proventricular adenocarcinoma in a Humboldt penguin (*Spheniscus humboldti*) and a great horned owl (*Bubo virginianus*); identification of origin by mucin histochemistry. *Avian Pathol* 33(1):77–81.

CASE 251

1 Which taxon is most commonly affected by bumblefoot? Raptors are most commonly affected, amongst whom falcons suffer the most, while hawks, owls, and eagles are rarely affected.

2 What are the risk factors most commonly responsible for this disease? Bumblefoot may occur after penetration of the foot by a thorn, talon, tooth, or other, especially if microorganisms enter the foot; however, this cause is responsible for a small percentage of cases. The vast majority of cases arise when excessive pressure is borne for an excessive period of time, mostly affecting the plantar aspect of the central pad or proximal digit four. Excessive pressure results in localized ischemia, the natural defense mechanism of the skin is broken down, and pathogens living on the skin enter the underlying soft tissues, resulting in a subcuticular cellulitis. The subcuticular tissue swells and yet the bird is obliged to continue to stand on it, compromising any of the body's attempts to control the infection and heal the tissues.

The risk factors are: colonization of the bird's skin from the handler with *Staphylococcus aureus*; inappropriate hard, smooth, or sharp perches; unsuitable perch material (not spreading the bird's weight); unsuitable perch size or design; poor perch or glove hygiene; poor nutrition; excessive weight bearing due to trauma to the contralateral leg; repeated trauma to the foot by grabbing aviary wire, hitting quarry hard, bating when tethered to a perch; inappropriate aviary size, so that braking in flight prior to landing is impossible and there is excessive trauma in landing; poor quality furniture (e.g. brass eyelets on Aylmeri jessies being too large and causing repeated trauma to digits); talons too long, so that the bird takes too much weight on the balls of the feet as the digits cannot grip the perch; talons overlong in aviary birds, so increased risk of talon penetrations of the feet when catching the bird in the aviary; falconer fails to check bird's feet daily (as aviary bird, or too many birds to look after) so that early changes are not detected and treated.

3 Why is that bumblefoot cases are often said not to respond to treatment? Often veterinarians are accused of failing to cure bumblefoot cases, while in truth, in the vast majority of cases, the cause of the bumblefoot is a husbandry problem. If the veterinarian fails to unravel and address the cause of the bumblefoot it will reoccur, therefore the original cause of the problem must be addressed.

Further reading

Bailey T, Lloyd C (2008) Raptors: disorders of the feet. In: *BSAVA Manual of Raptors, Pigeons and Passerine Birds*. (eds. J Chitty, M Lierz) British Small Animal Veterinary Association, Gloucester, pp. 176–189.

CASE 252

1 What two physical examination findings are present? There is a defect on the rhinotheca (keratinized portion of the beak over the maxilla), right of center, that appears to be partial thickness (only involving the keratin or horny portion of the beak) and not full thickness (exposure of the underlying bone). The coloration of the beak (dark in color) occurs as the bird is young, while adult male eclectus parrots have a bright orange colored beak.

2 What can you tell the client about the expected clinical progression of the physical examination findings? The keratin of the beak is created by the germinal epithelium at the rostral aspect of the cere or nares (fleshy area surrounding the nares). The defect in the beak will migrate rostrally (towards the tip) over time and eventually grow out. The color pattern of the beak will also change over time and the new beak growth at the germinal epithelium will begin to create the adult orange coloration.

Further reading

Cooper JE, Harrison GJ (1994) Dermatology. In: *Avian Medicine: Principles and Application.* (eds. BW Ritchie, GJ Harrison, LR Harrison) Wingers Publishing, Lake Worth, p. 607.

CASE 253

1 When should physical therapy be initiated? Physical therapy should be started as soon as the first postoperative recheck (24 hours). With adequate fixator rigidity, beginning gentle range of motion exercises on day one postoperatively and continuing on a regular basis will decrease morbidity.

2 Describe the approach to physical therapy. A gentle stretch and hold process should be used while extending each joint to the point of resistance. The propatagium and other soft tissues should be lightly massaged to improve circulation and gently stretched, the stretch being repeated 5–10 times. Frequency of physical therapy sessions should be balanced with patient stress and handling. Two sessions per week may be adequate for an uncomplicated case in a wild bird, although those with limited range of motion may need more frequent attention. A goniometer can be used to measure the range of motion of the joints and monitor response to therapy. The use of coaptation will increase the need for frequent physical therapy. As the bird increases its use of the limb, the need for physical therapy sessions will be decreased.

3 What ancillary therapeutics should be considered during physical therapy? Appropriate use of sedation or anesthesia and anti-inflammatory plus pain management, especially in the early postoperative period, are indicated for pain and stress management. The use of low-level laser therapy and therapeutic ultrasound has been reported anecdotally as adjunct therapy during physical rehabilitation in birds.

Further reading

Redig PT, Ponder J (2016) Management of orthopedic issues in birds. In: *Avian Medicine*, 3rd edn. (ed. J Samour). Mosby, St. Louis, pp. 312–350.

CASE 254

1 What would be the most likely differential diagnosis? The most likely differential in this case is iron storage disease (ISD). This condition may lead to hepatic necrosis, bile duct obstruction, cirrhosis, and fibrosis. A liver biopsy would show accumulation of a dense basophilic substance in the histiocytes and Kupffer cells, consistent with iron or hemosiderin. Hepatic iron concentration may be quantified to confirm the diagnosis. A primary genetic basis for iron overload in mynahs is suspected as mynahs have much higher uptake and retention of dietary iron and demonstrate high levels of expression of the intestinal iron transporters DMT-1 and intestinal Ireg1 (ferroportin). Natural diets for which 'sensitive' species have evolved are low in bioavailable iron, leading to selection for enhanced iron uptake and storage. Diets in captivity that provide too much available iron may exacerbate primary ISD. It can also be contributed to by other dietary factors such as high vitamin C content that support iron absorption. A thorough dietary history may help identify sources of iron and vitamin C in the diet.

2 What species are most commonly affected by this condition? Several bird species may suffer from ISD, particularly frugivorous species of the families Sturnidae, Paradiseadae, and Ramphastidae. There are also several descriptions in the literature of the disease in hawk-headed parrots (*Deroptyus accipitrinus*).

3 What would be your nutritional management plan for this patient? Nutritional management would include dietary iron restriction and vitamin C restriction. Low iron commercial (<50 ppm) pellets are recommended for maintenance feeding in these species. As many owners provide their toucans with fruits and vegetables as treats, it is important to consider that these may vary greatly in their vitamin C and iron content. Some high iron and vitamin C products include dark leafy greens such as spinach and kale, and fruit such as mulberries. Low vitamin C and iron products include pears, cantaloupes, peaches, and bananas.

Further reading

Drews AV, Redrobe SP, Patterson-Kane JC (2004) Successful reduction of hepatocellular hemosiderin content by dietary modification in toco toucans (*Ramphastos toco*) with iron-storage disease. *J Avian Med Surg* **18(2)**:101–105.

CASE 255

1 What is the most likely causative agent, and which special stain should be used for initial postmortem diagnosis? The most likely causative agent is *Mycobacterium* spp. In this particular case, *M. avium* subsp. *avium* was identified. Ziehl–Neelsen (ZN) stain, also known as acid-fast stain, may allow identification of the *Mycobacterium* organisms.

2 What diagnostic tests have the highest sensitivity? In general, antemortem diagnosis of mycobacteriosis can be challenging and ancillary blood test abnormalities may be limited and are generally nonspecific. In ring-necked doves, mycobacterial culture, ZN staining, and single-amplification PCR assay have been compared. Results showed that the use of one single test did not allow identification of all infected birds. For liver biopsy and bone marrow aspirate samples, culture had the highest sensitivity, while PCR assay and/or ZN staining had lower sensitivity. Splenic biopsy may have the greatest potential for antemortem diagnosis of mycobacterial infection; in one study, 88.24% sensitivity and 100% specificity were achieved. Western blot analysis was used to detect *M. avium* subsp. *avium* infection in ring-neck doves.

3 What are the treatment options? Treatment of avian mycobacteriosis is generally based on human protocols and involves combinations of antituberculosis drugs as resistance to a single drug can develop rapidly. Protocols include the combination of several antibiotics, such as ciprofloxacin, clarithromycin, clofazimine, ethambutol, isoniazid, rifabutin, rifampin, moxifloxacin, and streptomycin, for several months to years. In experimental *M. avium* subsp. *avium* infection in budgerigars, where treatment with clarithromycin, moxifloxacin, and ethambutol was given, although significant improvement was noted, the 4-month therapy was not sufficient for the complete recovery of all birds. Specifically in ring-neck doves, 180 days of treatment using azithromycin, rifampin, and ethambutol had poor efficacy. Furthermore, at the end of the experimental period, two mycobacterial isolates were resistant to ethambutol, intermediately sensitive to rifampin, and sensitive to azithromycin.

Further reading

Gray P, Saggese M, Phalen D *et al.* (2008) Humoral response to *Mycobacterium avium* subsp. *avium* in naturally infected ring-neck doves (*Streptopelia risoria*). *Vet Immunol Immunopathol* **125:**216–224.

Ledwoń A, Dolka I, Dolka B *et al.* (2015) Multidrug therapy of *Mycobacterium avium* subsp. *avium* infection in experimentally inoculated budgerigars (*Melopsittacus undulatus*). *Avian Pathol* **44:**470–474.

Lennox AM (2007) Mycobacteriosis in companion psittacine birds: a review. *J Avian Med Surg* **21:**181–187.

Saggese MD, Tizard I, Gray P *et al.* (2014) Evaluation of multidrug therapy with azithromycin, rifampin, and ethambutol for the treatment of *Mycobacterium avium* subsp. *avium* in ring-neck doves (*Streptopelia risoria*): an uncontrolled clinical study. *J Avian Med Surg* **28:**280–828.

Saggese MD, Tizard I, Phalen DN (2010) Comparison of sampling methods, culture, acid-fast stain, and polymerase chain reaction assay for the diagnosis of mycobacteriosis in ring-neck doves (*Streptopelia risoria*). *J Avian Med Surg* **24**:263–271.

CASE 256

1 What are the anatomic landmarks for a left lateral coelioscopy – where exactly is the telescope inserted? The anatomic landmarks are the last rib cranially, the pubic bone caudally, and the flexor cruris medialis muscle dorsally. The telescope is most commonly inserted behind the pelvic limb, which is secured craniad; however, older techniques have described drawing the limb caudad with the telescope inserted cranial to the limb, behind the last rib. In larger birds it is often possible to insert the telescope through an intercostal space if direct access to the cranial thoracic air sac is required, taking care to avoid intercostal vessels.

2 On entering the coelomic cavity via the landmarks described above, which air sac is most commonly entered in a psittacine? The caudal thoracic air sac.

3 Name the structure. What are the differential diagnoses for enlargement of this organ? Can this organ be biopsied? The spleen. Differential diagnoses for splenomegaly include bacterial diseases (e.g. chlamydiosis, mycobacteriosis), neoplasms (e.g. hemangiosarcoma), mycoses (e.g. aspergillosis), and viral infections (e.g. Pacheco's disease, polyomavirus). A splenic biopsy can be safely obtained endoscopically using 5-Fr biopsy forceps, with minimal hemorrhage, often undertaken to further differentiate the disease process.

Further reading

Divers SJ (2010) Avian diagnostic endoscopy. *Vet Clin North Am Exot Anim Pract* **13(2)**: 187–202.

Hernandez-Divers SJ, Wilson H, Lester VK *et al.* (2006) Evaluation of coelioscopic splenic biopsy and cloacoscopic bursa of Fabricius biopsy techniques in pigeons (*Columba livia*). *J Avian Med Surg* **20(4)**:234–241.

CASE 257

1 Name this foot arrangement. Zygodactyl.

2 This foot arrangement is particularly useful to a group of small parrots from South East Asia that hang upside down from branches. What is the name and the genus of this group? Hanging parrot, from the genus *Loriculus*.

3 The foot arrangement also allows parrots to perform what particular everyday task efficiently, which proves so useful during feeding? Grasping small objects. In addition, this foot arrangement allows parrots to grasp branches of different diameter and to perch efficiently.

Further reading

King AS, McLelland J (1984) (eds) *Birds: Their Structure and Function*. Baillière Tindall, Eastbourne.

CASE 258

1 What abnormalities are present in this image? Proventricular, ventricular, and duodenal impaction. A large matt of coarse grass is present in the proventriculus and ventriculus, and extends through the pylorus into the duodenum. The surface of the koilin has a dark red appearance suggestive of hemorrhage. Duodenal contents also have a red discoloration and there is necrotic material at the pylorus.

2 How common is this problem in ratites? Gastrointestinal impaction and foreign body ingestion are important diseases in ratites. Chicks are most frequently affected, but the condition can occur in adult birds as well. A wide range of often apparently insignificant management changes can predispose to gastric impaction, and birds may actively seek out foreign objects while foraging.

3 What options are available for diagnosis and treatment of affected birds? Diagnosis can be difficult and generally requires a combination of palpation, plain and/or contrast radiographs, or ultrasound. A history of management changes or recent construction activities (for foreign material) would be suggestive. In the majority of cases, surgical intervention to remove the impacted/foreign material is required.

Further reading

Smith DA (2007) Ratites. In: *Hand-Rearing Birds*. (eds. LJ Gage, RS Duerr) Blackwell Publishing, Ames, pp. 55–65.

CASE 259

1 In which Order of birds is the head of the spermatozoa characteristically spiral in shape? Passeriformes. The spermatozoa are characterized by a longitudinal spiral head in Passeriformes, while in nonPasseriformes the spermatozoa are characterized by a smooth longitudinal head.

2 What are the main characteristics of the semen of birds of this Order? The semen is brown in color and pasty in consistency. These seminal characteristics appear to be a common feature in all Passeriformes.

3 The semen of members of this Order is stored at 4°C lower than the body temperature in what anatomic structures? The seminal glomera. The seminal glomus (pl. glomera) is integrated by convolutions of the ductus deferens.

This structure is a unique anatomic feature and can be found in all Passeriformes and the budgerigar.

4 How do aviculturists use these structures to determine the sex of the birds? During the nuptial phase of the breeding cycle, the seminal glomera tend to increase considerably in volume, bulging on both sides of the cloaca, making sex determination relatively easy.

Further reading

King AS, McLelland J (1984) Male reproductive system. In: *Birds: Their Structure and Function*. (eds. AS King, J McLelland) Baillière Tindall, Eastbourne, pp. 166–174.

CASE 260

1 What is the cause of the problem? The chick has aerophagia. This is typically seen in a chick that is 'failing to thrive', but equally it can just be a very keen feeder who, in his readiness to take feeding formula, is gulping air before food is available or while food is being slowly delivered.

2 What is the initial recommended treatment for this condition? In many cases the air can be 'burped' back up and as soon as the crop is empty the crop is filled with food. In troublesome cases the affected chick is fed first, using a gavage needle. Once fed the aerophagia typically ceases, until the next meal is due. In time, the issue normally settles.

3 What further treatment may be necessary if the initial treatment fails? In persistent cases, following general anesthesia, a stent may need to be sewn into the proximal crop wall (i.e. to create a permanent valve, to allow air out in the event that excessive air is swallowed in). A stent may be readily manufactured from a section of sterile syringe barrel, with the edges of the aperture sutured around the outer diameter.

Further reading

Flammer K, Clubb SL (1994) Neonatology. In: *Avian Medicine: Principles and Applications*. (eds. BW Ritchie, GJ Harrison, LJ Harrison) Winger's Publications, Lake Worth, pp. 806–838.

CASE 261

1 What is the main differential for this lesion? Squamous cell carcinoma (SCC) of the uropygial gland. Other differentials include other types of neoplasia such as adenocarcinoma.

2 What is a potential predisposing factor for this lesion? Chronic inflammation from feather picking/ulceration, hypovitaminosis A, ultraviolet light exposure.

3 What are treatment options for this lesion? Complete surgical excision is indicated where possible (typically involving tail amputation when the uropygial gland is involved), which may result in resolution as these tumors are typically locally invasive but rarely metastasize. These lesions are generally slow/chronic to progress. The best chance to cure this lesion is complete surgical excision. If complete excision is not possible, adjunct therapy should be considered. Adjunct therapies to treat SCC in avian patients include intralesional chemotherapy, cryotherapy, radiation therapy, NSAIDs, and phototherapy. The prognosis is good in the case of complete surgical excision. Recurrence is likely in the case of incomplete surgical resection but adjunct therapy may slow progression of the lesion.

Further reading

Zehnder A, Graham J, Reavill D *et al.* (2016) Neoplastic diseases in avian species. In: *Current Therapy in Avian Medicine and Practice.* (ed. BL Speer) Elsevier, St. Louis, pp. 107–141.

CASE 262

1 What bacterial etiologies are compatible with the observed clinical signs? Chlamydiosis (zoonotic) has been associated with large-scale mortality events in waterfowl including mallards and domestic ducks. The disease can be acute, subacute, or chronic and clinical signs vary: lethargy, anorexia, ruffled feathers, weight loss, conjunctivitis, serous or infraorbital sinusitis, mucopurulent nasal and ocular discharge, green to yellow feces frequently with diarrhea, emaciation, dehydration, and death. Mortality up to 30% in ducks and 55% in goslings has been reported. Infections by *Riemerella anatipestifer* may manifest with similar clinical signs. Clinical signs associated with infections by *R. anatipestifer* in ducks and geese include ocular discharge, diarrhea, neurologic signs, and as much as 10% mortality. *Mycoplasma* spp. are not normally associated with ocular signs in ducks or geese.

2 What viral etiologies are compatible with the observed clinical signs? Viral infections have been also associated with upper respiratory signs in ducks and geese. Domestic ducks can be a key factor in the regional spread of H5N1 highly pathogenic avian influenza (HPAI) (zoonotic) virus in Asia. In domestic ducks inoculated intranasally with two H5N1 HPAI viruses, keratitis and corneal edema appeared more frequently than neurologic signs and mortality. Corneal ulceration and exophthalmos were rare findings. Avian paramyxoviruses types 1, 4, 6, 8, and 9 have been associated with infections in waterfowl. Infected ducks and geese are generally considered to be apathogenic except for a few exceptions reported in which ocular signs were not observed. However, it should be remembered that these species could act as carriers of these zoonotic diseases. Infections with avian adenoviruses have been associated with respiratory problems in ducks and geese, but ocular signs were not reported.

3 What fungal etiologies are compatible with the observed clinical signs? Corneal candidiasis and ocular aspergillosis have been associated with ocular signs (e.g. epiphora, keratitis) in ducks but are considered to be secondary infections related with corneal damage. There is a particularly high incidence of ocular candidiasis in marine ducks kept on fresh water.

Further reading

Flammer K (1997) Chlamydia. In: *Avian Medicine and Surgery*. (eds. RB Altman, SL Clubb, GM Dorrestein *et al.*) WB Saunders, Philadephia, pp. 364–379.

Yamamoto Y, Nakamura K, Yamada M *et al.* (2016) Corneal opacity in domestic ducks experimentally infected with H5N1 highly pathogenic avian influenza virus. *Vet Pathol* 53(1):65–76.

CASE 263

1 Which protozoal parasite would you consider as the most likely differential diagnosis? *Trichomonas* spp.

2 How would you test the rest of the specimens housed in the same aviary? A representative sample of birds should be caught and sampled. A damp microbiology swab is inserted in the mouth and rolled against the crop wall, prior to mixing in warm saline on a microscope slide. Microscopic examination under high power of these fresh and warm wet smears from mucus of the mouth and oropharyngeal area will yield *Trichomonas* if present, seen as directionally motile flagellated protozoa. Special culture media may facilitate the isolation of the parasite in cases where low numbers are present. PCR testing will allow definitive identification.

3 What treatment and control measures would you use if other birds in the aviary are also affected? Metronidazole (50 mg/kg PO q12h for 5–10 days), carnidazole (20–30 mg/kg PO once), ronidazole (10 mg/kg PO q24h for 6–10 days), and dimetridazole (200–400 mg/L drinking water for 5 days) have been reported as effective therapeutic agents but drug resistance has been encountered. Increased hygiene in feeding and watering stations, preventing access by wild birds to the aviary, disinfection with 10% bleach, and avoiding contaminated (fresh) prey in carnivorous birds will contribute to reducing the prevalence.

Further reading

Forrester DJ, Foster GW (2014) Trichomonosis. In: *Parasitic Diseases of Wild Birds*. (eds. CT Atkinson, NJ Thomas, DB Hunter) Wiley-Blackwell, Ames, pp. 120–153.

CASE 264

1 Describe the different parts of the cervicocephalic air sac. What are their functions? The cervicocephalic air sac has one or two divisions: the cervical division and the cranial cephalic division (in some species). The cranial cephalic division reaches from the occipital region just behind the cere and is absent in many bird species (e.g. macaws). The cervical division originates in the tympanic area and extends in two columns bilaterally down the neck. The air sac communicates with the caudal aspect of the infraorbital sinus. In contrast to other air sacs, the cervicocephalic air sac does not play a major role in gas exchange, but is important for insulation for heat retention, control of buoyancy, reducing the force of impact with water in fish eating birds, and support of the head during sleep or flight.
2 Why does hyperinflation of the cervicocephalic air sac occur in some birds? Rupture and subsequent hyperinflation of the cervicocephalic air sac may occur subsequent to trauma or chronic respiratory disease (chronic sinusitis, airsacculitis, pulmonary disease, living in a chronically tobacco smoke filled environment). The condition is typically seen as localized subcutaneous emphysema in the neck region, but generalized emphysema has also been described.
3 How would you manage hyperinflation of the cervicocephalic air sac? The distended air sac can be decompressed with a needle or, under general anesthesia, with a scalpel or radiosurgery, creating a stoma. These are temporary treatments and if the underlying cause is not addressed, hyperinflation of the air sac is likely to reoccur once the skin heals. Techniques using stents for refractory cases have also been described. Obliteration of the dead space of the air sac by administering irritant agents (e.g. doxycycline) into the space, followed by temporary compressive bandages for a few days to enable the air sac membranes to adhere to each other, has been also reported with variable success.

Further reading

Antinoff N (2008) Attempted pleurodesis for an air sac rupture in an Amazon parrot. *Proc Ann Conf Assoc Avian Vet*, Savannah, pp. 437–438.
Doneley B (2010) Clinical anatomy and physiology and Disorders of the respiratory system. In: *Avian Medicine and Surgery in Practice: Companion and Aviary Birds*, 2nd edn. (ed. B Doneley) CRC Press, Boca Raton, pp. 7–39 and 185–190.
Forbes NA (2016) Soft tissue surgery. In: *Avian Medicine*, 3rd edn. (ed. J Samour) Elsevier, St. Louis, pp. 294–311.

CASE 265

1 Provide a common form of flight restriction used with the following types of bird: caged psittacines and passerines; companion psittacines; cranes; falconry birds; flamingos in an outdoor exhibit.

- Caged psittacines and passerines: keeping birds in small enclosures that restrict ability to fly.

- Companion psittacines: wing clipping/trimming remiges.
- Cranes: brailing.
- Falconry birds: tethering.
- Flamingos in an outdoor exhibit: pinioning.

2 **List three positive welfare opportunities that trimming the remiges of a pet bird could provide.** (1) The bird can roam freely around the house and can be taken outdoors (i.e. is less likely to be confined to a small cage). (2) Clipping a wing of a male breeding cockatoo may reduce its potential aggression towards its mate. Will maintain the bird's activity within easy access of caretaker/owner, thereby reducing the potential need for chase or capture. (3) Restricts a bird's access to potential household dangers such as flying into fans or fires.

3 **List negative welfare aspects of preventing a bird from flying. Welfare may include physical, medical, as well as behavioral aspects.**

- Prevents natural flight escape mechanism when startled or frightened, resulting in increased fear and frustration.
- Reduces its level of exercise; will increase the risk of obesity and cardiovascular disease.
- Is likely to increase the risk of boredom and development of abnormal behaviors.
- Prevents a bird from escaping from risks (e.g. cats, falcons, aviary mates, house fires).
- Wing clipping increases the risk of trauma if a bird is unable to fly from perch to floor safely.
- Wing clipping can prevent flight feathers growing back safely due to increased risk of breaking blood feathers, as these will be less supported by mature hard penned feathers.
- The sharp ends of cut flight feathers can cause irritation and result in feather destructive behavior.
- Flight impaired birds of larger species have reduced egg fertility levels due to increased difficulty in balancing when copulating (e.g. flamingos).
- A tethered raptor is more likely to be stolen than one free lofted in an aviary.
- A tethered raptor carries a risk of tibiotarsus fracture if it is frightened and bates away from its perch.
- Inability of the bird to balance itself as a result of a deflighting procedure may cause serious injuries as the bird may fall and harm itself.
- Deflighting results in marked physiologic changes in the flight musculature.

Further reading

Animal Welfare Act 2006. United Kindom.

Ellis DH, Dein FJ (1996) Flight restraint. In: *Cranes: Their Biology, Husbandry, and Conservation.* (eds. DH Ellis, GF Gee, CM Mirande) US Department of the Interior, National Biological Service, Washington, DC and International Crane Foundation, Baraboo, pp. 241–244.

Hesterman H, Gregory NG, Boardman WSJ (2001) Deflighting procedures and their welfare implications in captive birds. *Anim Welf* **10**:405–419.

Speer BL (2001) The clinical consequences of routine grooming. *Proc Ann Conf Assoc Avian Vet*, Orlando, pp. 109–115.

Van Zeeland YRA, Spruijt BM, Rodenburg TB *et al.* (2009) Feather damaging behaviour in parrots: a review with consideration of comparative aspects. *Appl Anim Behav Sci* **121**:75–95.

CASE 266

1 What is the standard management of a broken blood feather with active hemorrhage (266)? If there is active hemorrhage, apply firm steady pressure. On occasions controlling ongoing bleeding is facilitated by sedation or anesthesia. Provide pre-emptive analgesia since pressure must be applied to this sensitive area. After bleeding has stopped, the broken can be left to grow out, although it could be trimmed to reduce the risk of trauma and pain. Do not apply hemostatic agents, such as silver nitrate or styptic powder, to the feather follicle as these substances can permanently damage the follicle. If the control of hemorrhage is challenging, an alternative method is to tie suture material around the blood feather just below the bleeding point. The distal end is then trimmed off at the level of the damage. The inside of the calamus is dried of blood with a fine microbiology swab after which a drop of tissue glue is applied within the calamus. Once the feather is hard penned (i.e. the feather is mature and the blood supply has retracted), the feather may be trimmed down to 2 cm above the skin line, and a replacement feather 'imped' in place, similar to a hair extension. If this is to be done, care must be taken to sterilize the replacement feather in case it is contaminated with any pathogen (e.g. circovirus).

2 If bleeding has stopped or is minimal with a broken blood feather, how should the avian patient be managed? If hemorrhage has stopped or is minimal, take measures to minimize patient stress and lower blood pressure by confining the bird to an incubator. It is useful to enquire of the owner as to how much blood they believe may have been lost. Dim room lighting, minimize disturbances, and monitor the patient regularly. Also, trim the plumaceous part of the feather to minimize the risk of trauma and pain. If the feather is tied off, there is no risk of repeat or ongoing hemorrhage.

3 Management of a bleeding broken blood feather on the wing should only involve pulling the feather as a last resort. Why should the feather be left in place, if possible? The flight feathers are embedded in the periosteum, and the process of pulling a blood feather is undoubtedly extremely painful. There is also the possibility that pulling the feather can damage the dermal papilla from which the feather grows, such that a replacement feather never grows or is bent, short, or otherwise abnormal.

Further reading

Schmidt RE, Lightfoot TL (2006) Integument. In: *Clinical Avian Medicine.* (eds. GJ Harrison, TL Lightfoot) Spix Publishing, Palm Beach, p. 403.

CASE 267

1 List three advantages for a bird's welfare to be housed with one or more of the same species. Pair housing can increase activity levels and behavioral diversity, and reduce neophobia and fearfulness towards humans.

2 Parrot owners may be concerned that socially housed parrots will bond to the other birds rather than to humans. Has this concern been validated or invalidated? Invalidated. A study by Meehan *et al.* (2003) showed that pair-housed orange-winged Amazon parrots (*Amazona amazonica*) responded less fearfully than singly housed birds to humans with whom they were not familiar. Isosexual pair housing can be a form of environmental enrichment such that parrots housed in pairs will be more active and perform fewer abnormal behaviors.

3 Species-specific characteristics must be taken into account when considering pair housing. What psittacine species is notorious for being prone to aggressive behavior toward conspecifics? Male cockatoos, especially red-vented cockatoos (*Cacatua haematuropygia*) and lesser sulfur-crested cockatoos (*Cacatua sulphurea*), frequently become aggressive towards their mates. Severe and fatal mate trauma in which the male bird bites the face, neck, wings, and legs of the female can occur. Mate trauma has also been reported in other species of psittacines but is not a common problem.

Further reading

Evans M (2001) Environmental enrichment for pet parrots. *In Practice* **23**:596–605.

Leonard AL (2005) *Companion Parrots and Their Owners: A Survey of United States Households.* M.S. Thesis, University of California, Davis.

Meehan CL, Garner JP, Mench JA (2003) Isosexual pair housing improves the welfare of young Amazon parrots. *Appl Anim Behav Sci* **81**:73–88.

Romagnano A (2006) Mate trauma. In: *Manual of Parrot Behavior.* (ed. AU Luescher) Blackwell Publishing, Ames, pp. 247–253.

Seibert LM (2006) Social behaviour of psittacine birds. In: *Manual of Parrot Behavior.* (ed. AU Luescher) Blackwell Publishing, Ames, pp. 43–47.

CASE 268

1 Why is intermittent anisocoria frequently observed in some birds? The avian pupillary muscles (constrictor and dilator) are predominantly striated with varying amounts of nonstriated fibers. As a result, physiologic contraction of the iris is influenced by retinal stimulation and subject to voluntary control.

2 How do you explain and interpret the diagnostic procedure shown in the image? The image shows a potential lack of direct and indirect pupillary reflexes. Due to the complete decussation of optic nerve fibers at the optic chiasm, slight, intermittent, and dynamic anisocoria may be normal in birds. Consensual pupillary light reflexes are not expected.

3 Why may directing the light source to one eye result in miosis in the contralateral eye? An artifactual consensual reflex may be observed due to inadvertent stimulation of the retina of the nonstimulated eye through the thin interosseous septum separating the two orbits.

Further reading

Gum GG, MacKay EO (2013) Physiology of the eye. In: *Veterinary Ophthalmology*, 5th edn. (eds. KN Gellatt, BC Gilger, TJ Kern) Wiley-Blackwell, Ames, pp. 171–207.

CASE 269

1 What are the toxic agents in chocolate? Theobromine and caffeine (both methylxanthines).

2 What are the expected clinical signs in cases of chocolate intoxication in birds? Adenosine receptors are most affected in the neurologic and cardiovascular systems of birds after chocolate ingestion. Antagonism of these receptors by methylxanthines causes tachycardia, ventricular arrhythmia, hypertension, hyperactivity, anxiousness, and sometimes seizures and hyperalgesia. Polyuria may also result from renal adenosine receptor inhibition. The few reported cases of chocolate intoxication in birds resulted in death.

3 How would you treat this bird in an emergency? Because of the poor prognosis, rapid preventive measures to prevent absorption are key. Crop and proventricular lavage and removal of large particles, assisted with endoscopy, are recommended to retrieve chocolate from the digestive tract. Afterwards, activated charcoal may be administered at 1–3 g/kg. Repeated administration may be required due to the enterohepatic cycle of the toxins. Symptomatic treatment may include anxiolytics such as midazolam 1–2 mg/kg (IV, IM, IN, or SC) as needed and anti-arrhythmic drugs. However, propranolol is not recommended as it slows the renal clearance of methylxanthines. Finally, fluid therapy (IV or SC) is also indicated to enhance elimination.

Further reading

Gartrell BD (2007) Death by chocolate: a fatal problem for an inquisitive wild parrot. *N Z Vet J* **55(3)**:149–151.

Lightfoot TL, Yeager JM (2008) Pet bird toxicity and related environmental concerns. *Vet Clin North Am Exot Anim Pract* **11(2)**:229–259.

CASE 270

1 What are the three main functions of feathers? Feathers are unique structures of the skin that provide insulation for controlling body temperature, aerodynamic power for flight, and colors for communication and camouflage. Feathers also perform secondary roles. Modified feathers are important in swimming, sound production, hearing, protection, cleanliness, water repelling, water transport, and tactile sensation.

2 Give a description of the function of the following feathers: flight feathers, down feathers, semiplumes, filoplumes, and bristles. The flight feathers of the tail attach to the pygostyle and function primarily in steering and braking during flight. Down feathers have loosely entangled barbules that trap air in a layer close to the skin, providing an excellent natural, lightweight thermal insulation. Powderdowns assist in cleaning the plumage. Semiplumes enhance thermal insulation, fill out the aerodynamic contours of body plumage, and serve as courtship ornaments. Filoplumes are hair-like feathers that monitor the movement and position of adjacent veined feathers, aiding aerodynamic adjustments. Bristles are specialized feathers with both sensory and protective functions (e.g. eyelashes of ostriches or facial feathers of raptors).

CASE 271

1 List key features to include in an avian welfare assessment. (1) Assessment of resources: considers the biological and physical needs of a bird. (2) Measures of the physical state of individual birds. (3) Measures of the mental state of individual birds.

2 Give examples of what resources can be objectively evaluated in an avian welfare assessment. Housing space, thermal zones, husbandry practices, diet, enrichment items, or activities.

3 Give examples of what the veterinarian can do to determine the physical state of individual birds. (1) Objective measurements such as weight, heart rate, respiratory rate, and recovery time after handling. (2) Note food and water consumption, feces and urate production, level of activity, and what the bird actually eats versus what food is provided. (3) Diagnostic evaluations such as CBC, plasma biochemistry values, and parasitic examination of the feces. (4) Subjectively scored parameters such as the bird's degree of responsiveness, body condition score, posture, and feather condition.

4 Evaluation of the mental state of a bird is the most abstract and subjective part of the overall welfare assessment. What kinds of questions are included in the assessment of a bird's mental state? (1) The person most familiar with a bird's temperament, preferences, behavior, and routine to be 'the voice' for that individual. (2) Use of free-choice profiling, which uses descriptive terms independently generated by several observers to score the bird, either by direct observation or by watching a video. (3) Determine if the bird is expressing behaviors driven by the positive emotional systems including seeking, play, and caring. (4) Determine if the bird is expressing behaviors driven by activation of the fear, rage, or panic systems.

Further reading

Paul-Murphy J (2015) Foundations in avian welfare. In: *Current Therapy in Avian Medicine and Surgery*. (ed. BL Speer) Elsevier Health Sciences, St. Louis, pp. 669–676.

Index

Note: References are to case numbers (questions and answers)

Index

Also available in the Self-Assessment Color Review series

Brown & Rosenthal: *Small Mammals*
Elsheikha & Patterson: *Veterinary Parasitology*
Forbes & Altman: *Avian Medicine*
Freeman: *Veterinary Cytology*
Frye: *Reptiles and Amphibians 2nd Edition*
Hartmann & Levy: *Feline Infectious Diseases*
Hartmann & Sykes: *Canine Infectious Diseases*
Keeble, Meredith & Richardson: *Rabbit Medicine and Surgery 2nd Edition*
Kirby, Rudloff & Linklater: *Small Animal Emergency and Critical Care Medicine 2nd Edition*
Lewis & Langley-Hobbs: *Small Animal Orthopedics, Rheumatology & Musculoskeletal Disorders 2nd Edition*
Mair & Divers: *Equine Internal Medicine 2nd Edition*
May & McIlwraith: *Equine Orthopaedics and Rheumatology*
Meredith & Keeble: *Wildlife Medicine and Rehabilitation*
Moriello: *Small Animal Dermatology*
Moriello & Diesel: *Small Animal Dermatology, Advanced Cases*
Obradovich: *Small animal Clinical Oncology*
Pycock: *Equine Reproduction and Stud Medicine*
Samuelson & Brooks: *Small Animal Ophthalmology*
Scott: *Cattle and Sheep Medicine 2nd Edition*
Sparkes & Caney: *Feline Medicine*
Tennant: *Small Animal Abdominal and Metabolic Disorders*
Thieman-Mankin: *Small Animal Soft Tissue Surgery 2nd Edition*
Verstraete & Tsugawa: *Veterinary Dentistry 2nd Edition*
Ware: *Small Animal Cardiopulmonary Medicine*